Oxford Medical Publications

Problem-orientated Clinical Microbiology and Infection

D1072878

Problem-orientated Clinical Microbiology and Infection

Second edition

by

Hilary Humphreys
Professor of Clinical Microbiology, The Royal College of Surgeons in Ireland and
Consultant Microbiologist, Beaumont Hospital, Dublin

and

William L. Irving
Professor of Virology, University of Nottingham and Honorary Consultant Virologist,
University Hospital, Queen's Medical Centre, Nottingham

With a Foreword by

C.A. (Tony) Hart
Professor of Medical Microbiology and Genito-Urinary Medicine, University of Liverpool
and Honorary Consultant Medical Microbiologist to the Alder Hey and Royal Liverpool
Hospitals

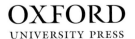

OXFORD
UNIVERSITY PRESS

OXFORD
UNIVERSITY PRESS

Great Clarendon Street, Oxford OX2 6DP

Oxford University Press is a department of the University of Oxford.
It furthers the University's objective of excellence in research, scholarship,
and education by publishing worldwide in

Oxford   New York

Auckland   Bangkok   Buenos Aires   Cape Town   Chennai
Dar es Salaam   Delhi   Hong Kong   Istanbul   Karachi   Kolkata
Kuala Lumpur   Madrid   Melbourne   Mexico City   Mumbai   Nairobi
São Paulo   Shanghai   Taipei   Tokyo   Toronto

Oxford is a registered trade mark of Oxford University Press
in the UK and in certain other countries

Published in the United States
by Oxford University Press Inc., New York

First edition published by Churchill Livingstone 1996
Second edition published by Oxford University Press 2004

A catalogue record for this title is available from the British Library

ISBN 0 19 851585 5 (Pbk)

10 9 8 7 6 5 4 3 2 1

Typeset by EXPO Holdings Sdn Bhd, Malaysia
Printed in Italy
on acid-free paper by
Giunti Industrie Grafiche

Foreword

Humans and microbes have had a long and sometimes turbulent interaction. Indeed, it could be argued that we are more microbe than man. The adult human comprises some 10^{13} human cells but these are greatly outnumbered by the 10^{14} bacteria, fungi, protozoa, multicellular parasites, and even insects that colonize us. In addition, some 3% of our genomes comprise complete retrovirus proviral DNA with another 5% being incomplete proviral footprints. Our mitochondria were originally symbiotic intracellular bacteria. From the above it is clear that we are all walking zoos.

Our normal flora, for this is what it is, usually has a neutral or beneficial effect. The genome, transcriptome, and proteome of our intestinal microflora greatly exceeds that of all our human cells together and its metabolome exceeds that of our livers. The normal bacteria help us by preventing more virulent bacteria from gaining access, and even by helping to produce essential nutrients and a strong immune system. However despite this apparently benign, and often beneficial interaction, it is also clear that things can go wrong and our 'normal' microbes can escape from their niche to cause disease or other microbes may be acquired from the external environment, animate or inanimate, to cause disease.

We are currently in a time of great advances in our understanding of the interactions between microbes and humans. The genome sequencing projects are providing the bedrock for further advances. Our understanding of how Gram negative bacteria cause disease by assembling secretion systems that inject effector molecules directly into human host cells, has led to the potential for new therapeutic interventions and vaccines as well as casting light on how human cells work. In addition, we have been discovering at least three 'new' pathogens each year over the last 30 years. Recent examples include the emergence of Nipah and Hendra viruses and the discovery of human metapneumovirus.

In this, the second edition of ***Problem-orientated Clinical Microbiology and Infection***, Professors Humphreys and Irving expand and improve on their very successful first edition. It is a most useful text for undergraduate medical students, providing logical access to information beginning with the patient presenting with infection, asking pertinent questions, and then providing the answers. For postgraduate doctors further in-depth information is provided which will, I am sure, also be of benefit for the interested undergraduate.

I commend the authors for this very useful clinically orientated text which fully reflects the excitement of the new 'era of the microbe'.

Professor CA (Tony) Hart
University of Liverpool
February 2004

Preface to the second edition

We are delighted to be able to update and extend the original version of this problem-orientated guide to microbiology and infectious diseases, first published in 1996. This has allowed us to take account of new developments in the subject such as the discovery of new infectious agents (e.g. human metapneumovirus, SARS coronavirus), the development of new modalities of antimicrobial therapy and prophylaxis (e.g. enfuvirtide, new antibiotics, and new vaccines), and of new management protocols (e.g. the routine screening of antenatal sera for evidence of hepatitis B and HIV infection). In addition to writing five new cases (needlestick transmission of blood-borne viruses, blood-borne virus infection in pregnancy, hepatitis C virus infection, *Clostridium difficile*, and orolabial herpes), we have reviewed all the subject matter and updated many sections. We have taken into account comments (both positive and negative) received on the first edition, and have re-ordered the cases into what we hope is a more logical sequence. We are grateful to our new publisher for allowing us to add over 60 new illustrations.

HH
WLI
November 2003

Acknowledgements

We are grateful to Professor Anthony Hart for his constructive comments during the draft stages of this book. We wish to thank the following for their helpful comments, input, support and encouragement: Ms Tracey Dillane, Professor David Greenwood, Ms Ann Shannon, and Dr Richard Slack. We appreciate the help of the following in the drafting of individual cases: Dr Immi Ahmed, Dr Mark Farrington, Dr E. (Nancy) Gallagher, Dr Gillian Murphy, and Dr Prith Venkatessen.

We acknowledge the following individuals or groups for supplying illustrations:

Dr B.R. Allan (Figs 1.1 and 1.2), American Academy of Pediatrics (Fig. 65.2), Dr A.P. Ball (Figs 6.1, 59.1), Dr Roger Bayston (Fig. 35.3), Dr Erwin Brown (Fig. 9.2), Dr Angie Browne (Fig. 49.2), Professor Mary Cafferkey (Fig. 41.5), Dr K.L. Dalziel (Fig. 2.1), Professsor Harminder Dua (Fig. 8.2(b)), Dr Dominic Dwyer (Fig 51.3), Dr R.T.D. Emond (Fig. 6.3), Dr Tony Egan (Fig. 11.1), Professor G. Enders (Fig. 62.1), Professor A.M. Emmerson (Fig.5.1), Dr Mark Everard (Fig. 21.4), Professor Roger Finch (Figs 12.1, 35.1), Professor David Greenwood (Figs 25.1, 30.3, 50.1, 55.1 and 55.2), Dr Andy Haynes (Fig. 66.1), Dr Martin Hewitt (Figs 42.1, 62.3), Dr Henry Irving (Figs 22.1, 26.2, 30.1), Professor David Isaacs (Figs 3.1, 3.2, 4.1, 6.2, 15.1), Dr Peter James (Fig 29.2), Professor Elaine Kay (Figs 33.1 and 33.2), Dr John Kurtz (Figs 17.2, 17.3, 17.4), Dr John V. Lee (Figs 19.1, 53.2), Professor Michael Lee (Fig. 13.2), Professor J. Lowe (Figs 46.1, 46.2), Dr Dan Peterson (Fig. 4.2 available at http://www.gentledentalcare.com/fever_blisters_2.html), Professor Stephen Porter (Figs 38.1, 51.1, 51.5), Dr M.W. McKendrick (Figs 7.1, 7.2, 28.1), The National Blood Authority (Fig. 29.1), Dr Colm O'Mahony (Figs 37.1, 40.1, 65.1), Dr G.W. Raborn (Fig. 8.2(a)), Professor N. Rutter (Figs 13.1, 61.1), Mr Andrew Shelton (Figs 24.1, 24.2), Dr Tony Simmons (Fig 7.5), Dr Richard Slack (Fig. 10.1c), Dr Alan Stevens (Fig. 52.5), Mr S. Vernon (Fig. 8.1), X-ray and Radiology Department, Queen's Medical Centre (Figs 18.2, 43.1, 51.4, 52.1, 54.1).

Permission has been sought for the use of Figs 7.3 and 7.4 from the Wellcome Slide Collection "Herpes zoster slide kit" (by Dr M. Wood, published by Gower).

Contents

N.B. Throughout the book undergraduate material is presented in blue; postgraduate material in red. **UG** indicates cases which contain predominantly undergraduate material (but may also contain postgraduate material). **PG** indicates cases which are primarily aimed at postgraduates (but also contain material which will be useful to undergraduates). See 'How to use this book' on p. *xv* for more information.

How to use this book

Undergraduate medical education is undergoing considerable change with greater emphasis on a core curriculum, integration of subjects, and self-assessment. The developments in education in the UK and elsewhere have therefore guided the principles upon which this book is based. It is intended to be a microbiological and infectious diseases text for undergraduate medical students but should also be of considerable use to postgraduate medical students studying for exams such as the MRCP (UK).

There are essentially two components to the book. The body of the book is a series of 70 case presentations, each describing the patient's presentation and their subsequent diagnosis and management. The reader is asked questions in logical order that, when answered, lead to further questions and the 'story' unfolds providing a comprehensive overview of the case and the subject material. Our aims are to inculcate the basic principles involved in the investigation and management of patients with infection and to encourage the student to formulate his/her own thoughts in a logical fashion. The second part of the book comprises a series of appendices providing basic information that the student can refer to when attempting to answer the questions.

The cases are clustered together according to the organ or system that is infected and, if additional information is required, the reader is referred to other cases as appropriate. The book contains cases that the authors consider suitable for undergraduate students (Q&A, Tables, and Boxes in blue) and cases that are more appropriate for the postgraduate student (Q&A, Tables, and Boxes in red). At the end of postgraduate cases, there is a résumé for the undergraduate student. There are also cases that contain both undergraduate and postgraduate material and this is indicated by the change in colour as the reader moves from one to the other. We would encourage undergraduate students to also read the postgraduate cases, and postgraduate students to read undergraduate cases as revision.

We have chosen the cases on the basis of their importance to medicine generally but we appreciate that it is not possible to be completely inclusive. Thus, in addition to the linear evolution of each particular case, there are Tables and Boxes which allow us to discuss and enlarge upon the material covered. Our intention is that the Tables contain information directly relevant to the case in question, whilst the Boxes summarize subject matter which, although not directly concerned with the case, is nevertheless important, although on occassions it has been difficult to decide what should be in a Table and what in a Box! We hope these adjuncts to the main text will also serve as useful revision aids prior to examinations. The summaries at the end of each case aim to review succinctly the information and knowledge obtained. At the end of each series of cases for a system, e.g. respiratory tract, there are a number of self-assessment questions that the student can use to determine whether he/she has fully comprehended the material. Finally, at the end of the book there is a list of the cases and the subject material that they cover, to enable readers to find information on a particular topic, although reference to this list will clearly give away the diagnoses in advance of reading the cases.

It is clear from even the most casual perusal of newspapers and the occasional viewing of television, that infection and its diagnosis, treatment, and control remain hugely important and are of great interest to the general public. Consequently, we believe it is essential that doctors understand the principles of clinical microbiology and infection as these pervade all branches of medicine. We hope therefore that this book will be useful, stimulating, and of interest to those who use it. Whilst we acknowledge that not all will be as fascinated by the vagaries of parasites, fungi, bacteria, and viruses as we are, we hope that those who use the book will derive some degree of the enjoyment and pleasure that we have experienced in writing it.

List of abbreviations

A&E	accident and emergency
AIDS	acquired immunodeficiency syndrome
ALT	alanine aminotransferase
AP	alkaline phosphatase
ARDS	adult respiratory distress syndrome
ASOT	antistreptolysin O titre (test)
ATLL	adult T-cell leukaemia lymphoma
AZT	azidothymidine
BBV	blood-borne virus
BCG	bacille Calmette–Guérin (vaccine)
BHIVA	British HIV Association
BSE	bovine spongiform encephalopathy
BSI	bloodstream infection
CAPD	continuous ambulatory peritoneal dialysis
CDC	Centres of Disease Control (USA)
CDSC	Communicable Disease Surveillance Centre
CFT	complement fixation test
cfu	colony-forming unit
CJD	Creutzfeldt–Jakob disease
CMV	cytomegalovirus
CNS	central nervous system
COPD	chronic obstructive pulmonary disease
CPE	cytopathic effect
CRP	C-reactive protein
CS	Caesarean section
CSF	cerebrospinal fluid
CT	computerized tomography
DEAFF	detection of early antigen fluorescent foci (test)
DHF	dengue haemorrhagic fever
DPT	diphtheria–pertussis–tetanus (vaccine)

EBV	Epstein–Barr virus
ECG	electrocardiogram
EEG	electroencephalogram
EHEC	enterohaemorrhagic *E. coli*
ELISA	enzyme-linked immunosorbent assay
EM	electron microscopy
EMRSA	epidemic MRSA
EPPs	exposure-prone procedures
ESR	erythrocyte sedimentation rate
FBC	full blood count
FEV_1	forced expiratory volume in one second
FSH	follicle-stimulating hormone
FUO	fever of unknown origin
FVC	forced vital capacity
G6PDH	glucose-6-phosphate dehydrogenase
GGT	gamma-glutamyl transferase
GRE	glycopeptide (e.g. vancomycin) resistant enterococci (also VRE)
GUM	genitourinary medicine (clinic)
H (or HA)	haemagglutinin
HAART	highly active antiretroviral therapy
HACEK	haemophilus–actinobacillus–cardiobacterium–eikenella–kingella (group)
HAM	HTLV-1-associated myelopathy
HAV	hepatitis A virus
Hb	haemoglobin
HBcAg	hepatitis B core antigen
HBeAg	hepatitis B extractable antigen
HBIg	hepatitis B immunoglobulin
HBsAg	hepatitis B surface antigen
HBV	hepatitis B virus
HCV	hepatitis C virus
HCW	health-care worker
HDV	hepatitis D virus

HEV	hepatitis E virus
Hib	*Haemophilus influenzae* type b
HIV	human immunodeficiency virus
HNIg	human normal immunoglobulin
HRIg	human rabies immunoglobulin
HSE	herpes simplex encephalitis
HSV	herpes simplex virus
HTLV	human T cell lymphotropic virus (two types 1 and 2)
HPV	human papillomavirus
ICU	Intensive Care Unit
IFN	interferon
IM	infectious mononucleosis
ITU	Intensive Therapy Unit
IU	international units
IV	intravenous
IVU	intravenous urography
LFTs	liver function tests
LP	lumbar puncture
LRTI	lower respiratory tract infection
LUC	large unclassifiable cells
MCV	mean corpuscular volume
MDRTB	multidrug-resistant tuberculosis
MIC	minimum inhibitory concentration
MMR	measles–mumps–rubella (vaccine)
MRI	magnetic resonance imaging
MRSA	methicillin-resistant *S. aureus*
MSU	midstream urine (specimen)
N (or NA)	neuraminidase
NAT	nucleic acid testing
NNRTI	non-nucleoside analogue RT inhibitors
NPA	nasopharyngeal aspirate
NPC	nasopharyngeal carcinoma
NRTI	nucleoside analogue reverse transcriptase inhibitors
NSU	non-specific urethritis
OHL	oral hairy leucoplakia
OPD	outpatients department
PAS	para-aminosalicylic acid
PB	Paul Bunnell (test)
PCP	*Pneumocystis carinii* pneumonia
PCR	polymerase chain reaction

PEG-IFN	pegylated alpha-interferon
PEP	post-exposure prophylaxis
PGL	persistent generalized lymphadenopathy
PI	protease inhibitors
PID	pelvic inflammatory disease
PML	progressive multifocal leucoencephalopathy
PMNLs	polymorphonuclear leucocytes
PrP	prion protein
RSV	respiratory syncytial virus
RT	reverse transcriptase
SARS	severe acute respiratory syndrome
SBE	subacute bacterial endocarditis
SCBU	special care baby unit
SGOT	serum glutamic-oxaloacetic transaminase
SPAG	small-particle aerosol generator
SRSVs	small round structured viruses (noroviruses)
SRVs	small round viruses
SSPE	subacute sclerosing panencephalitis
STD	sexually transmitted disease
STI	sexually transmitted infection
SV40	simian virus 40
TNF	tumour necrosis factor
TSP	tropical spastic paraparesis
TSS	toxic shock syndrome
TSST-1	toxic shock syndrome toxin-1
UKAP	United Kingdom Advisory Panel
URTI	upper respiratory tract infection
US	ultrasound
UTIs	urinary tract infections
vCJD	variant CJD
VHF	viral haemorrhagic fevers
VZIg	varicella-zoster immune globulin
VZV	varicella-zoster virus
WCC	white cell count
XLP	X-linked lymphoproliferative syndrome
WHO	World Health Organization
ZN	Ziehl–Neelsen (stain)

1

CHAPTER 1

Skin and mucous membranes

Skin and mucous membranes

Case 1 Howard, a 10-year-old boy with scaly skin lesions

Howard, a 10-year-old boy, is referred to the dermatology outpatients because of skin lesions on his arm that have been present for 3–4 months. He has never previously been seriously ill, is on no medication, and there is no family history of eczema or any other skin disorder. On examination he is seen to be a fit and active child, and the lesions are scaly, with raised margins (see Fig. 1.1).

Q What is the diagnosis?

A These lesions are typical of tinea or dermatophytosis, which is most commonly seen during childhood. They are caused by filamentous fungi that invade the stratum corneum. Three genera are responsible: *Trichophyton*; *Microsporum*; and *Epidermophyton* (contains only one species, *E. floccosum*). Tinea is infectious.

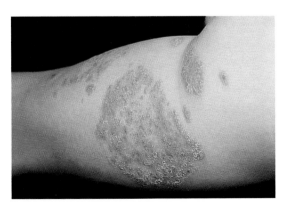

Fig. 1.1 Scaly lesion on Howard's arm.

Q What other questions might Howard or his parents be asked?

A Howard should be asked whether his brothers, sisters, or playmates have similar marks on the skin and whether there is a cat or dog at home, as some of the fungi are acquired from animals or on a farm. A history of a similar condition in other members of the family may reflect common exposure or increased genetic susceptibility, which may be mediated by differences in T-lymphocyte response.

Q Where else on the body might you look for tinea infections?

A Tinea infections may be found all over the body and are traditionally classified according to the anatomical location. Examples include:

- tinea pedis (feet): infects the interdigital spaces (also known as 'athlete's foot'), which may result in itching leading to blisters and secondary bacterial infections. Most commonly caused by *T. rubrum*, *T. mentagrophytes* (*interdigitale*)

- tinea cruris (groin): may present in genitourinary medicine clinics

- tinea corporis (body): classically referred to as 'ringworm', and may affect the arms, trunk, and legs. Most commonly caused by *T. rubrum*

- tinea capitis (head): infection of the scalp and hair. Characterized by scaling of the scalp, severe dandruff, and broken hairs. Rare in adults (see Fig. 1.2)

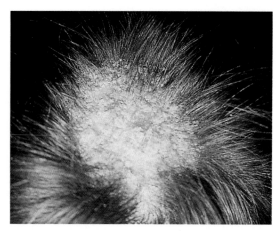

Fig. 1.2 Tinea capitis due to *M. audouinii*.

- onychomycosis: infection of the nailbeds, resulting in unsightly fingers and toes.

Q How may a diagnosis of tinea be confirmed?

A The classic appearance of the scaly lesions is diagnostic of 'ringworm' and frequently investigations are not conducted or warranted. Investigations will confirm the diagnosis and may indicate

a possible source, such as a domestic animal (see Box 1.1). Investigations include:

- ultraviolet light illumination of scalp (Wood's light): *Microsporum* infections fluoresce green. Not applicable, however, for other genera or other body sites
- microscopy: fungal elements may be seen following digestion of skin scales, nail clippings, or hairs in 10–20% potassium hydroxide. *Swabs are unsuitable*. Skin scales should be obtained from the *edge* and not the centre of the lesion
- culture: scales, hair, or nail clippings may be cultured for fungi on Sabouraud agar containing antibiotics and cycloheximide to suppress other flora. This may take up to 3 weeks, however.

A clinical diagnosis of tinea corporis was made, which was confirmed by the presence of fungal elements on microscopy and the isolation from skin scales of *T. rubrum*. Howard was prescribed a topical antifungal agent and, when he was seen again at the outpatients 1 month later, the lesions were almost gone.

Box 1.1 Classification of dermatophyte infections according to source		
Zoophilic	Acquired from animals such as cats, dogs, rodents, cattle	*M. canis*, *T. mentagrophytes* (rats), *T. verrucosum* (cattle)
Geophilic	Acquired from soil: more important in the tropics	*M. gypseum*
Anthrophilic	Acquired from siblings, playmates, school friends via desquamated skin scales, etc.	*T. rubrum* (most common), *E. floccosum*

Table 1.1 Commonly used agents to treat dermatophyte infections	
Azoles	Include clotrimazole (topical), miconazole (topical), ketoconazole (oral, a major advance in the treatment of nail infections), and itraconazole
Griseofulvin	Administered orally and preferentially deposited in newly formed keratin; therefore ideal for nail and hair infections. Only licensed agent available for children
Terbinafine	Allylamine agent administered orally. Appears to be as effective as griseofulvin over a shorter period, but not licensed for use in children
Whitfield's ointment	Consists of salicylic and benzoic acid. Inexpensive but very messy. Has largely been replaced by azoles

Q What options are there for the treatment of tinea infections?

A There are a limited number of drugs available (see Table 1.1). The mainstay of treatment is still a topical azole preparation, or griseofulvin taken orally. Skin infections require 2–4 weeks of therapy, whereas those affecting nails and hair may require 3–9 months of therapy.

Q What other non-bacterial infections or infestations of the skin may present with a rash or itching?

A These include:

- superficial candida: may affect skin, nails, or feet
- pityriasis versicolor: caused by the yeast *Malassezia furfur* and characterized by hypo- or hyperpigmented macules, which are not usually itchy. Very difficult to grow *in vitro* and diagnosis is made clinically and with microscopy
- scabies: caused by the insect *Sarcoptes scabiei* and is found worldwide, especially in immigrants and the homeless. Affects the clefts between the fingers, the hands, forearms, and genital area. Pruritus is characteristic. Scabies is quite infectious and may be acquired by close contact, such as during sexual intercourse, by a family member or even by a health-care worker during the care of an infested patient. Treatment with agents such as permethrin must be applied to the whole body and not just the affected area, bedclothes and clothing should be changed and washed, and all members of the household plus close contacts also treated
- lice: different types may infest the head, body, or pubic area (also known as crab louse). Common among vagrants and children
- viruses: a variety of viral illnesses may manifest with a skin rash or itchy lesions. These include herpes simplex (see Case 37), enteroviruses (see Case 3), measles (see Case 6), varicella zoster (see Case 7), rubella (see Case 59), and parvovirus (see Case 67).

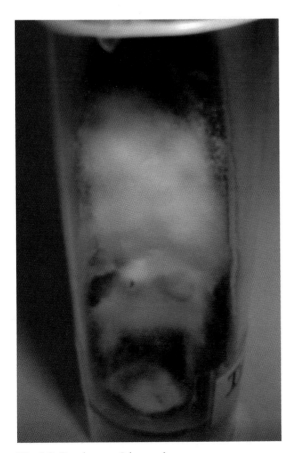

Fig. 1.3 *T. rubrum* on Sabouraud agar.

Summary: Tinea

Presentation

Scaling skin infections with a less inflamed centre. May also infect nails and hair. Contagious and may be acquired from domestic or farm animals

Diagnosis

Clinical presentation often diagnostic. Skin scales, nail scrapings, or hairs should be sent to the laboratory for microscopy and culture. Dermatophytes rarely isolated from swabs

Treatment

A topical azole for 2–4 weeks (skin infection) and oral griseofulvin or terbinafine for 3–9 months (nail or hair infections)

Case 2 Hannah, a 67-year-old widow with a leg ulcer

Hannah, a 67-year-old overweight widow, comes to the surgery because of a leg ulcer (see Fig. 2.1). Two weeks ago a swab was taken from the ulcer for culture and oral amoxycillin prescribed for 10 days. The result of the swab is as follows:

- heavy growth of *Escherichia coli* isolated
- moderate growth of *Proteus mirabilis* isolated
- moderate growth of *Enterococcus faecalis* isolated
- scanty growth of *Bacteroides* spp. isolated after 48 hours.

Hannah mentions that the ulcer has been increasing in size but there is little or no pain. On examination she is mildly hypertensive and has bilateral varicose veins. Examination of the leg reveals an ulcer with discoloration of the surrounding skin and some oedema. Arterial pulses are strong and there is no tenderness, pus, erythema, cellulitis, or lymphangitis.

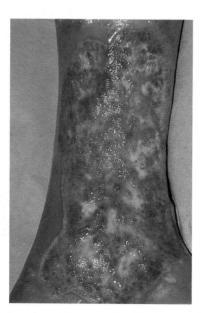

Fig. 2.1 Leg ulcer with surrounding discoloration of skin.

Q What kind of ulcer does Hannah have?

A The position of the ulcer, the presence of strong arterial pulses, the induration, oedema, and trophic changes as manifest by discoloration of the surrounding skin caused by haemosiderin deposition, the presence of varicose veins, and the absence of pain are all highly suggestive of a venous ulcer caused by inadequate superficial and deep venous drainage of the lower limb. Approximately 20% of elderly adults develop varicose or venous ulcers, but they are five times more common in females.

Q Is it surprising that the laboratory has not included the result of a Gram stain in the report?

A No. Most bacteriology laboratories do not routinely carry out Gram films on superficial swabs because the large number of mixed bacteria on the skin, especially in the ulcer base, often obscures the presence of pathogens, which may be detected following culture.

Q Which of the bacteria from the swab are likely to be clinically significant?

A It is highly unlikely that any of these bacteria are of pathogenic significance. Microbes recovered from the skin may be subdivided into two populations:

- normal resident flora, present on intact skin or in hair follicles. These include staphylococci (occasionally *Staphylococcus aureus*), micrococci, diphtheroids, and propionibacteria
- transient flora, removed by washing with soap or disinfectants such as chlorhexidine and originating from the general environment, contact with other individuals, or other parts of the body (e.g. the anus). Such flora are limited by the dryness of the normal skin and the secretion of inhibitory fatty acids, but often flourish in moist conditions or where there is a break in skin integrity. Transient flora include *S. aureus*, streptococci, enterococci (see Box 2.1), coliforms such as *E. coli* and *Proteus* (see Box 2.2) spp., *Pseudomonas aeruginosa*, and even *Candida* spp.

Box 2.1 Enterococci (faecal streptococci)

- May be haemolytic or non-haemolytic and some belong to Lancefield group D. Include *Enterococcus faecalis*, *E. faecium*

- Part of the normal upper respiratory and gastro-intestinal flora. Cause urinary infection (see Case 34), bacteraemia and endocarditis (see Case 49), and intraabdominal infection (see Case 26). Increasingly important as hospital pathogens

- Unlike other streptococci, resistant to most penicillins (except ampicillin, usually) and the cephalosporins
Glycopeptide (e.g. vancomycin) resistant entero-cocci, referred to as GRE or more commonly VRE (especially in the USA where teicoplanin is not licensed), are more prevalent in some hospitals, especially in the intensive care unit, where they can spread easily from patient-to-patient and persist in the environment

Box 2.2 *Proteus* spp.

- Oxidase-negative Gram-negative bacilli, e.g. *Proteus mirabilis*, *P. vulgaris*
  Grow well on most laboratory media but have a tendency to swarm (see Fig. 2.2)
  Urease production is characteristic

- Part of the normal gastrointestinal flora but may cause urinary infection (see Case 34) and bacter-aemia (see Case 47). Commonly colonize moist or broken skin, e.g. ulcers, otitis externa (see Case 13)

- Most isolates are sensitive to the penicillins and cephalosporins

Q Should sensitivities to antibiotics have been included in the report?

A No. The reporting of antibiotic sensitivities would be misleading as it would suggest that

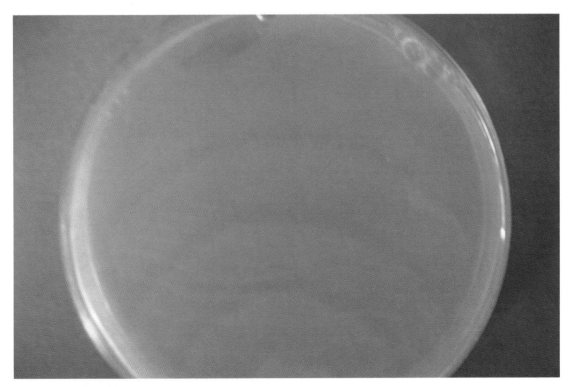

Fig. 2.2 *Proteus mirabilis* swarming on nutrient agar.

treatment with antibiotics was indicated. These organisms are unlikely to be pathogens here. Indeed, it would have been helpful if the report had included a comment to this effect!

Q Is this an infected ulcer?

A The absence of pain, erythema, pus, cellulitis, or systemic symptoms such as fever suggests that this is not an infected ulcer and that the bacteria isolated from the swab are colonizing the area of broken skin.

Q How may infected leg ulcers be classified?

A Most are secondarily infected rather than primary (where infection causes the ulcer).

1. Primary
   - Ecthyma gangrenosum, caused by *Pseudomonas aeruginosa*, usually in the immunosuppressed patient, and may be accompanied by bacteraemia
   - Syphilis, with a hard chancre usually on the external genitalia (see Case 36)
   - Tuberculosis, often in the form of lupus vulgaris, or associated with BCG administered subcutaneously to immunosuppressed patients
   - Anthrax, caused by infection with *Bacillus anthracis* due to contact with infected animals, hides, or other animal products. Generally occurs in farmers, vets, tanning workers, etc. Presents as a pimple leading to a pustule surrounded by inflammation (malignant pustule), with the centre becoming necrotic (see Case 10)
   - Parasitic, e.g. cutaneous leishmaniasis (see Case 55)
   - Anaerobic, e.g. *Bacteroides* spp. causing perianal ulcers with undermining of the edge and necrosis

2. Secondary
   - Associated with pressure sores, varicose veins, or arterial disease (e.g. peripheral vascular disease), and diabetes mellitus. Commonly colonized by Gram-negative bacilli (coliforms, *Pseudomonas*) but infections are usually caused by Gram-positive cocci (*S. aureus*, streptococci) and anaerobes

Q What investigations should routinely be carried out in patients with leg ulcers?

A When the ulcer is secondary to venous or arterial disease, with little or no evidence of local or systemic infection, no laboratory investigations are required. If there is erythema or cellulitis a swab should be taken to diagnose staphylococcal or streptococcal infection and, if the patient is systemically unwell, he/she should be admitted to hospital to exclude accompanying bacteraemia.

Where the ulcer is thought to be primary, dark-ground microscopy or serology (to exclude syphilis; see Case 36) and Ziehl–Neelsen stain and culture (to exclude tuberculosis; see Case 52) may be necessary, but these should be arranged in advance with a microbiology laboratory or advice sought from other specialist services, e.g. the genitourinary medicine department. A biopsy of the ulcer for histology, as well as microscopy and culture, should also be considered to diagnose some of the above conditions and to rule out malignancy.

Hannah's antibiotic is discontinued and she is advised about diet to lose weight, which is felt to be exacerbating the problem. She is also encouraged to exercise the leg, such as by ankle flexing to improve venous function. Following hydrocolloid dressings and compression bandages organized at the surgery, and with the assistance of the community nurse, her leg ulcer improves over the next 4 weeks. Her blood pressure returns to normal when she loses weight over the next 2 months.

Q Was oral amoxycillin the most appropriate antibiotic?

A No. As discussed earlier, an antibiotic was not indicated unless the ulcer looked infected, but in any case amoxycillin is not the agent of choice here.

Q Why is amoxycillin inappropriate here?

A Amoxycillin is active against aerobic and anaerobic streptococci, but most strains of *S. aureus* produce β-lactamase and hence will be resistant to penicillin and ampicillin (equivalent in its anti-bacterial activity to amoxycillin). Flucloxacillin alone, or in combination with amoxycillin, would be more appropriate pending the results of sensitivity testing. Alternatively, co-amoxiclav, which will cover both pathogens and is active against β-lactamase-producing isolates of *Bacteroides fragilis*, would also be appropriate.

Summary: **Leg ulcers**

Presentation

Breaks in the skin associated with venous or arterial disease in most cases

Diagnosis

Clinical. Microbiological investigations usually not necessary unless the ulcer looks infected (i.e. presence of swelling, erythema, and tenderness) or a less common aetiology is suspected

Management

Correction of the underlying disease, e.g. varicose veins, weight loss, or surgery with dressings/bandages and occasionally antibiotics

Case 3 Victoria, 4 years old, with painful mouth ulcers

A mother brings her 4-year-old daughter, Victoria, to see you. For the past 2 days, Victoria has complained of a painful mouth and a sore throat and has been unable to eat properly. Her past medical history is unremarkable, and she has received the standard childhood vaccinations, including measles, mumps, rubella (MMR). Two weeks ago, she started attending a playgroup, and her mother reports that a number of children at the playgroup have suffered a similar illness. On examination, she has a fever of 38.5°C, and in her mouth a number of vesicles and ulcers can be seen on the palate, tonsils, and tongue (see Fig. 3.1).

Q What is the differential diagnosis?

A The three most common causes of painful oral ulceration in a young child are primary orolabial herpes, herpangina, and hand, foot, and mouth disease.

On more careful examination of Victoria, you note that she has a few vesicles on her fingers and on her feet (see Fig. 3.2).

Q What do you think is the causative agent of her illness?

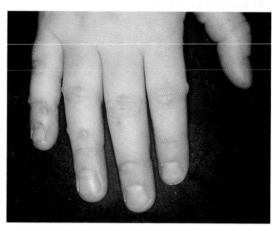

Fig. 3.2 Vesicles on fingers.

A The diagnosis is now one of hand, foot, and mouth disease. It is not uncommon for outbreaks of this to occur in child-care settings. This is a manifestation of infection with a coxsackie virus, usually a coxsackie A strain.

Q To which genus of viruses do the coxsackie viruses belong, and what are the other members of this genus?

A The genus of enteroviruses contains, polioviruses, coxsackie A and B viruses, echoviruses, and one or two others (see Box 3.1). There are a large number of enteroviruses that infect humans, and the somewhat

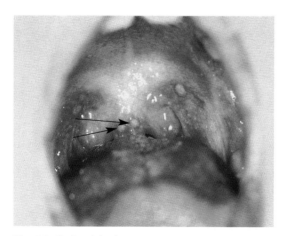

Fig. 3.1 Oral vesicles (e.g. arrows).

Box 3.1 The enteroviruses

- Polioviruses (types 1, 2, and 3)
- Coxsackie A viruses (23 types, numbered A1–A24, as Coxsackie A23 is the same virus as echovirus 9)
- Coxsackie B viruses (types B1–B6)
- Echoviruses (31 types, numbered 1–33, as echoviruses 10 and 28 have been reclassified into other virus families)
- Enteroviruses (types 68–71)

ad hoc nomenclature makes them rather confusing. Coxsackie is the name of a town in the USA where an outbreak of polio-like paralytic disease was caused by a hitherto unidentified virus—hence the name of the coxsackie viruses. These are split into A and B groups on the basis of their culture properties. Echo stands for entero cytopathic human orphan, and arises from the isolation of viruses from faeces that produced a cytopathic effect in tissue culture, but were not initially associated with disease. More recently discovered enteroviruses are now simply given the prefix EV, and a number. The value of remembering that all these viruses are enteroviruses lies in the fact that this gives an indication of their mode of spread—they enter through the mouth and are excreted in the faeces.

Table 3.1 Consequences of enterovirus infections

General

Asymptomatic infection	The most common sequela of infection
Infection in the newborn	Neonatal enteroviral infection can be life-threatening, owing to the multisystem nature of the infection in this patient group (e.g. myocarditis, hepatitis, encephalitis). Outbreaks may occur in neonatal units

Skin and mucous membranes

Fever and exanthem	Non-specific illness, often in the summer months
Herpangina	Usually coxsackie A viruses. Discrete small vesicles on the posterior pharynx, palate, tonsils, tongue
Hand, foot, and mouth disease	Coxsackie A or B viruses. Intraoral lesions are ulcerative; the lesions on hands and feet usually vesicular
Conjunctivitis	Coxsackie A 24 and EV 70 associated with epidemics of acute haemorrhagic conjunctivitis in Africa, the Americas, and the Far East

Musculoskeletal system

Pleurodynia (Bornholm disease or epidemic myalgia)	Usually coxsackie B viruses. Chest pain may mimic myocardial infarction

Central nervous system

Poliomyelitis	This is a syndrome of flaccid paralysis resulting from lower motor neuron damage, usually due to polioviruses, but can rarely be caused by other enteroviruses
Meningitis	The enteroviruses are one of the 2 most common causes of aseptic meningitis—the other being mumps virus
Encephalitis	May represent spread of infection from the meninges or rarely occur in the absence of meningitis

Respiratory system

Upper respiratory tract infection	For example, common-cold-like illness, pharyngitis
Lower respiratory tract infection	For example, bronchiolitis, or pneumonia, usually in young children

Cardiovascular system

Acute myo- and pericarditis	Coxsackie B viruses (see Fig. 3.3)

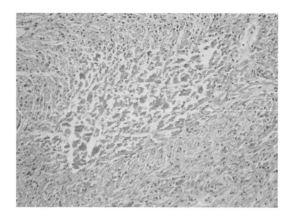

Fig. 3.3 Coxsackie-virus-induced myocarditis.

Q What other diseases are associated with infection with enteroviruses?

A These viruses give rise to a wide range of clinical syndromes, outlined in Table 3.1. Enteroviruses are an important cause of morbidity and mortality, and appear in the differential diagnosis of a number of the case histories presented in this text. However, despite their name, they have not been proven to cause disease of the gastrointestinal tract itself. Note that infection with one enterovirus does not induce protective immunity against any of the other enteroviruses.

In addition, there are a number of important diseases in which enteroviral infection has been suggested to play an aetiological role, including polymyositis and dermatomyositis, the chronic fatigue syndrome, dilated cardiomyopathy, and diabetes mellitus. However, the links between enterovirus infection and these diseases have not yet been conclusively proven.

Q How would you prove that a patient has an enterovirus infection?

A Traditional laboratory diagnosis is by isolating virus in cell culture. However, not all members of the enteroviral family will grow in standard cell cultures, so this approach may not always yield a positive result. Indeed, the likely cause of Victoria's hand, foot, and mouth disease, a coxsackie A virus, does not grow well, so this is essentially a clinical diagnosis.

Q Which samples should you send to the laboratory for virus isolation?

A Remember the name of this virus family—virus will be present in the throat and also in the faeces. Thus, at the very least, you should send a throat swab in viral culture medium, and a stool sample to the laboratory for viral isolation. Other samples may also yield virus, e.g. cerebrospinal fluid (CSF) in a patient with enteroviral meningitis, myocardial biopsy in a patient with myocarditis.

Q What other diagnostic approaches may be taken?

A Serological diagnosis may be possible by demonstrating a rise in enteroviral antibody titres, or by detection of enterovirus-specific IgM, although these tests are usually only performed in reference laboratories. A more modern approach is to demonstrate the presence of enteroviral RNA by a genome amplification technique, e.g. reverse transcription polymerase chain reaction (RT/PCR) assay. RT/PCR assay on CSF may soon become the standard method of diagnosis of enteroviral meningitis.

Q Is there any specific treatment for enteroviral infections?

A No.

Q How may enteroviral infections be prevented?

A Poliovirus vaccines are effective in preventing infection with the three serotypes of poliovirus, but do not provide cross-protection to infection with the other members of the genus. There are two types of vaccine available. Both are effective, and both have been adopted as prophylaxis by different countries. The major advantages and disadvantages of each are indicated in Box 3.2. There is a World Health Organization (WHO)-sponsored programme of worldwide vaccination with the aim of global elimination of poliomyelitis. Although the campaign is slightly behind time in achieving this laudable target, huge progress has taken place. In 2003, there are fewer than 10 countries remaining with endemic wild-type poliovirus infections.

Box 3.2 Poliovirus vaccines

- Component of routine childhood vaccination schedule
- Two types

Live attenuated (Sabin) vaccine

- Contains attenuated strains of all three poliovirus serotypes
- Given orally, therefore provides mucosal immunity
- May revert to virulence, resulting in vaccine-associated poliomyelitis
- Contraindicated in immunosuppressed patients

Killed (Salk) vaccine

- Given by intramuscular injection; therefore less effective in inducing mucosal immunity and hence herd immunity
- No risk of reversion to virulence
- Vaccine of choice in immunosuppressed individuals

Summary: Enteroviruses

Genus consists of polio-, coxsackie A- and B-, echoviruses

Presentation

Wide range of clinical manifestations including meningitis, myocarditis, poliomyelitis, rashes, upper and lower respiratory tract infections; do not cause diarrhoea

Diagnosis

Viral culture of throat swab, faeces, CSF; serology; genome amplification

Management

No specific therapy yet; polio is preventable by vaccination

Case 4 Albert, 4 years old, with painful mouth and sore throat

A mother brings her 4-year-old son, Albert, to see you. For the past 2 days, Albert has complained of a painful mouth, a sore throat, and being unable to eat properly. His past medical history is unremarkable, and he has received the standard childhood vaccinations, including MMR (measles, mumps, and rubella). On examination of Albert's mouth, a number of vesicles and ulcers can be seen on the palate, tonsils, tongue, lips, and adjacent skin (see Fig. 4.1).

Q What is the differential diagnosis?

A Albert has a very similar presentation to that of Victoria, in the previous case. As indicated in her case, the three most common causes of painful oral ulceration in a young child are primary orolabial herpes, herpangina, and hand, foot, and mouth disease.

Unlike Victoria, Albert has no lesions on his hands or feet. The extensive nature of his oral disease, with the spread of vesicles on to the adjacent skin, makes you strongly suspect orolabial herpes.

Q What other physical signs are likely to be present in a child with orolabial herpes?

A In addition to the extensive local disease in the mouth, such children also have evidence of systemic upset, e.g. a fever, being generally unwell, and tender cervical lymphadenopathy.

Q What is the causative agent of this infection?

A Herpes simplex virus (HSV) type 1 or 2. At the molecular level, these viruses are very closely related to each other. As a broad generalization, HSV-1 is responsible for the majority of herpetic infections above the waist (i.e. in the mouth), whilst HSV-2 is responsible for the majority of herpetic infections below the waist (i.e. genital herpes). However, this distinction has become blurred in recent years as more HSV-2-associated oral and HSV-1-associated genital herpes infections have appeared due to safe sex practices.

Q To which virus family do these viruses belong, and what are the other members that infect humans?

A HSV types 1 and 2 are two of the eight herpesviruses (or *herpesviridae*, to give them their Latin monicker) thus far discovered to infect humans. The members of this group are listed in Box 4.1.

Q All herpesviruses exhibit the phenomenon of latency. What is meant by the term 'latency'?

A This means that infection with any one of these viruses is followed by lifelong carriage, with the virus establishing a latent infection at some site

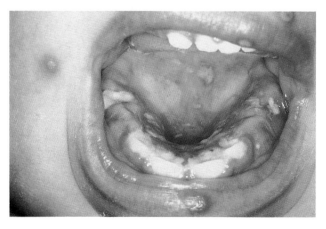

Fig. 4.1 Extensive oral ulceration and vesicles.

- Herpes simplex type 1
- Herpes simplex type 2
- Varicella zoster virus
- Epstein–Barr virus
- Cytomegalovirus
- Human herpesvirus type 6
- Human herpesvirus type 7
- Human herpesvirus type 8 (Kaposi's-sarcoma-associated herpesvirus)

within the body. In the latent state there is no viral replication or damage to the cell in which the virus exists. However, latent virus can be reactivated (i.e. start to replicate) at any stage in later life, thus giving rise to a secondary/reactivated/recurrent infection. Individuals can also be re-exposed to the virus, and become reinfected. It is therefore possible to undergo the following types of infection with a herpesvirus:

1 primary, i.e. the very first exposure to the virus

2 secondary, which can either be
- reactivation of endogenous latent virus or
- reinfection with exogenous virus

The clinical features of primary and secondary herpesvirus infections are very often quite distinct in an immunocompetent host, as the former occur in an immunologically naive host, and therefore may cause widespread severe and relatively long-lasting disease, whilst the latter occur in a host whose immune system has seen the virus before, and are thus in general much more trivial, localized, and quicker to resolve.

On closer examination of Albert, you note that he has a fever of 38.8°C and tender swollen cervical lymph nodes.

Q Which type of infection do you think Albert has?

A Primary orolabial herpes. The evidence in support of this includes:

- the extensive nature of his oral disease—throughout the oral cavity
- the spread of disease on to adjacent skin
- the systemic upset (fever) and cervical adenopathy

Q What, then, would be the typical features of secondary, or recurrent, orolabial herpes?

A The site of latency of HSV is the nerve cell body. Thus, during Albert's primary infection in the mouth, virus will enter the trigeminal nerve and travel up to the trigeminal ganglion. If virus reactivates from this site, it will travel back down the nerve to the periphery. The disease caused by this is more commonly known as a cold sore (see Fig. 4.2). The salient features of this secondary disease, in comparison to those of the primary infection listed above, are:

- the lesion usually consists of only one or two blisters, highly localized to one lip only
- there is no spread on to adjacent skin
- there is no systemic upset or cervical adenopathy

These differences arise largely because reactivation is occurring in a host whose immune system has had prior exposure to the virus, and is therefore able to exert control over local cell-to-cell spread of the virus.

Q How would you prove the diagnosis of orolabial herpes in Albert?

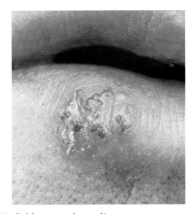

Fig. 4.2 Cold sore on lower lip.

A Albert's lesions will contain very high titres of virus. Thus, the easiest way to make the diagnosis is to send a swab of an ulcer base, or of vesicle fluid if there are any intact vesicles, to the laboratory for viral culture (note: the swabs should be broken off into viral transport medium to ensure survival of the virus on its way to the laboratory). HSV is a fast-growing virus. The laboratory should be able to confirm your clinical suspicions within 48 hours.

Q What complications may arise as a result of Albert's infection?

A These are listed in Table 4.1.

Q How should you manage Albert?

A HSV replication can be completely inhibited by aciclovir and the derivatives thereof (see Appendix 3). This is clearly indicated in a patient with primary disease, where the natural history of infection will take 2–3 weeks to resolve. Treatment will reduce time to cessation of new lesion formation, and time to healing by 7–10 days. Treatment is also indicated if there is a risk of severe complications (see Box 4.2), i.e. in immunodeficient patients or in patients with eczema.

Table 4.1 Complications of primary orolabial herpes

- Self-inoculation of virus to other sites, e.g. eyes (see Case 8), genitals, nail beds (herpetic whitlow)
- Secondary bacterial infection, e.g. staphylococci, streptococci
- In immunodeficient patients viraemic spread may occur, with internal organ involvement. These patients suffer more frequent and extensive recurrences
- In patients with eczema, the damaged nature of the skin may allow extensive contiguous spread of infection. This is known as *eczema herpeticum*. Can arise from primary and/or secondary infection. Access to bloodstream through damaged skin may lead to infection of internal organs, e.g. hepatitis, pneumonitis

---

Q Should you recommend antiviral therapy for a patient with a cold sore?

A Controlled clinical trials have demonstrated very little benefit of antiviral therapy in the treatment of recurrent oral herpes, e.g. 24 hours reduction in time to healing at best. This is because the natural history of the disease is to resolve in 5–6 days. In principle, it is not a good idea to use antiviral (or antibacterial) agents unnecessarily, as such use may encourage the emergence of drug-resistant organisms. Thus, antiviral therapy should *not* be recommended in this circumstance.

Q Do all patients who suffer from cold sores give a history of orolabial herpes similar to that in Albert?

A No. This is an important point. Although symptomatic primary disease can be very dramatic and debilitating, in fact most primary infections are asymptomatic. Presumably, the balance between disease/no disease is dependent on the infecting dose of virus and the speed/magnitude of the host immune response. However, even during asymptomatic infection, virus will enter the trigeminal nerve and go latent. Thus, most patients who have cold sores will not give a history of primary orolabial herpes. The same principle applies in genital herpes, where most patients with recurrent disease do not recall a symptomatic primary infection (see Case 37).

The consequences of infection with herpes simplex virus types 1 and 2 will crop up at several points during this book. This illustrates that HSV infection is common and can give rise to a multiplicity of disease states. The diverse manifestations of HSV infection are presented in Box 4.2.

Box 4.2 **Manifestations of herpes simplex virus infection**

Asymptomatic seroconversion

Orolabial herpes (this case)

Eczema herpeticum (this case)

Herpetic conjunctivitis (see Case 8)

Genital herpes (see Case 37)

Herpetic whitlow (see Case 10)

Herpes simplex encephalitis (see Case 42)

Neonatal herpes (see Case 63)

Summary: Orolabial herpes

Caused by HSV infection. Usually in young children but can be seen in older individuals

Primary disease
Extensive, systemic upset; 2–3 week duration

Secondary disease
Localized cold sore; no systemic upset; 5–6 day duration

Complications
Inoculation of distant sites; bacterial superinfection; bloodstream spread can be life-threatening in immunodeficient patients or patients with eczema

Treatment
Antiviral therapy (aci-, valaci-, famciclovir) for primary disease or complications

Case 5 Jamie, a 5-year-old with a troublesome graze

Jamie, a 5-year-old child, is seen in the accident and emergency department. Four days previously he was playing with his two sisters when he fell and sustained a graze over his left elbow. This was dressed and looked after by his mother, who is now concerned that the wound is infected. She claims that Jamie now cries whenever she or anybody else goes near it. In the past Jamie has been a healthy child and has received all his vaccinations to date, including tetanus and haemophilus. On examination Jamie is apyrexial but a little irritable, and screams when the doctor approaches his elbow. There is a small area of erythema with some tenderness surrounding the graze (Fig. 5.1), but there is no pus, lymphangitis, or lymphadenopathy. Movement of the elbow is not restricted.

Q What is the diagnosis and the likely aetiology?

A Jamie has cellulitis, as evidenced by the erythema and tenderness, which is most probably caused by a β-haemolytic streptococcus or possibly *Staphylococcus aureus* (see Case 54) acquired following the injury.

Q How are streptococci classified?

A Streptococci are Gram-positive cocci that appear in chains/pairs under microscopy but unlike staphylococci are catalase-negative. Streptococci are found as part of the normal flora of the upper respiratory, gastrointestinal, and lower genital tracts. Classification is based upon the ability of many streptococci to produce exotoxins, i.e. haemolysins, capable of breaking down red blood cells. Streptococcal haemolysis (see Table 5.1 and Fig. 5.2) may be:

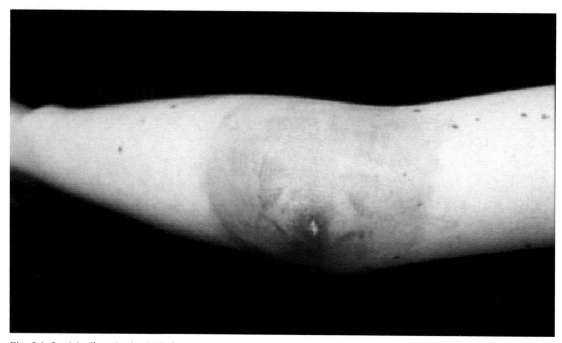

Fig. 5.1 Jamie's elbow in the A&E department.

Table 5.1 **Guide to streptococci (excluding anaerobes) and their clinical importance**

Group	Haemolysis	Examples	Infections
streptococci α or viridans	α	*S. mutans S. mitior, S. sanguis*	Bacteraemia, Infective endocarditis (see Case 49)
		S. pneumoniae	Pneumonia (see Case 18), meningitis (see Case 41)
β streptococci	β	*S. pyogenes*	Superficial and deep infection, including bacteaemia
γ streptococci	None	*S. salivarius*	Dental disease
Enterococci	α or β or γ	*E. faecalis*	Urinary tract infections (UTIs), endocarditis

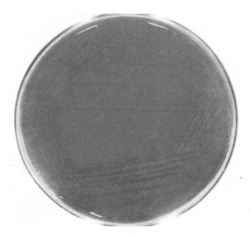 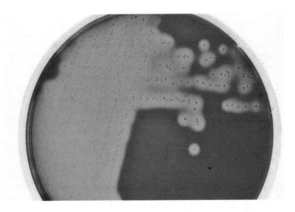

Fig. 5.2 Alpha (left) and beta (right) haemolytic on blood agar.

- α, partial haemolysis with a surrounding area of green coloration
- β, clear zone of haemolysis (often can read through the agar plate!)
- γ, no haemolysis

Q How are the β-haemolytic streptococci subdivided?

A These streptococci are subdivided on the basis of the Lancefield groups, which reflect differences in carbohydrate antigens of the cell. This grouping can be carried out on isolates in the diagnostic laboratory with appropriate antisera by precipitation or latex agglutination. Within the different groups there may be one or more species:

Group	Species
A	*S. pyogenes*: may be subdivided according to Griffith types (M, T, R) based upon surface antigens
B	*S. agalactiae*: causes infection in the mother and neonate during the postpartum period (see Case 58)
C	*S. equi* and *S. equisimilis*: very similar to group A but probably less virulent

D   includes the enterococci such as *E. faecalis, E. faecium* (see Case 2)

F   *S. anginosus* (previously known as *S. milleri*): part of the normal gastro-intestinal flora but may cause liver, lung, and brain abscesses (see Case 43)

G   very similar to A and C

Q How do group A streptococci cause disease?

A Group A streptococci are capable of producing an array of extracellular enzymes and toxins (many also produced by other β-haemolytic streptococci) that are considered to be potent virulence determinants. These include:

- haemolysins
- erythrogenic toxins: production mediated by phages and responsible for the rash in scarlet fever; also implicated in streptococcal toxic shock syndrome (see Case 9)
- streptolysins O and S: induce lysis in red blood cells (haemolysis) and are cytotoxic to other cells, such as neutrophils
- streptokinase: converts plasminogen to plasmin
- deoxyribonucleases: at least four of these are known
- hyaluronidase: partly responsible for spread of infection in cellulitis and erysipelas.

The severity of disease may also be related to underlying disease such as diabetes mellitus, but severe infections may also occur in the young, fit, and healthy population.

Q Which streptococci cause cellulitis?

A Groups A, C, and G. Group A causes the most severe or life-threatening form.

Q What is the antibiotic of choice to treat cellulitis caused by β-haemolytic streptococci?

A Benzylpenicillin, as all group A streptococci are still very susceptible to penicillin. It is also the treatment of choice for infections caused by groups B, C, and G. Treatment for cellulitis should be continued for at least 10–14 days, as there is initially often a slow response. If severe or accompanied by systemic signs or symptoms, antibiotics should be administered intravenously initially. When oral therapy is appropriate benzylpenicillin may be substituted by amoxycillin. Alternatives include erythromycin, a cephalosporin, or clindamycin, especially in the penicillin-allergic patient.

Q Are the enterococci sensitive to penicillin?

A No. The enterococci are penicillin-resistant but are usually susceptible to ampicillin/amoxycillin, and this is the treatment of choice for enterococcal urinary tract infection. Systemic enterococcal infection requires a combination of a penicillin and an aminoglycoside, or a glycopeptide such as vancomycin or teicoplanin. Enterococci resistant to the glycopeptides (GRE) are increasingly reported in many hospitals, especially in intensive care unit (ICU) patients or patients with chronic illnesses requiring antibiotics periodically such as those on haemodialysis. Although isolation of these bacteria often represents colonization only, when infection does occur there are few options for therapy—linezolid, a new oxazolidinone agent, which can be administered orally as well as parenterally, and quinupristin–dalfopristin, which is not active, however, against one particular species of enterococcus, *E. faecalis*.

Jamie is discharged from the accident and emergency department on a course of amoxycillin for 10 days. Three days later, when he is reviewed, the area of cellulitis has decreased and is less tender. A report from the microbiology laboratory indicates that a group A streptococcus, sensitive to penicillin, has been isolated from a swab taken from the wound site.

Q What other infections are caused by group A streptococci?

A These include:

- tonsillitis: but streptococci much less common as a cause than viruses
- quinsy: peritonsillar abscess that requires drainage

- impetigo: common in childhood and associated with overcrowding; also caused by groups C and G β-haemolytic streptococci and *S. aureus*
- wound infection following surgery
- erysipelas: more superficial than cellulitis
- scarlet fever
- bacteraemia: often with multiple organ failure and a high mortality, even in young patients (see Case 47)
- necrotizing fasciitis: often associated with other pathogens, such as *S. aureus*, coliforms, and anaerobes.

Q What other measures should be taken in cases of group A streptococcal infections admitted to hospital?

A This bacterium is highly infectious and spreads by direct contact or by the airborne route (e.g. tonsillitis). Patients with tonsillitis, cellulitis, or wound infection who require admission to hospital should be isolated in a single room where at all possible until 48 hours of antibiotic treatment have elapsed. Plastic aprons and gloves are necessary for patient contact and hand-washing is essential.

Q Which bacteria cause wound infection?

A The bacteria that most commonly cause wound infection are:

- *S. aureus*, responsible for 50–60% (see Case 54)
- groups A, C, and G β-haemolytic streptococci
- aerobic Gram-negative bacilli, e.g. *Escherichia coli*, *Klebsiella pneumoniae*, etc. but colonization with these bacteria is more common than infection (see Case 2)
- anaerobes, e.g. *Clostridium perfringens*, *Bacteroides fragilis*
- less commonly enterococci, *Pseudomonas aeruginosa*, and perhaps *S. epidermidis* (difficult to distinguish from normal skin flora). These are usually hospital-acquired and occur in debilitated patients or following complicated procedures
- dog bites may lead to wound infection due to less common Gram-negative bacilli, e.g.

Capnocytophaga canimorsus and *Pasteurella multocida*, which can occasionally result in systemic infection such as bacteraemia.

Q What are the risk factors for contracting post-surgical wound infection?

A Specific factors that influence the risk of contracting infection following surgery include the type of surgery and the anatomical location (see Table 5.1), whether a drain is left *in situ* where there is residual infected material, the experience and expertise of the surgical team, the patient's age, underlying disease such as diabetes mellitus, and, finally, whether antibiotic prophylaxis was used (see Case 26).

Three weeks later Jamie is seen again by the family doctor because his parents have noticed a low-grade fever, generalized weakness, some swelling around the face in particular, and blood while passing urine over the last week. The graze and the surrounding area of cellulitis have healed, and there is no longer any tenderness.

Q What possible diagnosis must be considered now?

A Post-streptococcal glomerulonephritis, which may be confirmed by the detection of red blood cell casts in the urine and elevated serum urea and creatinine. This condition is due to a cross-reaction

---

Box 5.1 Classification of surgical wounds

Clean

No break in any viscus or hollow organ, e.g. inguinal hernia; infection rate < 2%

Contaminated

Involves incision into the gastrointestinal or respiratory tract, with possible spillage but no pus, e.g. cholecystectomy; infection rate 10–40%

Infected

Surgery where there is infected tissue or a collection of pus, e.g. incision and drainage of peritoneal abscess; infection rate > 50%

between certain streptococcus antigens and those of the host, e.g. on the basement membrane of the glomerulus, leading to deposition of immune complexes and infiltration with polymorphonuclear and eosinophil leucocytes within the glomerulus, as seen on renal biopsy. Complement activation leads to decreased C_3 of the complement cascade. Certain Griffith types of group A streptococci are associated with glomerulonephritis, and these include M12 (post-tonsillitis) and M49, M55, and M57 (post-impetigo).

Q Should Jamie be treated with another course of antibiotics?

A No. This is a post-infectious disease syndrome and antibiotics are not indicated once the precipitating cause, namely, the streptococcal cellulitis in the case of Jamie, has been treated. Post-streptococcal glomerulonephritis usually resolves with conservative management including diuretics.

Q Name another important post-streptococcal disease.

A Rheumatic fever (see Box 5.2) where the immunopathogenesis is similar but directed against cardiac antigens.

Q Are there any laboratory tests apart from culture that might indicate recent group A streptococcal infection?

A A number of serological tests that may indicate recent or previous infection are available in most diagnostic or reference laboratories. These include antistreptolysin O titre or ASOT (normal value, < 250), anti-DNAse B titre (normal value, < 320), and antihyaluronidase (normal value, < 300). One or more of these is usually considerably elevated in cases of rheumatic fever or post-streptococcal glomerulonephritis.

Box 5.2 Rheumatic fever

Clinical featuers

Fever, arthralgia, nodules, skin rash (erythema marginatum) 1–5 weeks after a streptococcal infection. Only 15–20% are culture positive for group A streptococci from throat or other site, e.g. wound

Diagnosis

High probability if two *major* criteria (carditis, polyarthritis, chorea, erythema marginatum, subcutaneous nodules) or one *major* and two *minor* criteria (previous history of rheumatic fever, arthralgia, fever, elevated erythrocyte sedimentation rate (ESR) or C-reactive protein (CRP), abnormal electrocardiogram (ECG) with laboratory evidence of recent streptococcal infection

---

Summary: β-haemolytic streptococci

Presentation

A variety of superficial (wound infection, tonsillitis, erysipelas, impetigo) and systemic (bacteraemia with multiple organ failure) infections. Immune-mediated complications may ensue

Diagnosis

Culture of appropriate specimens, e.g. throat or wound swab, blood, etc. Serology useful especially in immune-mediated disease

Management

Penicillin is the antibiotic of choice for treatment of infection

Case 6 Simon, 4 years old, develops a rash

You are asked to visit Simon, 4 years old, as he has developed a rash in the last 12 hours (see Fig. 6.1(a)). He has been unwell for the past 3 days, with a fever, runny nose, and an unproductive cough. His GP saw him yesterday, and prescribed amoxycillin. He has received all the routine childhood vaccinations except MMR (measles, mumps, and rubella), as his parents were worried about the possible link between this and autism. Until this illness, he has been fit and well, with no history of allergy, and on no regular medication. On examination he is generally miserable and febrile (39.2°C) with a respiratory rate of 30/min. His conjunctivae are inflamed and red. The rash is most florid on his face. There is no lymphadenopathy or evidence of lower respiratory tract disease.

Q What is the differential diagnosis?

A The salient clinical features of a prodromal illness with fever, cough, coryza, and conjunctivitis, followed by a facial rash, in an unvaccinated child are highly suggestive of measles (see Table 6.1). The grim visage of the patient seen here is typical,

(a)

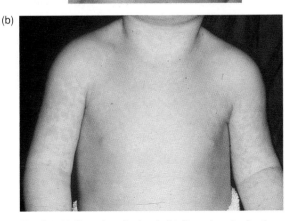

(b)

Fig. 6.1 (a) Simon's rash, day 1. (b) Simon's rash, day 3.

Table 6.1 Clinical course of uncomplicated measles infection

Transmission—droplet spread of respiratory secretions

Entry—through upper respiratory tract or conjunctiva

Incubation period—10–14 days; leucopenia develops as virus replicates in lymphoid tissue

Prodromal illness—2–4 days, as described above

Rash—appears first on face, spreads to body over 2–3 days (see Fig. 6.1(b)), then fades

Infectious period—from prodromal stage and for 4 days after onset of rash

---

Box 6.1 Roseola infantum (exanthem subitum, 6th disease)

Causative agent—primary infection with human herpesvirus types 6 or 7 (HHV6, HHV7)

Age—6 months to 2 years old

Clinical features—3–4 days pyrexia, without localizing signs, with morbilliform rash appearing as fever subsides

as children with measles are usually very miserable. Alternative diagnoses include:

- rubella, but prodromal illness is not a feature and posterior cervical adenopathy is usually more marked
- upper respiratory tract infection with an allergic reaction to ampicillin
- roseola infantum (see Box 6.1).

Q How can you confirm your diagnosis?

A By noting the presence of Koplik's spots on Simon's buccal mucosa. These small greyish-white lesions (see Fig. 6.2) are present during the prodromal stage, but fade once the rash appears. Laboratory diagnosis is by demonstration of measles-specific IgM antibodies in serum or saliva.

You diagnose acute measles virus infection and stop the antibiotics. Over the next few days, Simon's rash spreads to his trunk and limbs, then begins to fade, leaving a brownish discoloration. His respiratory symptoms improve, and his fever subsides. However, on day 7 after the onset of his rash, Simon complains of a headache, becomes increasingly irritable, and his fever returns.

Q What complication may now be developing?

A Acute measles post-infectious encephalitis. This serious complication usually presents with recrudescence of fever, headache, seizures, cerebellar ataxia,

and declining levels of consciousness, within 8–10 days of the onset of measles, in 1 per 1000–5000 cases of measles. Histology of affected brain shows demyelination and perivascular cuffing.

Q What is meant by the term 'post-infectious'?

A This refers to the pathogenetic mechanism underlying the disease. The damage appears not to be due to direct viral invasion of the brain, as neither whole virus nor viral antigens can be detected in affected brain tissue. The disease is therefore believed to arise from an aberrant immune response to the virus, which in some way cross-reacts with brain tissue, causing the pathology—hence the term 'post-infectious'. Post-infectious encephalitis may also be seen after varicella-zoster (see Case 7) and influenza virus (see Case 17) infections.

Q What is the prognosis of acute measles post-infectious encephalitis?

A Poor. There is no specific treatment, and corticosteroids have not been shown to be of value. Of cases, 15% are fatal; up to 40% of survivors suffer long-term neurological sequelae.

Q What are the other complications of measles infection?

A Most complications arise from secondary infection of the necrotic epithelial surfaces of the respiratory tract and include:

- bronchitis/bronchopneumonia
- otitis media
- purulent conjunctivitis
- laryngotracheitis
- giant cell pneumonia (rare)—a severe, protracted illness, often fatal, with characteristic multinucleate giant cells seen on histology. Due to direct spread of virus to the lower respiratory tract. Occurs usually in patients with underlying disease, e.g. leukaemia

Central nervous system complications include:

- acute measles post-infectious encephalitis (see above)
- subacute sclerosing panencephalitis (SSPE, see below).

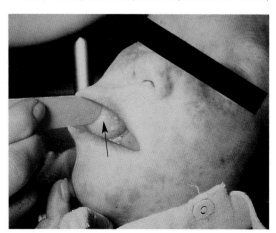

Fig. 6.2 Koplik's spots (see arrow).

Q How does SSPE differ from acute measles post-infectious encephalitis?

A The pathogenesis and clinical presentations of these two complications are quite distinct. The salient features of SSPE are shown in Box 6.2.

Q How does the epidemiology of measles differ in the developing world?

A The major differences are:

- The peak incidence of measles infection occurs earlier, e.g. at less than 2 years of age
- Measles is still a major cause of death, the mortality approaching 5–15%. WHO estimates there may be up to 1 million deaths per year arising from measles infection worldwide. Factors contributing to this are the immuno-suppressive effects of measles, due to infection and death of lymphoid cells, in a population that may already have reduced immunocompetence arising from malnutrition. Infection is therefore often complicated by life-threatening bacterial pneumonia (including tuberculosis) and severe diarrhoea

Q Is measles infection preventable?

A Yes, by means of a live attenuated vaccine. This is now incorporated into the MMR (measles/mumps/rubella) vaccine that should be given to all children at age 12–18 months. Measles is *not* a

---

Box 6.2 Subacute sclerosing panencephalitis

- Rare—1 per 10^6 cases of acute measles
- Presents *many years* (e.g. 5–10) after acute measles infection, with generalized intellectual deterioration, motor dysfunction, e.g. myoclonic jerks, dyspraxia
- Progressive—death in 1–3 years
- Measles virus *can* be isolated from affected brain tissue
- High measles antibody titres in both serum and CSF

---

trivial illness, and infection carries a significant risk of serious morbidity and mortality. Measles is highly infectious, and there have been outbreaks of disease in populations with respectable levels of vaccine coverage. Every effort should therefore be made to ensure and maintain high levels of vaccination.

Q What are the contraindications to measles vaccination?

A Genuine contraindications are few:

- acute febrile illness on presentation for immunization (vaccination should therefore be deferred)
- untreated malignant disease or altered immunity
- allergy to neomycin or kanamycin (these antibiotics are present in the vaccine)
- vaccine should not be given within 3 weeks of receipt of another live vaccine, or within 3 months of an injection of immunoglobulin
- allergy to egg, but only if this is manifested by an anaphylactic reaction. Even so, the vaccine is safe in over 99% of children with proven anaphylactic responses to oral egg challenge.

Q Why might measles vaccination not be as effective in the developing world as in the UK?

A Because of the difference in age-incidence of the disease. In developing countries, vaccination at 12–15 months of age may be too late to prevent much measles-associated mortality, which occurs mostly in younger children. Unfortunately, vaccination at a younger age, e.g. 9 months, is not as effective in inducing protective immunity. This paradox has yet to be satisfactorily resolved.

Q Were Simon's parents correct to refuse MMR vaccination because of a possible link with autism?

A No. There has been considerable adverse publicity in the lay press surrounding the MMR vaccine, with unproven claims of a causal link to the development of autism. There is an overwhelming body of epidemiological evidence that finds no link between rates of MMR vaccination and the incidence of autism. Whilst it may be impossible to rule out risks of very small magnitude, what is certain is that, if there is no change in MMR vaccination rates, many, many more children will die or suffer devastating long-term neurological sequelae from uncontrolled measles infection than might develop autism, not to mention the consequences of re-emergent rubella infection in pregnancy (see Case 59), or of mumps infection.

Measles vaccine is an effective vaccine and, in the UK, measles was a disappearing disease but, disappointingly, MMR vaccination rates in recent years have declined. They have dropped to a dangerously low level (below 80%), such that herd immunity may not be enough to prevent major epidemics of disease. It is sad to see the repeat of a medical tragedy from the 1970s, when over-publicized and incorrect scare-mongering about possible adverse reactions to whooping cough vaccines led to a dramatic reduction in vaccine uptake, with the all-too-predictable consequence of several whooping cough epidemics causing considerable morbidity and mortality.

Summary: Measles

Presentation
Prodome of upper respiratory tract symptoms, fever, and rash in an ill child

Diagnosis
Clinical (Koplik's spots, rash); serology; virus isolation

Complications
Secondary bacterial infections, acute post-infectious encephalomyelitis; giant cell pneumonia; subacute sclerosing panencephalitis (years later)

Management
No antiviral therapy. Preventable by vaccination

Case 7 Hayley, 8 years old, develops a rash

Eight-year-old Hayley has developed a generalized itchy rash that first appeared 2 days ago on her trunk as discrete red spots. These spots developed into small vesicles, and spread over her face and trunk, with lesions also appearing on her limbs. She has no other symptoms. There is no relevant past medical history, and she has not been on any medication recently. On examination, Hayley has a temperature of 37.9°C and the rash appears as shown in Fig. 7.1.

Q What is the diagnosis?

A The florid vesicular rash is characteristic of chickenpox, i.e. the manifestation of primary infection with varicella-zoster virus (VZV). In the early stages, or if the rash is less profuse, other possibilities would include herpes simplex virus infection or a drug reaction. The diagnosis is essentially a clinical one—the features of the chickenpox rash are given in Table 7.1. If necessary, the diagnosis can be confirmed by isolation of the virus from vesicle fluid or by demonstrating a rise in antibody titre in serum samples taken a few days apart.

Q What are the possible complications of chickenpox?

A These include:

1. secondary bacterial infection of vesicles

2. scarring—increased risk if lesions traumatized or infected

3. varicella pneumonia
   - usually in adults 2–3 days after onset of rash
   - chest X-ray shows diffuse patchy nodular infiltration
   - may also occur in neonates

4. encephalitis
   - uncommon. Usually 7–10 days after onset
   - cerebrospinal fluid (CSF) normal or increase in cells and protein
   - cerebellar syndrome most often seen. Hemiplegia also described

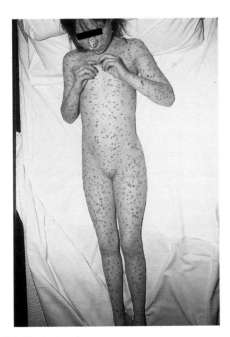

Fig. 7.1 Hayley's rash.

Table 7.1 Clinical features of chickenpox

Incubation period, 13–17 days

Rash usually appears first on the trunk and face, then spreads centripetally to involve scalp and limbs

Lesions evolve from macule to papule to vesicle in a few hours, to crust in 4 days

Usually several lesions in the mouth; pharynx and conjunctiva may also be involved

Cropping occurs over several days, so that lesions of differing ages may be present

Some generalized lymphadenopathy may occur

The rash is itchy in some, but not all patients

- recovery usually complete, but sequelae and fatalities may occur
- pathogenesis is post-infectious (see Case 6)

5. haemorrhagic varicella
   - rare. Usually associated with thrombocytopenia
   - bleeding from mucous membranes, into lesions, and into unaffected skin; often fatal

6. varicella in pregnancy
   - the complications of chickenpox in pregnancy are discussed in detail in Case 62.

Q Which patient groups develop chickenpox pneumonia?

A Adults, pregnant females, and immuno-compromised individuals. Pulmonary involvement is the most common life-threatening complication of varicella. This is extremely unusual in children, but may arise in 1–5% of immunocompetent adults with chickenpox. X-ray changes indicating involvement of the lungs are even more frequent (e.g. 10–15%). There is evidence to suggest that pregnant women are more susceptible than non-pregnant women (see Case 62). Patients of any age who are immunosuppressed (or immuno-immature, i.e. neonates), especially those with reduced cell-mediated immunity, are also at con-siderably increased risk of developing pneumonia, as they are less able to prevent spread of virus in the bloodstream.

Q What pathogenetic mechanism underlies the encephalitis that may follow chickenpox?

A Possible mechanisms of brain damage in viral encephalitis include direct spread of virus into the brain itself (see Case 42), and immune-system mediated damage due to an aberrant immune response to the virus cross-reacting with brain antigens (post-infectious encephalitis). The pathogenesis of varicella encephalitis is not known with certainty, but the timing, coincident with the development of a measurable immune response, suggests that this is a post-infectious encephalitis rather than the result of direct virus infection of the brain.

Q Should you offer any antiviral therapy to Hayley?

A VZV is sensitive to aciclovir and its derivatives (famciclovir, valaciclovir), although a higher dose is necessary to inhibit VZV replication compared to HSV. One would not hesitate to use such drugs intra-venously in life-threatening VZV disease, e.g. in a patient with chickenpox pneumonia. Also, chickenpox in any immunocompromised patient should be treated immediately, even if it appears mild at the time of diagnosis. The value of treating uncomplicated chickenpox in a child is arguable, as most children are not that sick with varicella. However, varicella in adults is often much more severe (even without the complication of varicella pneumonia), and some physicians would recommend treating all adults with such infection.

Despite Hayley's florid rash, she feels well in herself, and is keen to go back to school.

Q When should she be allowed to do so?

A Chickenpox is highly infectious, as patients excrete virus in droplets from their pharynx. In addition, the vesicles contain infectious virus in high titre. Hayley will have been infectious for a couple of days prior to the development of her rash, and will remain so until her last crop of vesicles have crusted over. She should not be allowed back to school until no new lesions have appeared for 2 days, provided the existing lesions have crusted.

By chance, the very next patient to enter your surgery has come to see you about a rash, very similar in appearance to Hayley's, but localized to an area of skin on his trunk (see Fig. 7.2). Roy is a 60-year-old hospital administrator, previously fit and well, who first noticed pain on his left side a week ago. This was followed by an odd sensation when he touched the area of skin involved, and, 3 days ago, by the emer-gence of several red spots. He has no other symptoms. In his social history, he says he has been under considerable stress recently in his job, and 2 weeks ago his mother died.

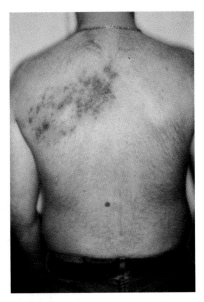

Fig. 7.2 Roy's rash.

Q What is the diagnosis?

A The vesicular appearance and dermatomal distribution of the rash are typical of herpes zoster, or shingles, involving a thoracic nerve root. This represents reactivation of latent VZV from within a dorsal root ganglion. The characteristic clinical features of an attack of shingles are listed in Table 7.2.

Table 7.2 **Clinical features of herpes zoster**
Malaise and pyrexia
Pain and tenderness over 2–3 adjacent roots precedes the eruption by a few days
Rash—groups of small, irregular, tense vesicles on an erythematous and oedematous area of skin; appear in crops
Lesions evolve to pustules to scabs in 5–10 days
Regional lymph nodes may be enlarged and tender
Most common sites—thoracic, cervical, and the ophthalmic branch of the trigeminal nerve (cranial nerve Va), in that order, but any segments may be involved

Q What is the relationship, if any, between this rash and that of Hayley?

A VZV, like all the human herpesviruses (see Case 4, Table 4.1), exhibits the phenomenon of *latency*. Thus, primary infection is followed by life-long carriage of the virus, which can then be reactivated at some later stage, resulting in a secondary, or recurrent, infection. The site of latency for VZV is within the nerve cell body, or ganglion. As primary VZV infection is a generalized phenomenon, latent virus may be found in multiple dorsal root ganglia around the body. Following reactivation from within a ganglion, virus tracks down the axon to the skin supplied by that particular nerve, resulting in the characteristic dermatomal distribution of zoster.

Q What are the risk factors for the development of herpes zoster?

A These are:

- Increasing age, presumably reflecting declining immunity to VZV; > 20% of individuals over the age of 80 will give a history of zoster
- Trauma (including surgery) to an area of the body may be followed by zoster appearing in that area some days later
- Psychological stress, e.g. a recent bereavement
- Immunodeficiency or immunosuppression results in increased frequency of reactivation of all herpesviruses. Bloodstream spread may result in a generalized zoster rash and life-threatening involvement of internal organs, e.g. lungs, liver, in this patient group

Q What are the possible complications of herpes zoster?

A These are to some extent dependent on which nerve is involved and are listed in Table 7.3.

Q How should you manage Roy's zoster rash?

A You should prescribe appropriate analgesia, and tell him that his shingles is likely to last for a few days only. You could consider giving him antiviral therapy (e.g. oral valaciclovir)—this has been shown in clinical trials to speed up recovery with

Table 7.3 Complications of herpes zoster

Postherpetic neuralgia

- Pain in the rash-affected area for more than 3 months after the rash itself has resolved
- Can be debilitating and result in clinical depression
- Likelihood of occurrence increases with increasing age, and with degree of severity of zoster rash

Motor nerve involvement

- e.g. C4 zoster may result in wasting of the deltoid muscle
- Facial nerve (cranial nerve 7) zoster may cause a facial (or Bell's) palsy

Ocular involvement

- Ophthalmic zoster (cranial nerve Va) may result in virus infection of the cornea i.e. keratitis (see Fig. 7.4)

Dissemination, with internal organ involvement (see Fig. 7.3)

- In the immunodeficient or immunosuppressed

Autonomic nerve involvement

- e.g. retention of urine in sacral zoster

Neurological (rare)

- Zoster encephalitis, transverse myelitis

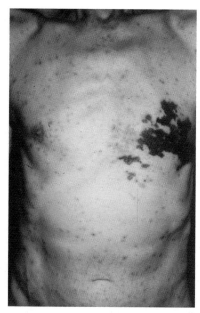

Fig. 7.3 Disseminated zoster rash.

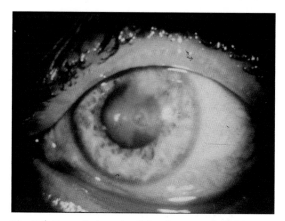

Fig. 7.4 Corneal ulceration following zoster keratitis.

shorter duration of pain, and there is evidence to suggest that antiviral therapy of an acute attack of zoster does reduce the risk and severity of postherpetic neuralgia. However, antiviral therapy is usually reserved for older patients (who are at increased risk of postherpetic neuralgia), any immunocompromised patient who develops shingles, no matter how mild the disease first appears (because of the life-threatening risk of dissemination and internal organ involvement—see Fig. 7.3), and patients with zoster that might lead to complications, e.g. ophthalmic zoster, where systemic antiviral treatment is mandatory in order to reduce the risk of zoster keratitis (see Fig. 7.4).

10 days later, Roy returns to your clinic, as his rash shows no sign of resolving—in fact, it is becoming more extensive, with areas of coalescent necrosis.

Q What should you consider now?

A In the immunocompetent host, VZV reactivation is a self-limiting disease. The continued appearance of new lesions in any patient raises the possibility of an underlying immunodeficiency

Table 7.4 Predisposing factors for severe herpes zoster

HIV infection

Malignancy, especially of the reticuloendothelial system, e.g. chronic leukaemias, multiple myeloma, lymphomas

Immunosuppression for transplant recipients

Chemotherapy

High-dose steroid therapy

Radiotherapy

disorder. A severe attack of zoster can be the presenting feature of a number of diseases, all of which have in common an element of immune dysfunction—see Table 7.4. Roy should be investigated accordingly. This applies to all cases of unusually aggressive, prolonged, or atypical zoster—making the diagnosis of zoster is not the end of the story, but only the beginning, as the patient must then be investigated for an underlying cause. An example of an atypical, aggressive zoster rash in a patient with underlying lymphoma is shown in Fig. 7.5.

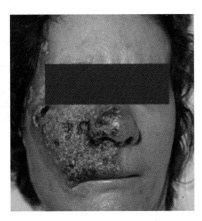

Fig. 7.5 Coalescent necrosis in zoster rash.

After further investigation, Roy was, in fact, diagnosed as having chronic lymphocytic leukaemia.

Q Can VZV infection be prevented?

A Yes. There is a live attenuated VZV vaccine (the Oka strain) that has been shown to prevent the serious complications of primary VZV infection when given to children in remission from leukaemia. It is available in the UK on a named-patient basis for such children. In the USA, the vaccine is now licensed and recommended for use as a universal childhood vaccine.

Summary: Varicella-zoster virus

Presentation

- Primary infection: varicella, i.e. chickenpox; generalized vesicular rash, usually in a child
- Secondary (reactivated) infection: herpes zoster, i.e. shingles; vesicular rash in dermatomal distribution

Diagnosis

Clinical. If any doubt, demonstrate virus in vesicle fluid by electron microscopy, culture, antigen detection

Complications

- Primary infection: pneumonia; post-infectious encephalitis; internal organ involvement in the immunosuppressed
- Secondary infection: postherpetic neuralgia; ocular involvement; motor nerve involvement; dissemination

Treatment

Aciclovir or derivatives—for immunosuppressed patients or complications, e.g. pneumonia

Case 8 Steven, a 42-year-old accountant with a red, painful eye

Steven, a 42-year-old accountant, has a routine eye check-up by his local optometrist, who notes that his intraocular pressure is on the high side and suggests he should seek ophthalmological advice. Steven therefore presents to the Eye outpatients department (OPD), where he is fully examined, but tonometry is normal. He is reassured and discharged. One week later, he notices a gritty sensation initially in his left eye, and pain when looking into bright light. He develops a watery discharge from both eyes, which become puffy and red (see Fig. 8.1), so he returns to the Eye OPD. Examination of the left eye reveals oedema of both conjunctivae and eyelids, and subconjunctival haemorrhage and punctate epithelial lesions are seen following fluorescein staining. Similar, but less marked changes are seen in the right eye. Bilateral enlarged preauricular lymph nodes are also noted.

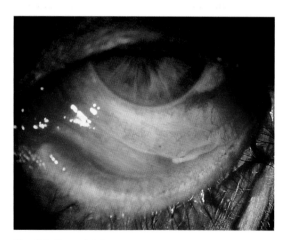

Fig. 8.1 Steven's left eye.

Q What is the likely diagnosis?

A The inflamed conjunctivae, together with the corneal lesions, indicate a keratoconjunctivitis. The acute onset is highly suggestive of an infectious aetiology. Viral infections of the eye are common and the absence of visible pus also makes bacterial infection less likely in this particular case.

Q How should you manage this patient?

A An eye swab should be taken, broken off into viral transport medium, and sent to the virology laboratory for virus isolation in cell culture. A second swab to be sent for bacterial culture should also be taken. Steven should be given topical chloramphenicol ointment to prevent secondary bacterial infection. He should also be instructed about scrupulous hand-washing to prevent accidental spread of infection. The presence of corneal lesions means that referral to an ophthalmologist is mandatory. Treatment of the acute episode may include a cycloplegic agent (e.g. cyclopentolate) to relax the ciliary body and iris, which will relieve his pain.

Q What is the likely outcome of Steven's infection?

A His symptoms should improve over the next 7–14 days. However, as the conjunctivitis resolves, epithelial opacities, which may impair vision, may become prominent. Steven will require long-term outpatient follow-up, as these lesions may take months or years to disappear.

Q What are the common infectious causes of conjunctivitis?

A These are:

1. Viruses
   - Adenoviruses. The most likely infection in this case. The cornea may also be involved (keratitis)

- Herpes simplex virus—see Box 8.1. HSV keratitis is the most common infectious cause of corneal blindness in the UK
- Varicella-zoster virus. Involvement of the ophthalmic division of the trigeminal nerve is common in herpes zoster, and virus may spread on to the cornea (see Case 7)
- Enteroviruses (see Case 3) particularly coxsackievirus A24 and enterovirus 70, associated with epidemics of acute haemorrhagic conjunctivitis in Africa, the Americas, and the Far East
- Measles. Conjunctivitis is a common manifestation during the prodrome (see Case 6)

2. Bacteria. Involvement of the cornea is unusual in bacterial infection unless secondary to virus infection, trauma, or in association with contact lens use
   - *S. aureus*. Gives rise to 'sticky eye' in neonates
   - *H. influenzae*
   - *Str. pneumoniae*
   - *Chlamydia trachomatis*. Causes conjunctivitis and trachoma (see Case 61)
   - *N. gonorrhoeae*. Causes ophthalmia neonatorum (see Case 61)
   - *Ps. aeruginosa*. Opportunist infection, e.g. after trauma

(a)

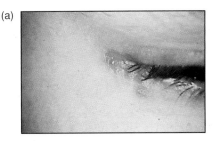

(b)

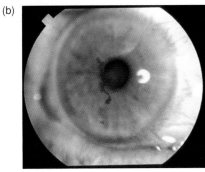

Fig. 8.2 (a) Herpetic lesions around eye. (b) Dendritic herpetic keratitis.

3. Other
   - Fungi, e.g. Candida, in immunosuppressed patients
   - Acanthamoeba. Severe keratitis associated with contaminated contact lenses
   - Worms. *Onchocerca volvulus*, giving rise to river blindness

10 days after Steven's second visit to the Eye OPD, the Virology laboratory issues a preliminary report of the eye swab stating 'Adenovirus isolated—type to follow'. There was no growth from the swab sent for bacterial culture. Two weeks later, a further report is issued, 'Adenovirus type 8 isolated'.

Q How might Steven have acquired his adenovirus infection?

A The incubation period of adenoviral keratoconjunctivitis is of the order of 7 days. Steven visited the Eye OPD 7 days before the onset of his illness. The worry here is that Steven's infection may have been nosocomially acquired, i.e. the adenovirus was introduced into Steven's eye during his first visit to the Eye OPD.

Q How do nosocomial outbreaks of adenoviral keratoconjunctivitis occur?

A Adenoviruses are difficult to remove by disinfection—the absence of a lipid envelope and the presence of a tight-knit protein capsid render such viruses stable to most of the commonly used disinfectants. Thus, unless appropriate agents (chloramine T or 1% sodium hypochlorite) are used for disinfection, virus may be passed from patient to patient via contaminated instruments, e.g. tonometers. The skin of staff handling these instruments may also become contaminated with virus. Staff may therefore inadvertently spread virus to otherwise sterile instruments, and thence into patients' eyes.

Q In what other way might infection be spread from patient to patient in an Eye OPD?

A Through the use of multidose vials, e.g. to administer local anaesthetic or fluoroscein dye to the eye. The use of such vials should be banned for this reason. All of the above routes of spread are highly efficient, as virus is inoculated directly into the recipients' eyes.

Q How might the hospital infection control team investigate a nosocomial outbreak of adenovirus eye infection?

A The first task is to gather evidence that such an outbreak has occurred. A continuous record of adenovirus isolates and typing results from eye swabs should be maintained, so that any increase in isolation rates, or the emergence of new or unusual serotypes, can be identified quickly. The dates of the eye swabs should be carefully noted, and whether those particular patients were attending the Eye OPD for the first time (in which case their infections were community-acquired) or were re-attenders. During a nosocomial outbreak, most patients will fall into the latter category, suggesting that the virus was acquired from their first visit.

Q What are the principles of management of a nosocomial outbreak?

A These consist of reviewing and tightening-up infection control policies within the unit. The importance of basic precautions such as rigorous hand-washing by all staff between patients must be emphasized. Disinfection protocols must be checked to ensure efficacy. All multidose vials should be abandoned—the increased costs of single-dose vials will be more than offset by the reduction in infections. Infected patients should also be educated about the possibility of spread to household and other casual contacts.

Q How are adenoviruses classified?

A There are currently 49 serotypes of adenoviruses, grouped into six subgenera (A–F), that may infect humans. Subgenus F contains serotypes 40 and 41, which behave somewhat differently to the other adenoviruses (see below).

Q What diseases do adenoviruses cause?

A Adenoviruses give rise to a number of distinct clinical syndromes.

1. Upper respiratory tract infection (see Case 14)
   - Usually in young children; adenoviruses 1–7 give rise to pharyngitis, tonsillitis, adenoidal enlargement, conjunctivitis, nasal congestion, cough

2. Lower respiratory tract infection
   - Laryngo-tracheo-bronchitis; bronchiolitis; pneumonia
   - Accounts for 10% of pneumonia in children
   - Outbreaks may occur in young adults crowded together, e.g. military recruits

3. Infections of the eye
   - Pharyngoconjunctival fever describes one particular syndrome
   - Follicular conjunctivitis may appear as a separate entity
   - Epidemic keratoconjunctivitis, as described in this case. Type 8 is the most common cause

4. Gastroenteritis
   - Mainly in young children (see Case 24). May or may not be associated with respiratory symptoms. Associated

particularly with types 40 and 41 (subgenus F) which are thus referred to as enteric adenoviruses.

5. Rare syndromes
   - Acute haemorrhagic cystitis—dysuria and haematuria (see Case 39)
   - Meningitis, encephalitis
   - Hepatitis in the immunosuppressed, e.g. bone marrow recipients

Q What techniques are available for the laboratory diagnosis of adenovirus infections?

A These are:

- Virus culture. May take up to 3 weeks to grow in laboratory tissue culture. Enteric adenoviruses do not grow on routine laboratory cell substrates
- Electron microscopy (EM). Enteric adenoviruses are excreted in large amounts in stool, and can be visualized under EM
- Antigen detection. Cells from, e.g. a nasopharyngeal aspirate, can be stained with monoclonal anti-adenovirus antibodies, the binding of which can be detected by immunofluorescence (see Case 21)
- Serology. A rising titre of antibodies may be detected in a pair of acute (i.e. taken at presen-

tation) and convalescent (i.e. taken 7–10 days later) sera

Q What specific antiviral therapy is available for serious adenovirus infections?

A No agent has undergone clinical trials, but there are anecdotal reports of the successful use of ribavirin in the treatment of life-threatening adenoviral infections. Some of the new phosphonate nucleotide analogues (e.g. adefovir; see Appendix 3) show activity against adenoviral DNA polymerase.

Summary: : Viral keratoconjunctivitis

Presentation
Painful red eye

Causes
Adenoviruses (may be nosocomial, may result in corneal opacities); herpes simplex virus (may recur, leading to corneal blindness)

Diagnosis
Viral culture of eye swab

Treatment
Requires ophthalmological expertise; topical aciclovir for HSV

Case 9 Extensive rash, headache, fever, and myalgia in Avril, a 20-year-old woman

It is the middle of July; 20-year-old Avril is brought to hospital by her boyfriend and two flatmates. The history from her friends is that up to a couple of days ago she had been fit and healthy and had even enjoyed a day out by the sea in the sun. Avril initially complained of feeling hot, with a frontal headache, loose bowel motions, and muscle aches and pains, for which she had taken some paracetamol. As far as is known she has never been seriously ill before or required admission to hospital, and is on no medication. There has been a steady deterioration in her condition over the last 24 hours, and this morning she is confused and clearly quite ill. On examination Avril has a temperature of 40°C, a pulse rate of 120/min, and a blood pressure of 90/60 mmHg. There is a widespread erythematous rash over the trunk, mild conjunctivitis, and inflamed mucous membranes of the mouth, but there is no meningism.

Q What is the differential diagnosis?

A The combination of confusion, a high fever, and hypotension suggests a serious systemic infection. The presence of the rash might suggest sunstroke due to the history of being in the sun during July, but hypotension would be unusual unless severe. The following should also be considered.

- Meningococcaemia: the absence of meningism does not exclude this but the skin rash is not typical of this condition, which is usually characterized by a purpuric rash (see Case 41)

- Gram-negative infection: a high fever, gastro-intestinal symptoms (loose bowel motions), and low blood pressure may indicate endotoxic shock (see Case 47) and must be considered. A rash does not usually occur with this condition, however

- Gram-positive infection: staphylococcal and streptococcal bacteraemia or certain toxin-mediated diseases may give rise to a high fever, a rash, and other features, e.g. depression of myocardial muscle function

- Leptospirosis (Case 53): the absence of a history of contact with rats or jaundice should not exclude infection caused by *Leptospira interrogans*, especially in the presence of conjunctivitis. Again the rash is atypical

- Viral illness: adenoviruses (see Case 8) and enteroviruses (see Case 3) may occasionally present like this in children, but are less common in adults and are usually characterized by a maculopapular rash

- Stevens–Johnson syndrome: a widespread erythematous rash accompanied by painful erosive lesions in the mouth and palate is a feature of this condition, which may be caused by drugs (e.g. sulphonamides, barbiturates) or herpes simplex infections (see Case 37)

- Kawasaki syndrome: an erythematous rash of the hands and feet, a strawberry tongue, conjunctivitis, and lymphadenopathy are diagnostic of this condition, which is usually seen during childhood. The aetiology is uncertain, but death may occur due to arrhythmias arising from cardiac involvement

- Rickettsial disease: many tick-borne diseases that are geographically defined, such as Rocky Mountain Spotted Fever, caused by *Rickettsia rickettsii*, may cause a systemic illness with a widespread rash, which is, however, usually macular.

Further questioning of Avril's female friends reveals that she had started her menses the previous day. A tampon is discovered on vaginal examination that, when removed, reveals a red and inflamed vaginal mucosa. Initial investigations reveal a leucocytosis of $18 \times 10^9/l$, thrombocytopenia ($60 \times 10^9/l$), abnormal liver function tests, and elevated urea (24 mmol/l) and creatinine (198 μmol/l).

Q Which microbiological investigations should be done?

A At least two sets of blood cultures should be taken to exclude bacteraemia, and other specimens essential for culture include urine (to exclude a urinary tract infection with bacteraemia), faeces (to exclude *Salmonella* or *Campylobacter* infection), and a high vaginal swab, not forgetting the tampon (to exclude toxic shock syndrome (TSS)). Acute serum should also be taken for serological studies (a convalescent serum later when available) and, where appropriate, to exclude rickettsial disease.

Q How should this case be managed initially?

A Irrespective of the aetiology, certain general principles apply. Intravascular fluid replacement in the form of saline or colloids is essential, and this should go some way towards normalizing the blood pressure. Organ support in an intensive care unit may be required, especially if the patient is hypoxic and requires ventilation or if there is myocardial dysfunction necessitating inotropic support. A broad-spectrum antibiotic, e.g. cefotaxime, to cover both Gram-negative and Gram-positive bacteria should be administered intravenously. An appropriate alternative would be a combination of penicillin, flucloxacillin, and gentamicin. Renal support in the form of haemofiltration or dialysis and parenteral nutrition may be required if initial attempts at resuscitation are unsuccessful.

Avril is transferred to the intensive care unit that evening for observation and a Swan–Ganz catheter is inserted to observe closely her haemodynamic status. Intravascular fluid replacement with colloid is started and intravenous cefotaxime commenced, but ventilation is not required. The next day her temperature is down to 38.5°C, serum creatinine is 140 μmol/l, and she has become more lucid.

Table 9.1 Diagnosis features of the toxic shock syndrome

- Temperature > 38.9°C
- Hypotension and/or decreased urinary output
- Widespread rash, usually erythematous with desquamation later
- Involvement of three or more organ systems, including gastrointestinal tract (e.g. diarrhoea), kidneys (elevated creatinine), mucous membranes (red, inflamed), respiratory tract (e.g. hypoxia), liver (abnormal function tests), blood (e.g. thrombocytopenia), and central nervous system (e.g. confusion)
- Negative serology for Rocky Mountain Spotted Fever (where appropriate), leptospirosis, adenovirus infection, etc.

Q What is the most likely diagnosis?

A The combination of a high fever, an extensive skin rash, hypotension, other organ involvement, and the finding of an inflamed vaginal mucosa with a tampon suggests the toxic shock syndrome (see Table 9.1).

Q Which pathogen is likely to have been responsible?

A *Staphylococcus aureus* is the most likely cause of toxic shock syndrome, although group A β-haemolytic streptococci (see Case 5) may also cause a similar syndrome. These bacteria may produce an array of extracellular enzymes, such as coagulase used to differentiate *S. aureus* from other staphylococci (Fig. 9.1), and toxins. Both toxic shock syndrome toxin-1 (TSST-1) and enterotoxins produced by *S. aureus* are implicated in toxic shock syndrome, and many of the isolates recovered from TSS cases belong to phage group I when typed using bacteriophages (viruses that induce lysis, often according to well-recognized patterns).

Staphylococcus aureus, resistant to penicillin but sensitive to flucloxacillin, is isolated from the vaginal swab and the tampon. On subsequent referral to a reference laboratory the isolate is

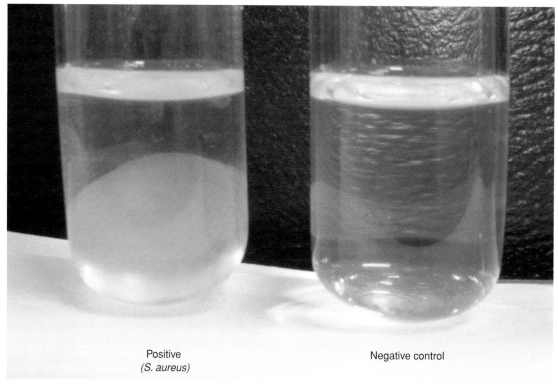

Positive
(S. aureus)

Negative control

Fig. 9.1 Coagulase used to differentiate *S. aureus* from coagulase-negative staphylococci such as *S. epidermidis*.

TSST-1-positive. Blood cultures are sterile, examination of faeces reveals no pathogens, and serological investigations are negative. The cefotaxime is changed to flucloxacillin and over the next couple of days there is a marked improvement in Avril's condition. She is transferred to a medical ward on day 3, and subsequently widespread skin desquamation becomes evident, especially on the palms of the hands and the soles of the feet (see Fig. 9.2).

Q What factors are important in the pathogenesis of the toxic shock syndrome?

A When the toxic shock syndrome was first described, it was believed to be confined to menstruating women from whom *S. aureus* was isolated, usually from the vagina or a tampon. It is now rec-

ognized, however, that this is just one form of the disease, and non-menstruating cases, e.g. following skin infection, may outnumber those associated with the menses in females. The relevant pathogenic factors appear to be:

- *Staphylococcus aureus*, usually from phage group I, capable of producing TSST-1 or one of the enterotoxins. Streptococcal toxic shock has also been described associated with the erythrogenic or pyrogenic toxins (see Case 5). These particular staphylococcal and streptococcal toxins are now considered to be superantigens (antigens that react non-specifically with T lymphocytes, leading to their activation and the release of cytokines that is both overwhelming and inappropriate). Bacteraemia is unusual as this is a toxaemic state

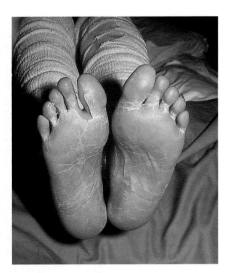

Fig. 9.2 Desquamation of the feet in toxic shock syndrome.

Q What other conditions associated with *S. aureus* are toxin-mediated?

A Both staphylococcal food poisoning/gastro-enteritis (see Case 23) and the scalded skin syndrome are due to the production of specific toxins rather than systemic or localized infection. The main features of these conditions are:

- Gastroenteritis is due to preformed enterotox-ins in food. There are seven enterotoxins, the most commonly implicated ones being entero-toxins A and B. These induce a self-limiting disease characterized by a short incubation peri-od, vomiting, and diarrhoea (see Case 23)

- Scalded skin syndrome is caused by epider-molytic toxins that induce skin desquamation and is most commonly seen during childhood. Histologically, there is cleavage of the middle layers of the epidermidis with bulla formation.

- tampons. First reports were associated with the use of certain makes of tampon in 70–80% of cases. It is believed that these tampons, which were hyperabsorbable, facilitated the local growth of *S. aureus* and the expression of TSST-1. This may have been due to the presence locally of an aerobic environment or magnesium binding by the tampons. In non-menstruating cases similar factors may be important, but it is not clear how they arise

- antibodies to TSST-1. More than 85% of patients with toxic shock due to *S. aureus* have low titres of antibodies to TSST-1 compared with healthy controls, 88% of whom have high titres. Healthy controls probably acquire antibodies through asymptomatic contact with toxin-producing strains. Patients who develop toxic shock and fail to mount a serological response are also at greater risk of relapse

---

Summary: Toxic shock syndrome

Presentation
Toxic state characterized by an extensive skin rash with multiple organ involvement. Not confined to menstruating women

Diagnosis
Clinical features accompanied by the isolation of a TSST-1 or enterotoxin-producing *S. aureus* from vagina or other site. Less commonly, a β-haemolytic streptococcus, group A, is involved. Bacteraemia is unusual

Management
Intravenous fluids, organ support, removal of infect-ed focus, e.g. tampon, and antibiotics, i.e. flucloxacillin for *S. aureus* or penicillin for strepto-cocci

Case 10 Mr Emmerson, Ms Lake, and Mr Palmer, all aged 30, with blisters

Mr Emmerson, Ms Lake, and Mr Palmer, all aged 30, come separately to your dermatology clinic, complaining of the vesicular lesions shown in Fig. 10.1. They are otherwise fit and well, with no past medical histories of note, and none of them are taking any regular medication. Mr Emmerson is a sheep farmer, Ms Lake is a dental nurse, and Mr Palmer is an abbatoir worker. Mr Emmerson's lesion is painless, while Ms Lake's is acutely tender and painful. There are no other abnormal physical signs in these two patients. Further details of Mr Palmer's lesion are provided below.

Q What are the diagnoses for Mr Emmerson and Ms Lake?

A The major clue in these cases, apart from the appearance of the lesions themselves, lies in the occupational histories.

Mr Emmerson (Fig. 10.1(a)) is suffering from orf. This is a zoonotic infection acquired from sheep, caused by a pox virus, and is therefore an occupational hazard of farm and slaughterhouse workers, and veterinarians. Parapox viruses include orf and pseudocowpox viruses. These are widespread in sheep, goats, and cattle. The lesions they cause in humans are essentially the same, but go under a

(a)
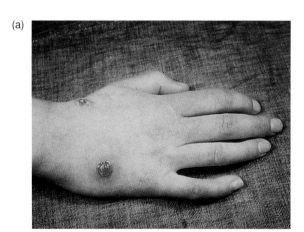

(b)
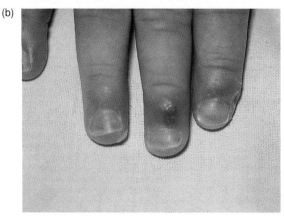

(c)
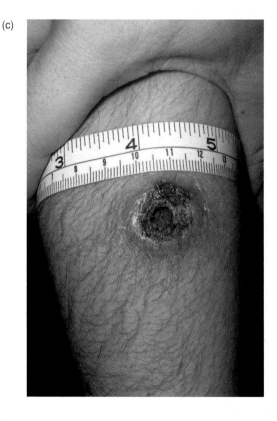

Fig. 10.1 (a) Mr Emmerson's hand; (b) Ms Lake's finger; (c) Mr Palmer's arm.

number of different names. The nomenclature of human disease is based on the identity of the host from which the infection was acquired:

Mode of spread	Resulting human disease
Cattle to humans	Pseudocowpox, paravaccinia, or milker's nodes
Sheep or goats to humans	Orf or contagious pustular dermatitis

Lesions are surprisingly painless, a useful diagnostic feature, and constitutional upset is slight. Diagnosis is usually based on the history, but can be confirmed by demonstration of pox viral particles by electron microscopy in fluid exuded from the nodule. Infection does not induce a protective immune response, and recurrent lesions (due to re-infection, not re-activation) may occur.

Ms Lake's finger (Fig. 10.1(b)) shows a herpetic whitlow, i.e. infection of the nail-bed with herpes simplex virus (HSV). Intact skin is an effective barrier to HSV but, if the contiguity of the dermis is broken, HSV can gain access. Thus, dental workers are at risk of acquiring dermal infection in their hands because of cuts and abrasions sustained during manipulations in the mouths of patients shedding virus. This is largely preventable by wearing gloves during dental and other procedures. Alternative modes of acquisition are by accidental needlestick injury with a contaminated needle (herpetic whitlows are therefore an occupational hazard of many health-care workers) or by auto-inoculation of nail folds in children with oral herpes who bite their nails.

The inflammatory response to HSV infection of the dermis gives rise to an acutely painful and tender swelling, as the tightness of the skin of the fingers resists expansion. Single or multiple vesicles appear, which coalesce into an oozing pustule or abscess, filled with a purulent-looking mixture of serum and debris. The differential diagnosis includes bacterial infection of the skin. Healing occurs gradually over a period of 2 or 3 weeks. If this is the patient's first exposure to HSV (i.e. a primary infection), then the whitlow may be accompanied by evidence of systemic upset—fever and lymphadenopathy. As with other forms of HSV infection, recurrences may occur at the same site—these are re-activations of virus, not re-infections (compare with orf, above).

Mr Palmer (Fig. 10.1(c)) first noticed an itchy papule, like an insect bite, but this developed over 2–3 days into a painless ulcer with surrounding vesicles containing serous fluid. A black centre then arose, with underlying oedema and induration. He complains of a headache and feeling unwell.

Q What is the diagnosis?

A This description is characteristic of cutaneous anthrax, also known as a malignant pustule. The central black lesion is known as an eschar and is due to coagulation necrosis. There may also be regional lymphadenopathy and systemic upset such as fever, malaise, and headache. After 1–2 weeks the eschar will dry and separate from the underlying skin, leaving a scar.

Q How would you confirm the diagnosis?

A In a straightforward case such as that of Mr Palmer, with an accompanying history of occupational exposure, a clinical diagnosis is often sufficient. If laboratory confirmation is required, a sterile swab should be rubbed in the vesicle fluid and sent to the laboratory. A film will reveal Gram-positive rods, and *Bacillus anthracis* can be easily grown on standard plates. However, any laboratory undertaking such diagnostic procedures must take precautions to prevent inhalation of the organism.

Q How may cutaneous anthrax be acquired, and who is at risk of infection?

A This is a zoonotic disease due to inoculation through the skin of material from infected animals contaminated with spores of *B. anthracis*. This is thus an occupational disease of workers in the leather and wool industries, who may be exposed to infected animal hides, especially from imported animals, and abbatoir workers and veterinarians, who may handle dead or dying animals.

Q Should Mr Palmer be treated?

A Yes. Antibiotic therapy will decrease the oedema and systemic symptoms, but probably does not alter the natural history of the skin lesion. Treatment is with penicillin, as β-lactamase-producing strains are rare.

Q Can anthrax be prevented?

A Yes. Simple precautions for at-risk workers include regular hand-washing and covering of cuts or abrasions. In addition, they may be protected by means of an alum-precipitated toxoid vaccine. However, this requires multiple doses, and frequent boosters, to maintain adequate levels of antitoxin antibodies.

Public interest in anthrax has been stimulated by the deliberate packaging of anthrax spores in letters sent around the USA in late 2001. Postal workers in particular were affected by this act of urban terrorism. A number of cases of cutaneous anthrax arose, none fatal. Unfortunately, there were deaths arising from inhalation of spores and subsequent pulmonary anthrax. If this agent were to be used in a large-scale deliberate attack, it is probable that an aggressor would use a strain genetically modified to be penicillin-resistant. Thus, recommended prophylaxis in such a situation is ciprofloxacin. The possibility of anthrax as a biological weapon has prompted research into the development of better vaccine preparations, e.g. recombinant antigens.

Summary: Vesicular lesions on upper limb

Differential diagnosis

- Orf—painless; re-infections may occur; occupationally associated (farm and animal workers)
- Herpetic whitlow—painful; recurrences may occur; occupationally associated (health-care workers)
- Hand, foot, and mouth disease—coxsackie virus infection; usually in a child (see Case 3)
- Cutaneous anthrax—itchy papule evolves into painless ulcer with surrounding vesicles; rare in the UK; occupationally associated due to exposure to contaminated animal material

Diagnosis

- Clinical: hand, foot, and mouth disease; cutaneous anthrax
- Demonstration of viral particles in vesicle fluid by electron microscopy: orf; HSV
- Gram film and culture of ulcer base swab: anthrax

Case 11 Skin rash and arthralgia in Jane, a 25-year-old woman

Jane, a 25-year-old woman, presents in mid-September with a 1-week history of arthralgia of the small joints of the hands and a painful elbow. Examination reveals discrete skin lesions on the abdomen, arms, and legs at various stages, which have been present for 3–4 days (Fig. 11.1). Three weeks earlier Jane and her boyfriend Tony had spent a 2-week holiday camping and fishing in the New Forest, England. Both reported being bitten on numerous occasions by insects and ticks, but he remains well.

Q What do the history and skin rash suggest?

A The combination of tick bites, a migrating skin rash, and arthralgia is consistent with a diagnosis of Lyme disease caused by *Borrelia burgdorferi*, a spirochaete transmitted by the *Ixodes* tick. Although first described in North America, this condition is now recognized in Europe and elsewhere. The initial clinical picture is characterized by erythema chron-icum migrans, myalgia, arthralgia, and lymph-adenopathy. The disease may go undiagnosed and later present with a variety of manifestations, including those of the nervous (meningoencephalitis) and cardiovascular systems (see Fig. 11.2).

Q What other infective conditions are tick-borne?

A A number of viral, bacterial, and rickettsial conditions are tick-borne and are often travel-associated (see Box 11.1).

Q How would you confirm the diagnosis of Lyme disease?

A Isolation of the bacterium from skin lesions is a specialized technique and largely confined to research centres. A polymerase chain reaction (PCR) assay may be available in some centres for the detection of bacterial DNA in tissue. Serology is the mainstay of diagnosis. A fourfold rise in antibody titres, or a single elevated titre in an enzyme-linked immunoassay (ELISA), confirmed by immunoblotting, clinches the diagnosis.

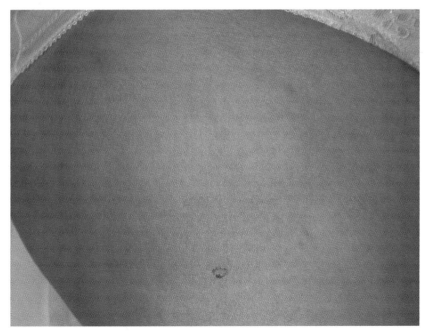

Fig. 11.1 Skin lesions like those described for Jane.

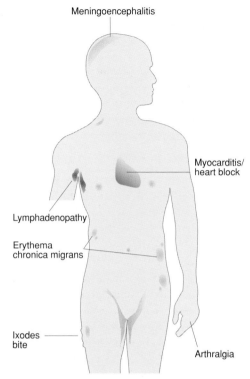

Fig. 11.2 Clinical features of Lyme disease.

Meningoencephalitis

Myocarditis/heart block

Lymphadenopathy

Erythema chronica migrans

Ixodes bite

Arthralgia

Q What is the treatment of choice?

A Penicillin, erythromycin, tetracycline, and the cephalosporins have all been used to treat Lyme disease. Doxycycline or amoxicillin to treat early disease are associated with fewer late complications, and should be continued for 10–20 days. Ceftriaxone, a third-generation cephalosporin with a prolonged half-life, has been used successfully to treat central nervous system (CNS) disease and has a lower failure rate than benzylpenicillin.

Q Should Jane's partner receive prophylactic antimicrobial chemotherapy?

A No. There is little evidence to suggest that antimicrobial agents administered after possible exposure either prevent or lessen the severity of disease. Those likely to be bitten by ticks in forests or elsewhere should minimize the skin surface area exposed, use insect repellents, and remove ticks likely to be caught in clothing as soon as they come indoors.

Q Is there an effective vaccine available for prevention?

A A recombinant vaccine is available in some countries, and has an efficacy of about 50% but is not routinely used. It may have a role for the protection of those most at risk, i.e. members of the public who live or work in tick-infested areas.

Summary: Lyme disease

Presentation
Variable, but skin rash following tick bite is the most common

Diagnosis
Clinical features confirmed by serology; paired sera usually required to demonstrate rise in antibodies

Management
Oral doxycycline but treatment of CNS infection more complex

Box 11.1 Other tick-borne conditions, with geographical distributions

Condition	Cause	Geographical distribution
Louping ill (encephalitis)	A flavivirus	UK
Omsk haemorrhagic fever	A flavivirus	Russia
Colorado tick fever	An orbivirus	North America
Relapsing fever	*Borrelia recurrentis*	Asia, Europe, Africa
Mediterranean Spotted Fever	*Rickettsia conorii*	Europe; North, Central, and South America
Tick-borne encephalitis	A flavivirus	Worldwide but vaccine-preventable

Case 12 Father Pat, a 45-year-old priest with a skin rash

Father Pat, a 45-year-old Roman Catholic priest, is referred to the dermatology outpatients clinic because of a skin rash on his right forearm. This has been present for some months, is associated with some skin discoloration, and is slowly increasing in size. Father Pat has spent most of the past 20 years teaching in a missionary school in Tanzania, but is currently home on holiday for 6 weeks. He has never been seriously ill in the past apart from occasional attacks of malaria. The rash is characterized by a pale area of skin over the forearm (see Fig. 12.1). There is some loss of feeling surrounding the lesion but general physical examination is normal.

Q What diagnostic test is indicated?

A A skin biopsy of the central and peripheral areas of the lesion should be taken and should also include some subcutaneous tissue.

Q What is the likely diagnosis?

A The history of residence in the developing world, the characteristic lesion, and the accompanying area of anaesthesia are very suggestive of leprosy. Histological examination using haematoxylin and eosin (to show the presence of granulomata) and a modified Ziehl–Neelsen stain (to detect the presence of acid-fast bacilli, see Case 52) is likely to confirm this. The causative agent of leprosy, *Mycobacterium leprae*, has never been grown in vitro.

Q How is leprosy spread?

A It is generally assumed that leprosy is spread by skin-to-skin contact—hence the tradition of ostracizing sufferers over the centuries. The epidermis of the skin is, however, usually intact and free of bacilli. It is more likely that the bacteria are shed from the nose. The number in nasal secretions may approximate to the numbers found in the sputum of patients with 'open' tuberculosis (see Case 52). The disease is almost exclusively confined to humans, but leprosy has been described in armadillos, chimpanzees, and monkeys. In endemic areas patients may have both leprosy and tuberculosis, and this has to be considered in diagnosis and management.

Q What are the complications of leprosy?

A The spectrum of disease varies from the lepromatous to the tuberculoid forms, with a number of stages in between (see Table 12.1). Hypersensitivity reactions are a feature of leprosy and these may be cell-mediated (type 4 hypersensitivity reaction), giving rise to swollen nerves, or characterized by immune complex formation (type 3 hypersensitivity reaction). Recognized complications include:

- erythema nodosum leprosum: more common in forms where bacilli are plentiful and consists of erythematous plaques or nodules with endarteritis, phlebitis, and leukaemoid reactions due to immune complexes

- physical deformities: nasomaxillary destruction and damage to upper and lower limbs, resulting from loss of sensory function and paralysis

- blindness: occurs in 5% of cases due to corneal ulceration or iridocyclitis

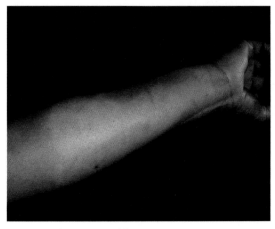

Fig. 12.1 Skin lesions of forearm.

Table 12.1 Features of lepromatous and tuberculoid leprosy

	Lepromatous	Tuberculoid
Clinical features		
Nasal destruction	+/−	+
Skin lesions	++	+/−
Nerves	Little damage	Extensive damage
Response to antimicrobial therapy	Poor	Good
Pathology		
Bacilli in lesions	++	+/−
Granuloma	−	++
Antibodies to M. leprae	++	+/−

Orchitis, periosteitis, cutaneous vasculitis (Lucio's phenomenon), and secondary amyloidosis may also occur.

The skin biopsy from Father Pat's lesion reveals mature epithelioid and Langerhans cells with granulomata, but no bacilli are seen. Cellular infiltration of the nerves and epidermis is seen, however, and it is concluded that Father Pat has a tuberculoid form of leprosy. He is started on antimicrobial chemotherapy and arrangements are made for him to be followed up when he returns to Tanzania.

Q What are the main drugs used to treat leprosy?

A Dapsone, a bacteriostatic agent, is the most useful drug. It is increasingly being used in combination because of the emergence of resistance. A 6–12-month course of dapsone and rifampicin is recommended for patients with tuberculoid forms. Two years' treatment or longer is necessary for lepromatous forms with two or more drugs such as daily dapsone and clofazimine (may cause discoloration of the skin) supplemented with monthly rifampicin. Surgery to correct deformities, such as a collapsed nasal bridge, and referral to an ophthalmologist may be appropriate in more advanced disease.

Résumé for undergraduate students

Leprosy is rare in the Western or developed world but it remains clinically important in tropical countries. *M. leprae* is an important member of the mycobacteria genus and the disease is of clinical significance when assessing the returned traveller with a skin lesion of undefined aetiology.

Summary: Leprosy

Presentation
Raised skin lesions with localized anaesthesia, but extensive destruction of limbs and nasomaxillary area seen in advanced disease

Diagnosis
Clinical features and skin biopsy

Management
Dapsone in combination with other agents for 6–12 months or longer, with surgical treatment of complications

Self-assessment

1. Which one of the following statements concerning measles is incorrect?
  - (a) The most common life-threatening complication is acute encephalitis
  - (b) Patients with measles are infectious before the onset of the rash
  - (c) There is usually a prodrome with upper respiratory symptoms
  - (d) Koplik's spots appear before onset of the rash
  - (e) Measles vaccine contains inactivated whole virus

2. Recognized complications of measles include all but which of the following?
  - (a) Pneumonia
  - (b) Encephalitis
  - (c) Otitis media
  - (d) Purulent conjunctivitis
  - (e) Meningitis

3. Match the following organisms with the appropriate diseases.
  - (a) Human herpesvirus 6
  - (b) Parvovirus B19
  - (c) Varicella-zoster virus
  - (d) Measles virus
  - (e) Rubella virus
  - (i) Slapped cheek syndrome
  - (ii) German measles
  - (iii) Rubeola
  - (iv) Chicken-pox
  - (v) Exanthem subitum

4. Adenovirus infection may give rise to all but which one of the following?
  - (a) Pneumonia
  - (b) Gastroenteritis
  - (c) Urethritis
  - (d) Tonsillitis
  - (e) Conjunctivitis

5. Which one of the following statements regarding viral conjunctivitis is not true?
  - (a) The clinical features may include preauricular lymphadenopathy
  - (b) The discharge is usually purulent
  - (c) May be caused by enteroviruses
  - (d) May be caused by adenoviruses
  - (e) May be spread nosocomially

6. Which one of these statements is *not* true?
  - (a) Orf and pseudocowpox viruses produce identical lesions
  - (b) Reinfections with orf are rare
  - (c) Recurrent herpetic whitlows are due to reactivation of virus
  - (d) Orf is an occupationally acquired disease
  - (e) Cutaneous anthrax is usually painless

7. Which one of the following statements is *not* a characteristic feature of chickenpox?
  - (a) The patient is infectious for 48 hours before the rash appears
  - (b) The rash is vesicular, starting on the trunk
  - (c) Encephalitis is the most common life-threatening complication
  - (d) New lesions continue to appear for up to 7 days after first appearance of the rash
  - (e) The disease is usually more severe in adults than in children

8. Recognized features of herpes zoster include which of the following? (More than one may be correct.)
  - (a) Increased incidence with increasing age
  - (b) Regional lymphadenopathy
  - (c) Pain and tenderness occurring before appearance of the rash
  - (d) Involvement of motor nerves
  - (e) Urinary retention

9. Which specimen is most appropriate to routinely diagnose tinea?

 (a) Dry skin swab

 (b) Skin swab in transport medium

 (c) Nasal swab

 (d) Skin scrapings

 (e) Skin biopsy

10. What is the agent of choice for the treatment of scabies?

 (a) Trimethoprim

 (b) Permethrin

 (c) Metronidazole

 (d) Fusidic acid

 (e) Whitfield ointment

11. Which of the following bacteria is least likely to be a pathogen when isolated from a swab taken from a leg ulcer?

 (a) *Staphylococcus aureus*

 (b) *Proteus mirabilis*

 (c) *Clostridium perfringens*

 (d) Beta-haemolytic streptococcus (BHS) Group A (*Strep. pyogenes*)

 (e) BHS Group C

12. Which antibiotic is most appropriate for the treatment of skin or soft tissue infection?

 (a) Ampicillin

 (b) Metronidazole

 (c) Trimethoprim

 (d) Ciprofloxacin

 (e) Co-amoxyclav

13. Which of the following bacteria is most likely to be alpha-haemolytic?

 (a) *Streptococcus pyogenes*

 (b) *Streptococcus agalactiae*

 (c) *Enterococcus faecalis*

 (d) *Strep. anginosus (S. milleri)*

 (e) *Streptococcus pneumoniae*

14. *Pasteurella multocida* soft tissue infections are associated with?

 (a) Swimming in tropical fresh water

 (b) Contact with cattle

 (c) Recent sexual intercourse

 (d) A dog bite

 (e) Infestation with body lice

15. What feature predisposes to the development of toxic shock syndrome?

 (a) *Staphylococcus aureus* bacteraemia or bloodstream infection

 (b) Female sex

 (c) Low antibody titres to TSST-1

 (d) Underlying malignancy

 (e) Methicillin-resistant *Staph. aureus*

16. In the differential diagnosis of toxic shock syndrome, which other infection should be excluded?

 (a) Chickenpox

 (b) Scabies

 (c) Rocky Mountain Spotted Fever

 (d) Gonorrhoea

 (e) Influenza

17. Leprosy is most likely spread by which route?

 (a) Nose-to-skin

 (b) Faecal–oral

 (c) Sexually

 (d) Bloodborne

 (e) Skin-to-skin

18. Which one of the following tick-borne infections is not caused by a virus?

 (a) Louping ill

 (b) Omsk haemorrhagic fever

 (c) Colorado tick fever

 (d) Kyasanur forest disease

 (e) Mediterranean spotted fever

19. Which antibiotic is the most appropriate for the treatment of Lyme disease with CNS involvement?

 (a) Ceftriaxone

 (b) Benzylpenicillin

 (c) Flucloxacillin

 (d) Rifampicin

 (e) Tetracycline

20. Which of the following anti-infective regimens are most appropriate for the treatment
of leprosy?

(a) 6 months of rifampicin, isoniazid, and
pyrazinamide

(b) 3 months of ciprofloxacin

(c) 6–12 months of dapsone and rifampicin

(d) 12 months of linezolid

(e) 3 months of ciprofloxacin

2

CHAPTER 2

Respiratory system

SECTION 2
Respiratory system

Case 13 Darren, a hot and irritable 12-month-old infant

A 12-month-old male child, Darren, is off form for 24–36 hours and is noticed by his parents to be hot and irritable. The illness fails to settle with paracetamol and he is therefore brought to his GP for assessment.

Q What should be looked for on examination?

A General examination should include vital signs, such as temperature, heart rate, and degree of irritability, and then specific signs. The absence of a purpuric rash and neck stiffness makes meningitis, especially meningococcal meningitis, less likely, but this could only be excluded following a lumbar puncture. Lower respiratory tract infection may be excluded by the absence of tachypnoea, difficulty with breathing, increased respiratory secretions, or abnormal signs on auscultation. Tenderness over the ear (easier to assess in the older child, who may complain of earache) might suggest an ear infection, but whether this sign is present or absent, auroscopy should be performed.

Examination reveals a bulging, opaque eardrum (Fig. 13.1). A presumptive diagnosis of otitis media (to be distinguished from otitis externa; see Box 13.1) is made, ampicillin to be given by mouth is prescribed, and Darren's parents are instructed to bring him back if he does not settle.

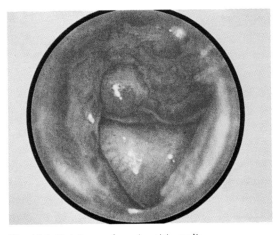

Fig. 13.1 Bulging eardrum in otitis media.

> ### Box 13.1 Otitis externa
>
> - Skin condition of the external auditory meatus, in any age group, characterized more by inflammation than infection, i.e. a form of local dermatitis
> - Often chronic or relapsing
> - Gram-negative bacilli (including *Proteus* and *Pseudomonas* spp.) and fungi such as *Candida* or even *Aspergillus* may be isolated from swabs
> - Aural toilet with or without topical antibiotics such as polymyxin, sometimes combined with topical steroids, is the first approach to management
> - Infection with *Pseudomonas aeruginosa* in the elderly diabetic patient may lead to deep infection of the bone and meningitis (malignant otitis externa)

Q Should the GP have taken any specimens for microbiological confirmation?

A The management of uncomplicated otitis media does not usually warrant investigations. A Gram stain of pus or drainage fluid and culture is possible and to be recommended if the eardrum has perforated or if a myringotomy is carried out. Blood cultures should be done if the child is toxic or to exclude another possible focus of infection, especially if admission to hospital is required.

Q What are the most common causes of otitis media?

A In order of frequency these are:

- *Streptococcus pneumoniae*
- *Haemophilus influenzae* (non-capsulated)
- β-haemolytic streptococcus groups A (*S. pyogenes*), C, and G
- *Staphylococcus aureus*
- Respiratory viruses such as parainfluenza virus, respiratory syncytial virus (RSV)
- Less commonly, *Moraxella catarrhalis*, coliforms such as *Escherichia coli*, other viruses, and *Mycoplasma pneumoniae*

Q Is oral ampicillin a good choice here?

A Ampicillin, or preferably amoxycillin (better absorbed), is most commonly prescribed in this setting or while awaiting the results of culture and sensitivity tests. Penicillin V (oral penicillin) is poorly absorbed and inactive against Gram-negative bacilli. Increasingly, national and other guidelines suggest holding off giving antibiotics unless symptoms persist or the child appears systemically ill, as is the case with Darren.

Two days later Darren is only marginally better and, as the swelling of the eardrum has worsened, he is referred to hospital, where fluid from the middle ear is aspirated and sent to the microbiology laboratory for culture. *Haemophilus influenzae* (see Table 13.1), resistant to ampicillin/amoxycillin, is isolated and, following a 7-day course of co-amoxyclav (amoxycillin/clavulanic) acid, Darren makes an uneventful recovery.

Table 13.1 *Haemophilus influenzae*

- Small Gram-negative bacillus
- Human pathogen only
- Requires X (iron-containing pigment) and V (coenzyme) factors for growth *in vitro*
- 50% of healthy people are carriers; 5% carry capsulated strains
- Recent viral infection facilitates colonization and infection

---

Q What is clavulanic acid?

A This is a β-lactam antibiotic that has a broad spectrum of activity but low potency. It inhibits β-lactamases produced by some bacteria, a common mechanism of resistance. It is used in a fixed ratio with amoxycillin or ticarcillin.

Q How common is ampicillin-resistant *H. influenzae*?

A The majority of isolates are ampicillin-sensitive but approximately 15–20% are resistant, usually owing to the production of β-lactamase, which can be counteracted by the addition of clavulanic acid as discussed above. Apart from ampicillin and ampicillin/clavulanic acid, other agents useful in the blind therapy of otitis media include oral cephalosporins (cefaclor, cefixime) and trimethoprim. Macrolides, especially erythromycin, are not used due to poorer activity against *H. influenzae*. Tetracyclines are contraindicated in the growing child because of deposition in teeth (resulting in staining) and bone.

Q Should Darren have been vaccinated against *Haemophilus influenzae*?

A Yes. The vaccine protects against infection with capsulated type b strains. This is a non-live conjugate vaccine in which the haemophilus capsular polysaccharides are linked to proteins that enhance immunogenicity, especially in children less than 1 year of age. It should be offered to all infants from the age of 2 months and is administered by deep subcutaneous or intramuscular injection in three doses, with an interval of 1 month between doses. It will reduce the incidence of invasive disease

Box 13.2 **Conditions associated with** *Haemophilus influenzae*, **type b, and non-capsulated** *H. influenzae*

H. influenzae, type b	Non-capsulated *H. influenzae*
Meningitis (see Case 41)	Otitis media
Epiglottitis	Sinusitis (see Fig. 13.2)
Bacteraemia (see Case 47)	Bronchitis (see Case 20)
Pneumonia (see Case 18)	Conjunctivitis
Septic arthritis and osteomyelitis (see Case 54)	
Cellulitis (see Case 5)	

due to type b (see Box 13.2), which occurs more frequently in children under 5 years, but will not affect the incidence of otitis media, which is caused by non-capsulate strains.

Q What complications may ensue from otitis media?

A Most cases resolve spontaneously, but a delayed diagnosis or inadequate treatment may result in:

- chronic suppurative otitis media—chronic discharge of pus with hearing loss

- glue ear—mucinous effusion in the middle ear, with fluctuating hearing loss and delayed childhood development

- mastoiditis—may proceed to meningitis and brain abscess (see Case 43).

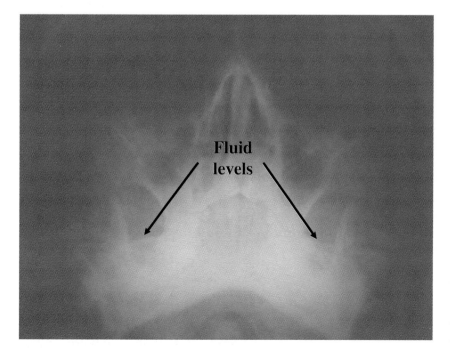

Fluid levels

Fig. 13.2 Skull X-ray of fluid level (arrows) indicative of sinusitis, commonly caused by *Haemophilus influenzae*.

Summary: Otitis media

Presentation
Fever, irritability, painful ear, inflamed eardrum in infants and young children

Diagnosis
Bulging tympanic membrane on auroscopy (fluid + blood for culture if severe)

Management
Antipyretics; antibiotics (amoxycillin, co-amoxy-clav, trimethoprim, oral cephalosporin) if does not settle; occasionally myringotomy. Hearing tests on follow-up if severe or complicated

Case 14 Susan, a 21-year-old with a runny nose and imminent exams

Susan, a 21-year-old university student, complains of a runny nose and headache. She was well until yesterday, when she began sneezing and felt some irritation at the back of her throat, which has now progressed to a cough and sore throat. She is anxious as she has heard that there is a lot of 'flu' about, and she has an important examination to sit in 1 week's time. There are no abnormal physical signs, she is apyrexial, and has no lymphadenopathy.

Q What is your diagnosis?

A Rhinitis (runny nose), headache, sore throat, and cough are all features of the common cold (coryza). The absence of systemic symptoms and signs (e.g. fever, myalgia) distinguish this syndrome from classical influenza (see Case 17).

Q What can you tell Susan about the likely course of her illness?

A Headache, sneezing, and sore throat usually disappear after 2–3 days. A clear and watery nasal discharge usually becomes mucopurulent and tenacious after a few days. These nasal symptoms tend to be more persistent and severe than other symptoms. Cough also peaks after 4–5 days, and may persist. This is a composite view of the common cold syndrome, and it should be noted that individuals vary in their perception of the relative severity of their different symptoms. There is little or no fever, and systemic manifestations are rare. Overall, patients are most miserable after 3–5 days, but have recovered completely by 7–10 days.

Q How may respiratory tract infections be classified?

A There are a number of ways, e.g. by aetiological agent or anatomical site affected. Clinically, the most important distinction is between *upper* and *lower* respiratory tract infections (URTI and LRTI, respectively). In general, the former are considerably more common but are associated with less morbidity than the latter, which may be life-threatening. URTI include the syndromes of otitis media, rhinitis or common cold, sinusitis, conjunctivitis, pharyngitis, laryngitis, croup, and laryngo-tracheo-bronchitis. The relative frequencies of these syndromes differ with age. Whilst some syndromes are distinctive (e.g. otitis media), there is considerable clinical and aetiological overlap between many others, e.g. a patient with a sore throat may be classified as having a cold, a pharyngitis, or a glandular-fever-like illness depending on the presence of other symptoms or signs and the degree to which the sore throat is the dominant symptom.

Q What is the aetiology of the common cold?

A Rhinoviruses and coronaviruses are the two most common causative agents, accounting for around 50% of illnesses, although the syndrome may arise from infection with a wide range of other viruses including respiratory syncytial virus (RSV), parainfluenza viruses, human metapneumovirus, enteroviruses, and adenoviruses.

Q Why is the common cold so common?

A Quite simply because there are so many causative agents. There are over 100 serotypes of rhinoviruses, different serotypes circulate in different years, and infection with one serotype does not induce protective immunity against other serotypes. On average, in the UK, common colds occur at the rate of almost one per person per year, although this varies with age, being higher in the first few years of life.

Q Should you prescribe antibiotics for Susan?

A No. Antibacterials are not indicated as her illness is viral in aetiology and indiscriminate antibiotic use in this setting may result in increased antimicrobial resistance and superinfections, e.g. oral candidiasis.

Q Which antiviral agents may be used to treat a cold?

A None. There have been intensive efforts to develop an effective antiviral agent for the treatment of the common cold—from the point of view of a pharmaceutical company, this would seem like a very lucrative target. Recently, pleconaril, a drug with activity against picornaviruses (i.e. the rhinoviruses and enteroviruses), has been shown to be of potential use, but it is not yet licensed. Pleconaril is a canyon-blocking agent, so-called because it binds to a canyon-shaped structure in the viral outer protein, thereby blocking binding of the virus to cellular receptors. Alternatively, patients may achieve at least some symptomatic relief with appropriate analgesics, sympathomimetic nasal decongestants, antitussives, and antihistamines. A range of over-the-counter medicines are available, although hot whisky or other home-brewed cocktails may be just as effective!

Q What complications may arise from an acute rhinovirus infection?

A These are:

- Sinusitis. Radiological evidence of involvement of the epithelium of the sinuses is common. Rhinoviruses have been isolated from sinus fluid, but of greater clinical importance is secondary bacterial sinusitis, the key features of which are shown in Box 14.1

Box 14.1 Acute sinusitis

- **Clinical features**: facial pain, nasal discharge, localized tenderness over affected sinus
- **Causative organisms**: common bacteria include *H. influenzae*, *S. pneumoniae*, beta-haemolytic group A streptococci (*S. pyogenes*). Anaerobes may also be involved
- **Management**: definitive diagnosis is by aspiration of pus from affected sinus, but this is not usually performed. Amoxycillin is first-line therapy
- **Complications**: chronic sinusitis. Rarely may lead to osteomyelitis, or cerebral abscess (see Case 43), especially if frontal sinuses involved

---

- Otitis media. The role of rhinoviruses is unclear. Secondary bacterial infection may occur (see Case 13)
- Exacerbations of asthma and chronic bronchitis. Recent studies suggest that the common cold viruses are responsible for a large majority of wheezy attacks in children. The pathogenetic mechanisms underlying this association are the subject of current research
- Lower respiratory tract infection, such as bronchiolitis or pneumonia, but this is rare

Q What is croup?

A Croup is more properly known as acute laryngo-tracheo-bronchitis, and is therefore a URTI.

Q What are the clinical features of croup?

A Croup is usually seen in children aged 6 months to 3 years. Clinical presentation is with coryzal symptoms for 1–2 days, followed by development of an inspiratory stridor (due to passage of air through an inflamed and partially obstructed larynx) and a 'croupy' or 'barking' cough that is worse at night. There is little constitutional disturbance, with only a mild pyrexia. On examination, supraclavicular and sternal recession may be evident, as well as use of accessory muscles of respiration.

Q What are the causes of croup?

A Several viruses can cause croup of which the parainfluenza viruses are the most common. Rhinoviruses, RSV, influenza, and measles viruses may also give rise to this syndrome.

Q How is a child with croup managed?

A Hospital admission may be necessary, depending on the degree of stridor. Important differential diagnoses of stridor to consider are acute epiglottitis and inhalation of a foreign body. Management of croup is to keep the child as settled as possible. Antibiotics, humidified air, and routine oxygen are of no proven benefit. Corticosteroids may have a place in the management of severe cases and, with imminent exhaustion of the child, intubation may be necessary. With expert care, the overwhelming majority of cases of croup make an uneventful recovery.

Summary: Upper respiratory tract infections

Presentation
Variable, depending on age and the anatomical site involved

Aetiology
Viral: rhino-, corona-, parainfluenza-, entero-, adeno-, and respiratory syncytial viruses

Diagnosis
Clinical

Management
No specific antiviral therapy

Prognosis
Excellent

Case 15 Peter, a 19-year-old student with a sore throat

Peter, a 19-year-old student, gives a 4-day history of a sore throat, difficulty in swallowing, and general malaise. His past medical history is unremarkable, and he is not taking any form of medication. On examination, he has a temperature of 38.6°C. His pharynx is obviously inflamed, and there is a patchy whitish membrane over his tonsils—see Fig. 15.1. He has marked cervical adenopathy.

Q What is the differential diagnosis?

A This is a young man with severe pharyngitis. A number of acute infections can present in this way:

- viruses: Epstein–Barr virus; cytomegalovirus; adenoviruses; enteroviruses

- bacteria: groups A,C, and G streptococci; *Corynebacterium diphtheriae* (see Box 15.1); mycoplasma; chlamydia

On closer examination, you decide that Peter's conjunctivae have a tinge of yellow and, in addition to the cervical adenopathy, you palpate axillary nodes and a spleen tip, but no liver.

Q How do these new findings influence your clinical diagnosis?

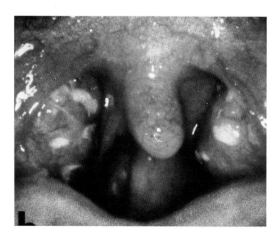

Fig. 15.1 Peter's pharynx.

A You have now elicited evidence of systemic disease, with generalized lymphadenopathy. These clinical findings are best described as a 'glandular fever' or 'infectious mononucleosis' (IM) syndrome. Note that the IM syndrome is not an aetiological diagnosis; it is a syndrome, i.e. a constellation of certain symptoms and signs. The most common cause of this syndrome is infection with Epstein–Barr virus (now referred to as EB virus, or EBV). Other infectious causes include acute infection with cytomegalovirus, *Toxoplasma gondii*, or human immunodeficiency virus (HIV; the so-called seroconversion illness, see Case 38). Malignant disease, particularly of the reticuloendothelial system (lymphoma, leukaemia), cannot be excluded at this stage.

Box 15.1 Bacterial causes of a severe sore throat

Diphtheria

- Severe sore throat with a 'false membrane' caused by *Corynebacterium diphtheriae*

- Exotoxin responsible for complications, which include polyneuritis, myocarditis/heart block, pneumonia, otitis media

- Laboratory diagnosis requires specialist media, e.g. tellurite, and confirmation of toxin production

- Toxoid is part of dipphteria–pertussis–tetanus (DPT) vaccine administered universally in childhood

Streptococcal sore throat

- Lancefield group A the most common cause of bacterial pharyngitis. Group C + G less common and less severe

- Exudates often seen on the tonsils. Marked fever and cervical lymphadenopathy not unusual

- Penicillin is the treatment of choice but should be continued for 10–14 days to prevent relapse or complications (see Case 5)

Direct questioning of Peter reveals no risk factors for HIV infection.

Q What investigations should you perform?

A A full blood count including differential and film, liver function tests (especially in view of the possible jaundice noted above), a 'Monospot' or Paul Bunnell test, and viral serology will help to distinguish between the common causes of glandular fever listed above. A throat swab for bacterial culture is also indicated.

The next day you receive the following results.

*   haemoglobin (Hb), 12.6 g/dl
*   white cell count (WCC), 14.3 × 10⁹/l
    polymorphonuclear leucocytes (PMNLs), 30%
    lymphocytes, 53%
    monocytes, 6%
    large unclassified cells (LUC), 11%
*   film shows atypical mononuclear cells (see Fig. 15.2)
*   platelets, 400 × 10⁹/l
*   alanine aminotransferase (ALT), 86 U/l (normal range, up to 50)
*   bilirubin, 41 mmol/l (normal range, up to 17)

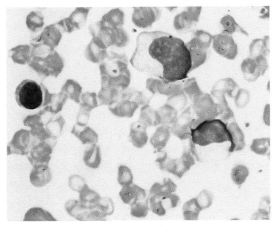

Fig. 15.2 Two atypical mononuclear cells (and one normal lymphocyte). Features of atypical mononuclear cells include large size relative to normal lymphocyte, increased cytoplasm:nucleus ratio, and indented, kidney-shaped nucleus.

*   alkaline phosphatase, 43 U/l (normal range, 40–120 U/l)

Q How do you interpret these findings?

A The blood count and film, showing a lymphocytosis with the presence of atypical mononuclear cells, confirm the clinical diagnosis of infectious mononucleosis. The characteristic features of the latter cells include large size (relative to normal lymphocytes), lobulated nuclei eccentrically placed, and an increased amount of cytoplasm. The liver function tests indicate hepatic involvement.

Q What are the atypical mononuclear cells?

A Activated CD8-positive T lymphocytes. It is these cells that are reported in the differential WCC as 'large unclassified cells'. These arise in many acute viral infections, in relatively small numbers. However, if they constitute > 10% of the total WCC, EBV infection (see Table 15.1) is the most likely cause.

Q What is the basis of the Monospot and Paul Bunnell (PB) tests?

A These tests are unusual in that they are used in the diagnosis of a virus infection (specifically EBV) but do not detect antiviral antibodies. In fact, they are red cell agglutination tests. They detect the presence of antibodies that react with antigens expressed on foreign red blood cells. These are referred to as heterophile antibodies (antibodies that react with antigens other than the specific inducing antigen). EBV infection often results in the transient production of such antibodies, presumably as a result of EBV-induced polyclonal B cell activation (see Table 15.1). Hence the presence of these antibodies, as detected by either of the above tests, is highly suggestive of recent EBV infection. The Monospot test is slightly more sophisticated, as it involves an absorption step to distinguish heterophile antibodies that react with different species of red blood cells.

Further results from Peter are:

*   Monospot—negative
*   throat swab—commensals only

Table 15.1 Epstein–Barr virus

Classification

A herpesvirus—human herpesvirus 4

Sites of infection

- Oropharyngeal epithelial cells, resulting in release of infectious virus in saliva
- Circulating B lymphocytes—the site of EBV latency. Note that infection of B cells *in vitro* results in polyclonal B cell activation, i.e. antibody production, and transformation, i.e. immortalization of cells into a lymphoblastoid cell line

Transmission

Via saliva—'kissing disease'!

Outcome of infection

- Asymptomatic seroconversion—the usual outcome in the first few years of life
- Acute infectious mononucleosis—a disease of teenagers and young adults
- Chronic infectious mononucleosis—a controversial diagnosis. Prolonged time to recovery may be part of the natural history of acute EBV infection
- Oral hairy leucoplakia—occurs in immunodeficient patients (see Case 38)

Association with malignancy

- Lymphoproliferative disease in the immunosuppressed
- Burkitt's lymphoma
- Nasopharyngeal carcinoma (undifferentiated or anaplastic type)

Q Does a negative Monospot result exclude a diagnosis of acute EBV infection?

A No. Of individuals infected with EBV, 10% fail to produce heterophile antibodies, and are therefore Monospot- and PB-negative. Note that cytomegalovirus (CMV)-, toxoplasma-, and HIV-induced acute IM are all heterophile-antibody-negative, and therefore Monospot- and PB-negative.

Q What further tests should you order to confirm Peter's diagnosis?

A Tests for the presence of antibodies specific for EBV should be done. The presence of EBV-specific IgM antibodies in an acute serum sample is diagnostic of acute EBV infection. A rise in antibody titre to CMV or toxoplasma in paired serum samples, or the presence of specific IgM against either organism would confirm infection with those agents. The diagnosis of the HIV seroconversion syndrome is considered in Case 38.

The EBV IgM result is positive. Peter is suffering from EBV-induced infectious mononucleosis.

Q What are the complications of acute EBV infection?

A Complications include:

- hepatitis: 5–10% patients are jaundiced
- splenomegaly: splenic rupture may be fatal
- central nervous system (CNS) manifestations, e.g. encephalitis, meningoencephalitis, Guillain–Barré syndrome, cranial nerve palsies
- airway obstruction due to exudative pharyngotonsillitis: may also be fatal. Steroids may be life-saving in reducing the inflammation and hence the obstruction

Hepatitis and CNS involvement can occur in the absence of other features of acute IM, especially in older patients, leading to diagnostic difficulties.

Four months later, Peter returns to see you complaining that he still feels lethargic and unable to resume many of his normal daily activities. He is worried that he may be suffering from some underlying disease, and also that his academic performance is declining. On examination, all the abnormal physical signs present during the acute illness have resolved. Investigations conducted in the previous month showed that his white cell count had returned to normal and the atypical cells had disappeared.

Q How should you proceed?

A Acute infectious mononucleosis is not a trivial illness. Many patients describe taking months or even a year or two before they feel fully fit again. Peter should be reassured that his prolonged lethargy does not indicate some dreadful disease process, but is relatively common. It should also be made clear to him that he will eventually recover. A report should be sent to his university tutor indicating the diagnosis, as his illness should be taken into account in relation to his poor academic performance.

Q What other diseases are associated with Epstein–Barr virus infection?

A EBV infection is important in the development of a number of malignant diseases:

- lymphomas in the immunosuppressed, i.e. transplant recipients, AIDS patients. Initially these are polyclonal B cell proliferations that develop subsequently into monoclonal lymphomas. Pathogenesis is related to loss of potent T cell control of EBV-driven B cell proliferation
- Burkitt's lymphoma, discussed below
- nasopharyngeal carcinoma, discussed below
- Hodgkin's disease. EBV may be associated with 40% of cases of this lymphoma; the role of EBV in its pathogenesis is the subject of much current research
- X-linked lymphoproliferative syndrome (XLP), formerly known as Duncan's syndrome. This rare disease is due to an inherited defect in the immune response to EBV, resulting in uncontrolled lymphoproliferation in affected males following acute infection, with a high mortality

Q What is the evidence linking EBV infection to the development of Burkitt's lymphoma and nasopharyngeal carcinoma (NPC)?

A The evidence includes:

1. The tumour cells—B cells in Burkitt's lymphoma, and epithelial cells in NPC—contain multiple copies of the EBV genome (EBV was first isolated from a Burkitt's lymphoma biopsy)

2. Sera from patients with these tumours contain very high titres of antibodies to EBV, often directed against unusual viral antigens

3. Antibody titres parallel clinical events, i.e. chemotherapy-induced remission is associated with a drop in antibody titres, whilst recurrence of the tumours may be heralded by a rise in titre

4. As a result of (2) and (3), EBV serology can be used to screen patients for the presence of Burkitt's lymphoma and NPC, and to monitor response to therapy

5. EBV is tumourigenic in animal models (inducing lymphoma formation in tamarin monkeys) and can immortalize B cells in vitro.

However, EBV cannot be the only factor resulting in these malignancies, as 90% of the world's population are infected with EBV and yet these tumours are very geographically restricted in their distribution. Other co-factors must act together with EBV infection in their pathogenesis. One such co-factor in the development of Burkitt's lymphoma is the presence of hyperendemic malaria. Possible co-factors for NPC include a genetic predisposition, and chronic exposure of the nasopharynx to chemical carcinogens or physical irritants, e.g. salted fish (dietary exposure) or smoke or dust (occupational exposure).

Q What other virus infections are associated with the development of malignant disease?

A These include:

- Hepatitis B virus and hepatocellular carcinoma (see Case 28)
- Hepatitis C virus and hepatocellular carcinoma (see Case 29)
- Human T cell lymphotropic virus HTLV-1 and adult T cell leukaemia/lymphoma (see Case 66)
- Human papillomaviruses, particularly types 16, and 18, and carcinoma of the uterine cervix (see Case 40)
- Human herpesvirus type 8 and Kaposi's sarcoma and primary effusion lymphoma (see Case 51)
- SV40 and lymphoma (see Case 40)

Summary: Infectious mononucleosis

Presentation
Fever, pharyngitis, lymphadenopathy, with lympho-cytosis including atypical mononuclear cells

Causative agents
EBV, CMV, HIV, toxoplasmosis

Diagnosis
Full blood count and film; monospot/Paul Bunnell tests; serology; culture of throat swab

Complications
Hepatitis, splenomegaly, neuropathy, respiratory obstruction

Management
Symptomatic; steroids if respiratory obstruction

Case 16 Respiratory distress and fever in Catriona, a 1-year-old infant

A 1-year-old dehydrated female infant, Catriona, is brought to the accident and emergency department in respiratory distress. Her father reports that, following a period of increased nasal discharge and a slight pyrexia, which lasted for 3 days, she began breathing fast and developed a paroxysmal cough.

Q What other information should be elicited from the parents?

A Apart from assessing whether other siblings were affected the significant question here concerns the vaccination status of the patient. In particular, has the child been vaccinated against whooping cough?

Catriona is admitted to hospital and nursed in a side room. Vital signs are closely monitored and parenteral hydration is commenced. Over the next 2–3 days she becomes less distressed and the coughing resolves. It is subsequently learned that Catriona has not been vaccinated against whooping cough because her parents were concerned about reported side-effects.

Q What are the clinical features of whooping cough?

A Not all children with whooping cough have the 'whoop', the classic feature of this condition. The condition may present with severe cough, tachypnoea, and cyanosis, but in many instances the presentation may not be dissimilar to that of other respiratory infections.

Q What is the mechanism by which the 'whoop' is produced?

A The 'whoop' is caused by a series of expiratory bursts followed by an inspiratory gasp, i.e. the whoop. The whooping or spasmodic stage is preceded by the catarrhal stage, and is followed by a period of recovery when the paroxysms of coughing become less severe.

Q How may the diagnosis of whooping cough be confirmed?

A Whooping cough is a clinical syndrome most commonly caused by *Bordetella pertussis*, which can be cultured during the early stages of the illness, but the condition may also be caused by:

1. *Bordetella parapertussis*

2. viruses
   - respiratory syncytial (RSV)
   - parainfluenza
   - adenovirus

3. *Mycoplasma pneumoniae*

Isolation of *Bordetella* is best achieved from a pernasal swab (see Table 16.1 and Fig. 16.1). A pernasal swab on a flexibile wire is passed along the floor of the nose near the midline until there is some resistance as it reaches the posterior wall of the nasopharynx.

Q What is the antibiotic of choice to treat *Bordetella* infections?

A It is not clear whether antimicrobial treatment alters the natural history of infection, but erythro-

---

Table 16.1 Laboratory diagnosis of *Bordetella pertussis* and *B. parapertussis*

Specimen

Pernasal preferred to nasal swab, sputum, or nasopharyngeal swab. Cough plates may also be used but are less convenient

Media

Selective media such as Bordet and Gengou or charcoal–cephalexin. Specimen should be transported to the laboratory rapidly or transport medium used

Identification

Plates incubated for up to 5 days. Suspect colonies (mercury-like on charcoal, haemolytic on Bordet and Gengou) are tested for agglutination with polyvalent serum for confirmation

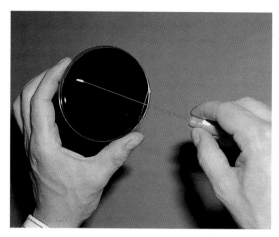

Fig. 16.1 Inoculation of pernasal swab on to charcoal blood agar.

mycin is usually prescribed in the hope of reducing infectivity. This may be important where there are non-vaccinated siblings.

Q What are the complications of whooping cough?

A Complications are most likely in children less than 1 year, and these include:

- apnoea leading to convulsions and possibly brain damage
- pneumonia, lobar collapse, and pneumothorax
- subconjunctival haemorrhage and epistaxis (due to convulsive coughing)
- hernias and rectal prolapse (due to convulsive coughing).

Q How may whooping cough be prevented?

A Pertussis vaccine (Table 16.2) is very effective in preventing whooping cough and, when immunization rates are low in the community, major outbreaks are likely. Treatment with antibiotics, such as a macrolide, e.g. erythromycin, may reduce infectivity and contribute to the resolution of symptoms, but often infection will have spread to other siblings by the time a laboratory diagnosis is made.

Table 16.2 Pertussis acellular vaccine

- Includes pertussis toxin, filamentous haemagglutinin, peractin, and fimbrial antigens
- Administered by deep intramuscular injection with diphtheria and tetanus in three doses, e.g. at 2, 4, and 6 months (booster 4–5 years later)
- Adverse reactions include swelling and redness at injection site, screaming and crying attacks, and fever

Q What are the contraindications to pertussis vaccination?

A Reasons for not vaccinating include:

- concurrent fever greater than or equal to 40°C or acute illness (postpone vaccination)
- recent convulsions or high-pitched screaming within the last 72 hours
- history of previous adverse local (severe) or general reaction

A personal or family history of allergy (e.g. to aspirin or penicillin) is not a contraindication, nor are stable neurological conditions such as cerebral palsy or previous febrile convulsions.

Q What are the side-effects of the vaccine?

A These include local swelling at the site of injection and crying. The most controversial and serious, however, with the previous vaccine used, i.e. the whole-cell vaccine (killed organism with adjuvant), were neurological including encephalopathy and prolonged convulsions, resulting in severe brain damage and even death. It was not possible to link the vaccine directly with the complications, however. More recent vaccines, i.e. the acellular vaccines, are considered safer with fewer local and lymph node side-effects, probably because of the absence of endotoxin unlike with the whole-cell vaccine.

Summary: Whooping cough

Presentation
Paroxysmal cough; respiratory distress

Diagnosis
Clinical features; pernasal swab for isolation of *Bordetella*

Management
Vaccination (prevention); rehydration; ventilation occasionally; erythromycin

Case 17 Mrs Carter, 32 years old, with a cough and generalized muscle aches and pains

Mrs Carter, a 32-year-old woman, complains of a febrile illness that began abruptly 3 days ago, on Christmas day, with a marked fever, headache, and shivering. Since then she has developed a non-productive cough, muscle aches all over her body, especially in the legs, and her eyes have become watery and painful to move. She is a non-smoker, previously fit and well, and on no regular medication. On examination, she is febrile (38.2°C) and has difficulty in breathing through her nose, but there are no other abnormal physical signs.

Q What is the diagnosis?

A These are the classic symptoms and signs of influenza. Clinically, the terms 'flu' and 'flu-like illness' should refer to more than just a simple common cold (runny nose, headache, irritating cough; see Case 14), i.e. there should be evidence of systemic upset, with fever, myalgia, and severe malaise. However, this terminology is often misused by the lay public, who may regard any upper respiratory tract symptoms as evidence that they are suffering from 'flu'. Although infection with influenza viruses A or B is the most common cause of this clinical syndrome, especially in winter, other infectious agents may be responsible, e.g. respiratory syncytial virus (RSV; particularly in the elderly), adenovirus, *Mycoplasma pneumoniae*, and *Chlamydia* species (see Case 19). In 2003, a new syndrome, severe acute respiratory syndrome (SARS), which bears many similarities to severe influenza virus infection, was described (see Box 17.1).

Q How are influenza viruses classified?

A A schematic diagram of an influenza virus is shown in Fig. 17.1. Influenza viruses are classified into *types* A, B, or C (*type* C is not a serious human pathogen) on the basis of the nature of the *internal* viral proteins (e.g. nucleocapsid protein). Influenza A viruses are further subdivided into *subtypes* on the basis of the nature of the two surface glycoproteins, i.e. the haemagglutinin (H or HA) and neuraminidase (N or NA). Influenza viruses are widespread throughout nature, and thus far 15 distinct H and 9 N molecules have been identified in influenza A viruses. Each H or N molecule differs by at least 20% in amino acid sequence from all other H or N molecules. It is customary, therefore, when referring to an influenza A virus, to indicate which subtype it is, i.e. which particular H and N molecules it possesses, e.g. influenza A H1N1.

Box 17.1 Severe acute respiratory syndrome (SARS)

Case definition

A person presenting with sudden onset of high fever (> 38°C), cough or difficulty breathing, a history of contact with a patient with SARS in the previous 10 days, with chest X-ray findings of pneumonia and no response to standard antimicrobial therapy

Causative agent

- SARS coronavirus, first identified in 2003

- Distinct from known human serotypes represented by coronaviruses 229E and OC43 previously associated with upper respiratory tract infection (see Case 14) and possibly viral gastroenteritis (see Case 24)

- Most probably arose from cross-species spread into humans in China, November 2002

Mortality rate

5% in under-60 age group; 15% in over-60s

Management

Requires intensive infection control procedures to prevent nosocomial spread

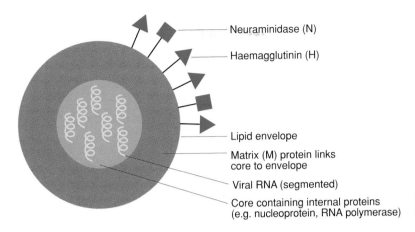

Neuraminidase (N)

Haemagglutinin (H)

Lipid envelope

Matrix (M) protein links
core to envelope

Viral RNA (segmented)

Core containing internal proteins
(e.g. nucleoprotein, RNA polymerase)

Fig. 17.1 Schematic diagram of
influenza virus.

(a)

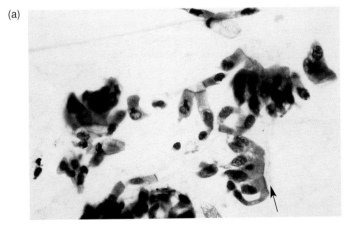

(b)

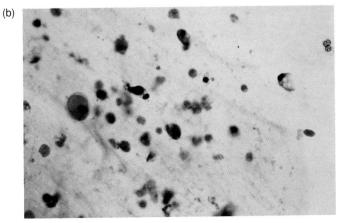

Fig. 17.2 (a) Sputum epithelial cells from
normal individual (arrow points to ciliated brush
border). (b) Sputum epithelial cells from
influenza-infected individual; all cells are
rounded up and dying/dead.

Q What is the pathogenesis of influenza virus infection?

A Influenza viruses are pneumotropic, i.e. they preferentially infect the epithelial cells lining the respiratory tract. All such cells, whether in the upper or lower respiratory tract, are susceptible. The infection is a lytic one, i.e. infected cells become rounded, swollen, and die. The virus therefore effectively strips away the lining respiratory epithelium. In this way, the ciliated cells (i.e. those bearing small hair-like structures, or cilia, on their luminal surface) are lost (see Fig. 17.2), as well as mucus-secreting glandular cells. In the normal course of events, inhaled particulate matter (including bacteria) becomes stuck in the respiratory mucus, and is then moved upwards by the coordinated beating of the cilia, to be expectorated in sputum. Loss of mucus-secreting and ciliated cells therefore removes an important defence mechanism in preventing such matter from gaining access to the lower respiratory tract.

The systemic symptoms of influenza—the fever and myalgia referred to above—are most probably due to virus-induced release of cytokines such as alpha-interferon, which circulate in the bloodstream. Viraemia (i.e. virus in the peripheral blood) is very difficult to demonstrate even during the acute stage of the illness.

Q What complications may arise from influenza virus infection?

A These include:

- Respiratory tract: tracheobronchitis, bronchiolitis, and pneumonia (see below) are the most common

- Myocarditis may arise, a serious complication especially in individuals with pre-existing cardiac disease

- Neurological: post-infectious encephalitis (see Case 6 for definition of this term), Guillain–Barré syndrome, and Reye's syndrome (precipitated by aspirin ingestion)

Q What aetiological types of pneumonia may complicate influenza virus infection?

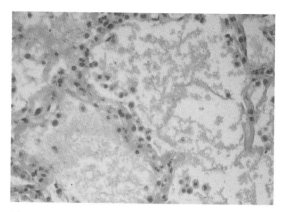

Fig. 17.3 Primary viral pneumonia—alveolar walls infiltrated with mononuclear cells.

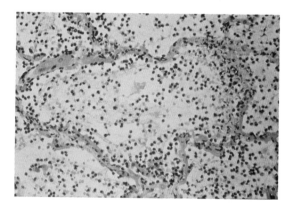

Fig. 17.4 Secondary bacterial pneumonia—alveolar space filled with polymorphonuclear neutrophil leucocytes (PMNLs).

A Primary viral or secondary bacterial pneumonia (see Figs 17.3 and 17.4 and Table 17.1).

Your initial management of Mrs Carter is conservative—advising bed-rest plus symptomatic relief with paracetamol (aspirin should be avoided in young children because of the risk of Reye's syndrome), as the infection usually resolves within 7 days, although many patients commonly complain of feeling listless and unwell for some time afterwards. However, when you visit her 2 days later, she still has a significant fever (38.5°C) and is feeling worse. Her cough has become more pronounced,

Table 17.1 Pneumonia following influenza infection

Primary viral pneumonia (Fig. 17.3)

- Causative agent—influenza virus
- Arises from direct spread of virus to the lower respiratory tract
- Can occur in previously fit and healthy persons
- Follows on from acute infection
- Alveolar space becomes filled with fibrinous material
- Mononuclear cell infiltrate into alveolar walls

Secondary bacterial pneumonia (Fig. 17.4)

- Causative agents, e.g. *Streptococcus pneumoniae*, *Haemophilus influenzae*, *Staphylococcus aureus*
- More common than viral pneumonia, especially in the elderly
- Many patients have underlying disease, e.g. chronic bronchitis
- May follow period of initial improvement of acute disease
- Alveolar space filled with polymorphonuclear cell infiltrate

although not very productive, and she complains of chest tightness and breathlessness on the slightest exertion. There are no signs of consolidation within the chest, but widespread rhonchi and crepitations are heard on auscultation. You admit Mrs Smith to hospital for further investigation and management.

Q What complication of influenza virus infection are you now worried about?

A Pneumonia. This is the most common life-threatening complication of influenza virus infection.

Q What microbiological investigations should you perform?

A Confirmation of the influenza virus infection should be sought by sending a nasopharyngeal aspirate (NPA) or throat swab in viral transport medium to the virology laboratory, and an acute serum sample for subsequent antibody assays. A sputum sample, for both bacterial and viral culture, is also mandatory. Blood cultures should be taken to diagnose bacteraemic pneumonia. *In extremis*, in a patient failing to respond to therapy where no diagnosis has been reached and where atypical pneumonia is a possibility (see Case 19), bronchoalveolar lavage fluid should be sent for microbiological analysis.

Q What tests would the virology laboratory perform on an NPA, sputum, or lavage fluid?

A In addition to inoculating appropriate tissue cultures for virus isolation, a rapid diagnosis can be attempted by immunofluorescent staining of cells obtained from the clinical material with monoclonal antibodies against a variety of organisms, e.g. influenza A virus, influenza B virus, RSV, parainfluenza viruses, adenoviruses, and chlamydia. The technique of immunofluorescence is explained in Case 21.

Mrs Carter's chest X-ray shows diffuse shadowing in both lung fields. Blood gases demonstrate hypoxia (p_aO_2 = 9.2 kilopascals), and a full blood count shows a normal white cell count and differential. You receive a phonecall that afternoon informing you that Mrs Carter's sputum was positive for the presence of influenza A virus by immunofluorescence. The next morning, bacterial culture of the sputum reveals commensals only.

Q What is your diagnosis?

A The clinical picture here is very suggestive of primary viral pneumonia, as evidenced by: illness in a previously fit non-smoker; failure to mount a neutrophil response; virus but no bacterial pathogens in the sputum sample.

Q What antiviral agents are available for the treatment of influenza virus infection?

A Until recently, the answer would have been amantadine (and its derivative, rimantadine) or ribavirin. Amantadine interferes with uncoating of virus within infected cells, is active only against influenza A virus, and has central nervous system side-effects such as insomnia, confusion, and restlessness that render it poorly tolerated, especially by the elderly. Ribavirin interferes with processing of viral mRNA, is active against both influenza A and B viruses and RSV, but must be administered by continuous inhalation for optimal effect. However, a new class of 'designer' drugs, the neuraminidase (NA) inhibitors, has now appeared, with zanamavir and oseltamivir the first members of this class to be licensed for use. NA is one of the two surface proteins of the influenza viruses. As new influenza virus particles bud from an infected cell, they remain bound to the cell surface through binding of the HA to sialic acid residues. It is the role of the NA to cleave these residues and thereby allow the virus particles to leave their cell of origin and seek out new cells to infect. These are 'designer' drugs in the sense that they were designed in the knowledge of the crystal structure of influenza virus NA, and specifically bind to (and inhibit) the active site of the enzyme. The two drugs mentioned have activity against all known subtypes of influenza NA.

Mrs Carter was treated with an NA inhibitor and cefuroxime (to cover undiagnosed bacterial pneumonia including *Staph. aureus*) and observed carefully. Her chest gradually improved, and she was well enough to be discharged 14 days after admission. No bacterial pathogen was ever isolated from her chest or blood cultures.

Q Should you have treated Mrs Carter sooner with antiviral drugs?

A The introduction of the NA inhibitors has created a controversial problem—should these drugs be given to patients with otherwise uncomplicated influenza? For the best therapeutic gain, they should be given as soon as possible. On the plus side, the drugs are effective—reducing time to recovery and days off work by perhaps 2–3 days. On the minus side, their widespread use would be expensive; their use would require an about-turn as to how influenza is currently handled in primary care, i.e. instead of encouraging patients to remain at home in bed, patients would need to come to the surgery as soon as possible for diagnosis and treatment; the drugs only work against influenza viruses so that prescription to patients suffering other infections would be useless. Not all patients with a 'flu-like' illness have influenza virus infection, and currently there is no 'bedside' diagnostic test to enable a rapid laboratory diagnosis to be made; there is always the worry that widespread use of any antiviral drug will encourage the emergence of drug-resistant viral variants (although there is little evidence thus far that this will be a problem with these particular drugs).

Current recommendations in the UK are to use NA inhibitors for the prevention and treatment of influenza-associated complications, rather than for uncomplicated influenza virus infection alone.

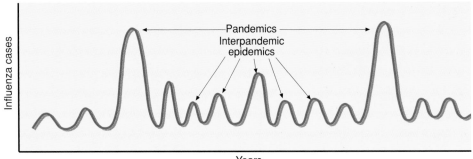

Fig. 17.5 Epidemiology of influenza.

Q What is understood by the terms 'pandemic' and 'interpandemic epidemic' influenza?

A The epidemiology of influenza is most unusual (see Fig. 17.5). Epidemics occur every winter in temperate climates, to a greater or lesser extent. However, every 20 years or so, a massive epidemic sweeps the globe, with hugely increased numbers of infected individuals and associated mortality. These occurrences are referred to as pandemics, and the smaller peaks of infection and morbidity occurring in between the pandemics are known as interpandemic epidemics.

Q What are the mechanisms underlying the emergence of influenza epidemics and pandemics?

Table 17.2 Antigenic drift

- Occurs in both influenza A and B viruses
- Caused by random spontaneous mutation of viral genes encoding H and N molecules
- Results in 1–2% differences in amino acid sequences of H and N molecules each year
- Mutations are clustered within key epitopes of the H and N molecules, thereby allowing virus to avoid some of the immune response induced by circulation of the previous year's virus

---

Table 17.3 Antigenic shift

- Occurs only in influenza A viruses
- Mechanism thought to involve genetic reassortment between human and non-human influenza viruses, leading to the production of new subtypes of influenza A, e.g.

    In 1957, H1N1 virus 'shifted' to H2N2 virus (Asian 'flu')

    In 1968, H2N2 virus 'shifted' to H3N2 virus (Hong Kong 'flu')

- Results in > 20% differences in amino acid sequences of H and/or N molecules and hence the emergence of new pandemic strains, against which the population has no pre-existing immunity

---

A Antigenic *drift* (see Table 17.2) is responsible for the generation of new epidemic strains each winter, whilst antigenic *shift* (see Table 17.3) gives rise to the pandemic strains every 20 years or so. These terms refer to changes that take place in the surface glycoproteins (i.e. the H and N proteins) of the viruses.

Since the last pandemic in 1976, three human influenza viruses have co-circulated each winter—influenza A viruses H1N1 and H3N2 and influenza B. In any one season, one of these three viruses tends to dominate, but the dominant virus may change from season to season. In 2001, the emergence of an A H1N2 strain was seen, presumably due to reassortment between H1N1 and H3N2 viruses. The emergence of a new pandemic subtype of influenza A is unpredictable. There was a major scare in 1997, with several cases of H5N1 infection of humans reported in Hong Kong. However, this outbreak appears to have arisen from direct transfer of an H5N1 virus directly from chickens to humans—all but one of the cases had a history of close contact with infected chickens, the one exception being a health-care worker. Thus, this virus was not a true reassortant, and by chance was not well suited for human-to-human spread. The outbreak was controlled by mass slaughter of all chickens in Hong Kong.

Q Is influenza virus infection preventable?

A Yes, by means of inactivated subunit vaccines. Vaccines must contain H and N molecules from each of the co-circulating viruses. Current vaccines are about 70% effective in protecting against infection.

Q For how long are the vaccines effective?

A One winter only, as the circulating viruses exhibit antigenic drift from year to year. Thus, the constituent vaccine viruses need to be altered and upgraded accordingly, and vaccinees need a dose of vaccine each autumn. The WHO monitors the antigenicity of circulating influenza viruses, and recommendations are made each year as to which would be the most appropriate strains to include in the vaccine.

Q Who should be vaccinated against influenza?

A The current policy in the UK is to protect those patient groups who are at increased risk of serious complications of infection, i.e. selective rather than universal vaccination. Immunization is strongly recommended for:

1. all individuals over the age of 65
2. all aged over 6 months in the following risk groups
   - chronic respiratory disease, including asthma
   - chronic heart disease
   - chronic renal disease
   - diabetes mellitus and other endocrine disorders
   - immunosuppression due to disease or treatment.

Immunization is also recommended for individuals within residential homes or other institutions where rapid spread is likely to follow introduction of infection.

Q Is there any alternative to vaccination, e.g. in those allergic to eggs (a contraindication to vaccination)?

A Yes. Amantadine given as prophylaxis has been shown to be effective in preventing influenza infection, but is poorly tolerated by many patients. This is useful in an outbreak setting, where there may not be sufficient time to allow the vaccine to work. Recent studies have shown that the NA inhibitors may also be effective when used prophylactically.

Summary: **Influenza**

Presentation

Coryza, cough, headache, fever, generalized myalgia

Diagnosis

Clinical; serology; virus detection in NPA, throat swab

Complications

Pneumonia (primary viral or secondary bacterial); myocarditis; post-infectious encephalitis

Management

Symptomatic; antiviral drugs if in high-risk group for serious complications; antibiotics if pneumonia

Prevention

Vaccination of high-risk groups

Case 18 Sarah, a 55-year-old woman with rigors, cough, and chest pain

Sarah, a 55-year-old pyrexial woman, is referred to the A&E department with a 24-hour history of cough, left-sided chest pain, and rigors. She has a cough productive of sputum most mornings, but this has become increasingly purulent. Until a myocardial infarction 2 years previously she smoked 40 cigarettes a day.

Q What physical findings might be elicited on respiratory examination?

A Physical signs of consolidation, i.e. dullness on percussion, an area of bronchial breathing with or without absent breath sounds, would suggest lobar pneumonia, whereas reduced breath sounds accompanied by crepitations would be more characteristic of bronchopneumonia.

On examination Sarah has a fever of 40°C, a tachycardia of 130/min, and is tachypnoeic, but her blood pressure is normal. Auscultation of the respiratory system indicates probable consolidation.

Q What is the clinical diagnosis and how may this be confirmed?

A A high fever, chest pain, productive cough, and the above findings on physical examination are very suggestive of pneumonia requiring admission to hospital. Chest X-ray, white cell count, sputum for microscopy and culture, blood cultures, and arterial blood gases will help in assessing the likely aetiology and the severity of the illness.

The peripheral white cell count is elevated, at $22 \times 10^9/l$ (90% polymorph neutrophils) and

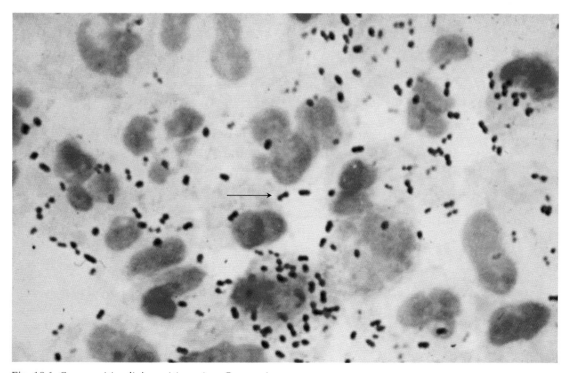

Fig. 18.1 Gram-positive diplococci (arrow) on Gram stain.

numerous pus cells and Gram-positive diplococci are seen in the Gram stain of the sputum
(Fig. 18.1). Chest X-ray confirms right lobar
pneumonia (Fig. 18.2(a)).

Q What does the Gram stain tell you?

A The presence of pus cells in the absence of
epithelial cells confirms that this is most likely a
specimen obtained from the lower respiratory tract,
and therefore culture may reflect the cause of the
infection. It is not possible to distinguish definitely the different types of inflammatory cell (i.e.

Table 18.1 *Streptococcus pneumoniae*

Microbiology

- Gram-positive coccus that may be in pairs or
  short chains
- α-haemolytic colonies on blood agar identified
  by sensitivity to optochin
- Virulence determinants include a capsule and
  pneumolysin

Diseases

1 *Systemic*
   - Pneumonia (also abscess and empyema)
   - Bacteraemia (see Case 47)
   - Meningitis (see Case 41)
   - Septic arthritis (see Case 54), peritonitis (pri-
     mary), etc.
2 *Localized*
   - Otitis media (see Cases 13 and 14)
   - Sinusitis/mastoiditis (see Case 13)
   - Bronchitis (see Case 20)
   - Conjunctivitis (see Case 8)

(a)

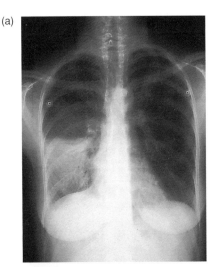

(b)

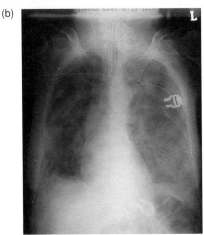

Fig. 18.2 Chest X-rays of (a) lobar pneumonia and
(b) bilateral bronchopneumonia.

polymorphs, lymphocytes, monocytes) seen with a
Gram stain, but in this instance these are likely to
be polymorphs. The organisms seen are likely to
be *Streptococcus pneumoniae* (pneumococcus; see
Table 18.1). The isolation of α-haemolytic streptococci (see Case 5) with typical colonial features and
sensitive to optochin (an antibiotic used for identification but not treatment) will confirm the cause.

Q What other investigations may be helpful?

A Many patients with pneumococcal pneumonia
are bacteraemic and therefore blood cultures are
important, especially where sputum is not available, e.g. in the elderly patient. The presence of
bacteraemia usually heralds a poorer prognosis.
Respiratory specimens obtained at bronchoscopy
are also useful if there is no sputum, if the diagnosis
is uncertain, or if an atypical pathogen (see Case 19)
is suspected. Urine may also be sent for pneumococcal and legionella (where suspected) antigen
testing, which is increasingly available in many

Table 18.2 **Aetiology of community- and hospital-acquired pneumonia**

Community-acquired	Hospital-acquired
S. pneumoniae	Enterobacteriaceae, e.g. *E. coli*, *Klebsiella*
Mycoplasma pneumoniae (young adults)	*Pseudomonas aeruginosa* (ICU)
Chlamydia pneumoniae	*Staphylococcus aureus*
Haemophilus influenzae	Anaerobes, e.g. *Bacteroides fragilis* (aspiration)
Moraxella catarrhalis	Fungi (less common), e.g. *Candida*, *Aspergillus*
Influenza	
SARS coronavirus (Case 17)	
Legionella spp.	

centres. Finally, paired sera (10–14 days apart) and pleural fluid for culture may also be helpful and indicated in certain circumstances.

Q What are the most common causes of pneumonia?

A *S. pneumoniae* is by far the commonest cause of community-acquired pneumonia, followed by *Mycoplasma pneumoniae*, but the aetiology of hospital-acquired infection is different, with *S. pneumoniae* encountered much less frequently (see Table 18.2).

Q Why is the aetiology of hospital-acquired pneumonia so different?

A Gram-negative bacilli and *Staphylococcus aureus* predominate in hospital because of increased colonization of the upper airways following hospital admission, administration of antibiotics, and invasive procedures. Polymicrobial infection may follow aspiration and, in severely immunosuppressed patients, viral (cytomegalovirus) and fungal (*Aspergillus*, *Pneumocystis carinii*) causes must be considered.

Q What is the treatment of choice for pneumococcal disease and community-acquired penumonia?

A Benzylpenicillin (minimum inhibitory concentration to *S. pneumoniae* is 0.03 mg/l) is the treatment of choice unless the patient has a definite history of penicillin allergy or the isolate is resist-

ant. Where the aetiology of pneumonia is unclear, amoxycillin or co-amoxyclav is preferred in the first instance to cover *H. influenzae* (more commonly a cause of acute bronchitis than pneumonia) as well as the pneumococcus. Erythromycin or clarithromycin should be added to cover other possible causes such as *Mycoplasma pneumoniae* and *Legionella* species if likely.

Sarah is started on intravenous benzylpenicillin, but 12 hours later she is transferred to the intensive care unit (ICU) for ventilation because of persistent hypoxia. *S. pneumoniae* is isolated from two sets of blood cultures taken on admission as well as from sputum. Three days later she still requires ventilation and her antibiotic is changed to cefotaxime, to cover against an ICU-acquired pneumonia. The white cell count is now over $35 \times 10^9/l$ and the chest X-ray shows deterioration, with increasing consolidation and a pleural effusion. Repeat respiratory specimens taken during bronchoscopy and blood cultures are sterile. On day 5 Sarah has a cardiac arrest and dies.

Q What factors are associated with an unfavourable prognosis?

A A high mortality from pneumococcal pneumonia is associated with:

- bacteraemia (20% versus 5% in non-bacter-aemic patients)
- accompanying extrapulmonary focus
- certain capsular types (typing of isolates not routine)
- underlying disease such as splenic dysfunction, cirrhosis

Q Is penicillin resistance amongst pneumococci common?

A This depends on geographical location. In the UK it is 5–10% but in other parts of the world such as South Africa or countries bordering the Mediterranean the prevalence can be as high as 40–50%. Many of these isolates are not fully resist-ant and therefore patients may respond to high doses of benzylpenicillin but, for meningitis, a third-generation cephalopsorin such as cefotaxime is recommended to ensure eradication and for phar-macokinetic reasons (see Case 41).

Q How may pneumococcal disease be prevented?

A A polyvalent vaccine derived from 23 capsular types is available and has an efficacy of 60–70%, especially in non-immunosuppressed adults. A single dose is administered intramuscularly or sub-cutaneously. Indications for vaccination are:

- splenic dysfunction such as sickle cell disease; before elective or following emergency splenec-tomy
- chronic heart, lung, liver, or renal disease
- diabetes mellitus
- immunosuppressed patients, including those with HIV infection

However, this vaccine is ineffective for children less than 2 years of age but new 7- or 9-valent conju-gate vaccines are now available and may ultimately replace the capsular-based vaccine.

Summary: Pneumococcal pneumonia

Presentation

Lobar (more characteristic) or bronchopneumonia with high fever, purulent sputum, chest pain, rig-ors, and signs of consolidation

Diagnosis

Physical findings on examination; chest X-ray; spu-tum or bronchoscopy specimens for microscopy and culture; and blood cultures

Management

Prevention by vaccination for at-risk groups; ben-zylpenicillin is the antibiotic of choice

Case 19 Dermot, a 57-year-old smoker with increasing dyspnoea and confusion

Dermot, a 57-year-old man, is admitted to hospital because of increasing dyspnoea and confusion. Five days previously he developed a non-productive cough, which has become worse, and he has become more housebound because of breathlessness. He smokes 20–30 cigarettes a day. His only medication is a thiazide diuretic for mild hypertension. On examination he is a little drowsy and disorientated in time. He has a respiratory rate of 22/min, a heart rate of 95/min, and his temperature is 37.5°C. Scattered crepitations, more marked on the left, are heard on auscultation. Neurological examination is grossly normal.

Q What relevant initial investigations should be carried out?

A The previous medical history and presenting symptoms suggest a possible cardiac cause, and consequently an electrocardiogram (ECG) and chest X-ray should be carried out immediately. Blood gases will indicate whether he is hypoxic and/or hypercapnic and, in a distressed patient with pyrexia, sputum (if available) and blood should be taken for culture.

The ECG is normal and the arterial oxygen pressure is low at 8 kPa (normal range, 11–13 kPa). Chest X-ray reveals a normal heart size but patchy consolidation in the left-mid and upper zones. Full blood count, urea and electrolytes, serum glucose, and calcium are normal. Despite nasal oxygen, Dermot remains hypoxic and within 18 hours of admission requires ventilation in the intensive care unit (ICU). His wife, Maura, is interviewed and she remarks that he has become more disorientated and confused in recent days, but that he had been well throughout their holiday in Greece, from which they returned a week ago. She also remarks that the illness started with generalized lethargy, nasal discharge, and a mild cough.

Q What diagnosis comes to mind following the collateral history from his wife?

A The clinical and radiological features of this case strongly suggest pneumonia, but the absence of a high fever, a productive cough, and marked physical findings on examination of the chest point to a diagnosis of so-called 'atypical pneumonia'.

Q What is 'atypical' compared with 'typical' pneumonia?

A The term 'atypical' is usually meant to refer to the less common aetiological agents that do not present with classical pneumonia but there is considerable clinical overlap between pneumonia caused by atypical agents and pneumococcal pneumonia (Case 18). The term 'atypical' refers to a number of issues:

- *Presentation*: flu-like illness, sometimes with few if any respiratory symptoms. Productive cough and a high fever, which are characteristic of pneumococcal pneumonia (see Case 18), are often absent

- *Diagnosis*: the organisms responsible are largely non-bacterial and therefore culture of sputum and blood will only serve to exclude more conventional causes of pneumonia, such as *Streptococcus pneumoniae* (see Case 18). Respiratory specimens obtained during bronchoscopy, specialized culture techniques, antigen detection, and serology are part of the work-up of such a patient

- *Aetiology*: bacterial, viral, chlamydial, and rickettsial causes have all been implicated, and many of these are associated with specific clinical and/or epidemiological features (Table 19.1)

- *Treatment*: failure to respond to β-lactam antibiotics such as a penicillin or a cephalosporin

Table 19.1 Aetiology and features of so-called 'atypical pneumonia'

Class of microbe	Organism	Features of infection
Bacteria	*Legionella pneumophila*	Ubiquitous in aquatic environment. Associated with travel abroad, air-conditioning system (e.g. in hotels)
	Mycoplasma pneumoniae	Cell wall-deficient bacteria. Most common cause of pneumonia in young adults
Chlamydiae	*Chlamydia psittaci*	May be associated with psittacine birds. Causes a severe pneumonia
	Chlamydia pneumoniae	Occurs in children or young adults. May recur
Rickettsiae	*Coxiella burnetti*	May be occupation-related, e.g. farmers. Also causes endocarditis (see Case 49). Also known as Q fever
Viruses	Influenza A and B (see Case 17)	Occur during epidemics, especially A
	Adenovirus	Important cause in the young, especially in institutions such as military barracks
	Coronavirus SARS (see Case 17)	History of travel to Far East or contact with known case

On admission to the ITU a bronchoscopy is carried out and the bronchi are noted to be inflamed, with increased secretions, especially on the left side. Following instillation of normal saline, lavage fluid is obtained and sent to the laboratory for routine culture, *Legionella* isolation, and direct antigen detection by immunofluorescence. Immunofluorescence is negative for *Legionella*, *Mycoplasma pneumoniae*, *Chlamydia* spp., adenoviruses, and influenza viruses.

Q Does a negative immunofluorescence result rule out infection with *Legionella*?

A No. Immunofluorescence is a highly specific test in the diagnosis of *Legionella* infection, but it is less sensitive than culture because a smaller volume of specimen can be examined. Patients who have recently been treated with antimicrobial agents active against *Legionella* may be negative on culture but positive for immunofluorescence, since the lat-

ter is not dependent on viable organisms. Antigen detection in urine may be useful in making a diagnosis early in the course of the illness. It is also possible that DNA probes that detect gene-specific ribosomal RNA will increasingly be used in diagnosis and, in some centres, polymerase chain reaction (PCR) is already available. Culture has the added advantage that it will not only isolate *L. pneumophila* serogroup 1, but also other serogroups or species, and susceptibility testing against various antimicrobial agents is possible.

L. pneumophila serogroup 1 is isolated from the bronchoscopy specimen and, although antibodies to *Legionella* are 1/16 on admission, these rise to 1/128 10 days later when repeated. It is therefore concluded that Dermot has Legionnaires' disease.

Q How useful is serology in making a diagnosis?

A Serology is negative—i.e. there is a failure to demonstrate a fourfold rise in titres—in up to 25%

of cases, and therefore a range of diagnostic approaches must be considered when investigating cases of legionella pneumonia or other causes of atypical pneumonia.

Q What other clinical features may be seen with Legionnaires' disease?

A Diarrhoea is present in about a quarter of cases. Changes in mental status, including encephalopathy, and peripheral neuropathy may also be seen. Remember, Dermot was confused and disorientated at the initial clinical presentation. A number of laboratory parameters are often abnormal, including liver function tests and hyponatraemia.

Q What is the antibiotic of choice for treatment?

A Legionellae, like chlamydia and rickettsiae, are resistant to the β-lactam antibiotics (penicillins and cephalosporins). Erythromycin or clarithromycin for two to three weeks is the agent of choice, with rifampicin added for severe cases requiring ventilation or organ support. A quinolone, e.g. ciprofloxacin, may also be used but studies demonstrating a better outcome have not been carried out. Erythromycin is also the drug of choice for *Mycoplasma pneumoniae* infections, but a tetracycline is generally preferred for the treatment of chlamydial and rickettsial infections. Because of the relative infrequency of many of these causes of pneumonia, large-scale comparative antibiotic trials have not been conducted and recommendations on treatment have arisen from individual and collective experience, *in vitro* studies on antimicrobial activity, and by general consensus.

Dermot is started on intravenous erythromycin and improves after 48–72 hours. Two days later he is transferred back to a general medical ward, and later the erythromycin is changed to oral administration for the remainder of his course. Dermot is subsequently discharged from hospital having made a full recovery. Maura, his wife, continues to remain asymptomatic.

Q How may infection with Legionella be acquired?

Table 19.2 **Legionella**

- Gram-negative rods poorly visualized on routine microscopy. Natural habitat is water, such as hot water systems, nebulizers, showers, and air-conditioning systems; 36 species, the most important being *L. pneumophila*

- Causes Pontiac fever (a mild flu-like illness) and pneumonia, which is more severe in patients with pre-existing lung disease

- Will not grow on routine laboratory media. Bronchoscopic specimens are superior to sputum for culture and antigen detection. Serology for antibody testing and urine for antigen detection are important in the absence of respiratory specimen

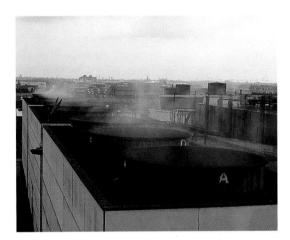

Fig. 19.1 Cooling towers—a possible source of *Legionella* infection.

A Legionellae are Gram-negative rods that are widely distributed in nature (see Table 19.2), especially in aquatic environments. They flourish in the water systems of buildings, such as potable water and cooling towers (see Fig. 19.1). It is possible that Dermot acquired the infection while on holiday in Greece, especially if the hotel in which the couple were staying had air-conditioning. Most community-acquired cases of Legionella infection are sporadic and no definite source is ever identified. Nosocomial infection is also described, most likely occurring during the summer months, and is associated with widespread and heavy contamination of water sources, conducting systems such as piping, or inadequately heated hot water. The facility of Legionella to survive inside protozoa, which may be found in many water systems and biofilms, partly explains their ability to persist in domestic and other water supplies.

Q What precautions should nursing and medical staff take while caring for this patient?

A Person-to-person spread of *Legionella* is not known to occur and therefore special precautions are not required to prevent transmission to other patients or staff. There is a possibility that Dermot's wife may have contracted *Legionella*, as she is likely to have been exposed to the same sources as her husband. She may not, however, develop symptoms because of having been exposed to a smaller inoculum, previous exposure to *Legionella* and some degree of immunity, or the absence of underlying disease such as emphysema due to smoking.

Summary: Legionnaires' disease

Presentation
Fever, dry cough, dyspnoea, but often without rigors or purulent sputum. Respiratory failure may be a feature in patients with underlying lung disease

Diagnosis
Clinical suspicion in a patient with so-called 'atypical' features of pneumonia; bronchoscopy specimens for culture and antigen detection; urine for antigen detection; paired sera for antibody testing

Management
High-dose erythromycin or clarithromycin with or without rifampicin in severe cases. Patients may require ventilation in an intensive therapy unit

Case 20 Dyspnoea, wheeze, and a productive cough in Charlie, a 55-year-old smoker

Charlie is a 55-year-old electrical wholesaler who complains of increasing breathlessness, wheeze, and a productive purulent cough for the last 3 days. He smokes 20 cigarettes a day, down from 30–40 a day since a previous admission to hospital 2 years ago for pneumonia, expectorates clear sputum most mornings, and is on no medication apart from a salbutamol inhaler, which he uses occasionally. He is examined by his GP, who notes that he has a pyrexia of 38°C and that he has scattered rhonchi throughout both lung fields.

Q What is the underlying disease?

A Chronic bronchitis.

Q What is chronic bronchitis?

A A diagnosis of chronic bronchitis is a clinical one and is made on a history of sputum produced on most days for at least 3 consecutive months for more than 2 consecutive years. Pathologically, chronic bronchitis is usually characterized by bronchial oedema, epithelial hyperplasia, increased mucus-secreting cells, and bronchospasm. It is closely associated with cigarette-smoking. In some patients emphysema is predominant; in others an asthmatic component, as described here, largely explains the symptomatology. This patient most probably has an acute exacerbation of chronic bronchitis superimposed upon chronic obstructive lung disease.

Q What clinical features would suggest an infective component?

A Acute bronchitis of infective aetiology is usually characterized by fever and a cough, with or without productive sputum, but acute exacerbations of chronic obstructive airways disease are not always necessarily due to infection. Increased sputum, accompanied by a change in colour from clear or mucoid to purulent (see Fig. 20.1) with or without a fever, indicates a probable infective component. A complaint of fatigue or other systemic symptoms also points towards infection. Non-infective causes include increased cigarette-smoking and environmental factors such as smog.

Charlie's GP advises him to reduce the number of cigarettes smoked, or preferably stop altogether, and prescribes inhaled salbutamol four times daily to reduce wheezing, and inhaled atropine to improve bronchospasm and inhibit the formation of mucus. She also prescribes a 5-day course of oral amoxycillin, but 1 week later his cough is no better, despite now smoking only 10 cigarettes a day. The sputum has also become more purulent.

Q What investigations, if any, are now required?

A A chest X-ray will help exclude other pathology in a smoker, including a lung neoplasm, pneumothorax, consolidation, or possible tuberculosis. If none of these is present the X-ray may reveal

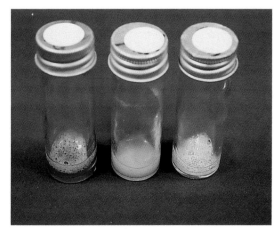

Fig. 20.1 Examples of (left to right) blood-stained, purulent, and mucoid sputa.

signs of chronic chest disease, such as emphysema and increased bronchiolar markings, but there are no characteristic radiological features of acute exacerbations of chronic obstructive airways disease.

Microscopy and culture of sputum is probably indicated because the sputum has become more purulent despite antibiotic treatment. A good-quality sputum should reveal numerous pus cells, few if any epithelial cells (which usually arise from the buccal mucosa), and bacteria, some of which may be responsible for Charlie's symptoms.

Q What microbes are responsible for acute exacerbations of emphysema and chronic bronchitis?

A Potential respiratory pathogens can be cultured from the sputum of most of these patients, unlike that of non-bronchitic patients. It may, however, be difficult to distinguish microbes representing colonization secondary to respiratory epithelial damage from those responsible for symptoms. *Streptococcus pneumoniae* and *Haemophilus influenzae* are the two most frequently implicated bacteria (see Table 20.1). However, potential viral causes are probably much underestimated.

A chest X-ray is unremarkable, but *Moraxella catarrhalis* is isolated in heavy growth from sputum. The isolate is reported as resistant to ampicillin/amoxycillin and trimethoprim but sensitive to co-amoxyclav, cefaclor, cefuroxime, and the quinolones. Following a 5-day course of co-amoxyclav (see Case 13), Charlie's cough improves and the sputum becomes much less purulent. Subsequently, however, Charlie returns to smoking over 20 cigarettes a day!

Q What is *M. catarrhalis*?

A This bacterium is a Gram-negative coccus, previously known as *Neisseria* and subsequently as *Branhamella catarrhalis*. It can be distinguished from *Neisseria* in the laboratory by a number of biochemical reactions and the production of DNAase. It may be part of the normal upper respiratory tract flora, but in recent years it has been increasingly recognized as a cause of upper (e.g. otitis media) and lower (e.g. pneumonia, bronchitis) respiratory tract infection, especially in patients with pre-existing chest disease. If clinically significant, it is usually present in heavy growth from purulent sputum. Scanty growth or isolation from mucoid or non-purulent sputum should not be considered clinically significant. Of isolates 50% or more are β-lactamase producers and consequently will be resistant to penicillin or ampicillin.

Table 20.1 **Microbial pathogens responsible for acute exacerbations of chronic bronchitis and emphysema**

Organism	Comment
Streptococcus pneumoniae	Common
Haemophilus influenzae	Non-encapsulated
Moraxella catarrhalis	Previously known as *Branhamella catarrhalis*
Staphylococcus aureus	Less common
Enterobacteria, e.g. *Escherichia coli*, *Klebsiella* spp.	Less common, may represent colonization following antibiotics
Mycoplasma pneumoniae	Occasional cause. Diagnosis by serology
Viruses, e.g. influenza, coronavirus, parainfluenza, rhinovirus, respiratory syncytial virus (RSV)	More common than appreciated and often precede bacteria

Table 20.2 Oral antibiotics used to treat exacerbations of chronic bronchitis

Ampicillin/amoxycillin	Active against *S. pneumoniae* and most isolates of *H. influenzae*. 50% of *M. catarrhalis* resistant
Co-amoxyclav	Also active against β-lactamase-producing *H. influenzae* and *M. catarrhalis*
Erythromycin	Poor activity against *H. influenzae* but the agent of choice for *M. pneumoniae* and *Legionella*
Clarithromycin	Also a macrolide; is often better tolerated and has some activity against *Haemophilus influenzae*
Trimethoprim	Less commonly used now. Fewer side-effects than co-trimoxazole but inactive against *M. catarrhalis*
Cefaclor/cefadroxil/cefixime	Broad-spectrum cephalosporins with enhanced activity against *H. influenza* Expensive
Ciprofloxacin/moxifloxacin/ levofloxacin	Second-line agents. Ciprofloxacin has relatively poor activity against *S. pneumoniae*
Tetracycline	Rarely used now. Indicated if penicillin allergy or mycoplasma/chlamydia infections likely

Q What is the antimicrobial agent of choice for the initial treatment of exacerbations of chronic chest disease such as this?

A There are a number of options available, but most would consider a penicillin such as amoxycillin initially (better absorption than ampicillin following oral administration). Factors influencing the choice of one agent over another are a history of recent antibiotic use, treatment failure, side-effects, and the results of antibiotic susceptibility tests. Where β-lactamase production among *H. influenzae* isolates is common (> 20%) amoxycillin is not appropriate. Options for antimicrobial therapy are outlined in Table 20.2.

Q What other measures should be considered to reduce infective exacerbations of chronic bronchitis?

A Apart from reducing smoking, losing weight, and regular exercise to improve general health and pulmonary function, vaccination against pneumococcal disease (see Case 18) and influenza (see Case 17) should be considered, especially if the patient is over 65. Prophylactic antibiotics have no role to play in minimizing either the frequency or the severity of exacerbations and, indeed, may result in the emergence of resistance. It may be appropriate for some patients, however, to have a course of antibiotics at home to take early during an exacerbation when the sputum changes colour, especially if there is likely to be a delay in seeing the GP.

Summary: Infective exacerbations of chronic bronchitis

Presentation

Increased sputum production with change in colour, wheeze, and breathlessness

Diagnosis

Essentially clinical. Chest X-ray to exclude other pathology and sputum microbiology to guide choice of antibiotic

Management

Cessation of smoking; bronchodilators; antibiotics (e.g. cefaclor, co-amoxyclav); vaccination against pneumococcus and influenza

Case 21 Shula, 5 months old, off colour, and feeding poorly

Shula, 5 months old, is brought to paediatric A&E during the week before Christmas. Her parents have noticed she has been 'off colour' for the past 72 hours with a runny nose, not eating well, and waking during the night with a non-productive cough. Her cough has become more pronounced in the past 24 hours. Her temperature last night was 38.5°C, so her parents gave her paracetamol syrup. This morning, they have noticed her breathing is very rapid.

Shula was born by normal vaginal delivery, weighing 7 lbs, and has subsequently hovered around the 30th centile for weight. She has received all the routine recommended vaccines for her age, the last set being given 3 weeks previously. She has two older siblings, aged 3 and 5 years, both of whom are well.

On examination, Shula is restless and distressed. She is febrile (38.4°C) and has a pulse of 160/min and a respiratory rate of 70/min. There is visible in-drawing of the chest-wall during inspiration. Diffuse wheezes and crackles are heard throughout both lung fields. Apart from the tachycardia, there are no other abnormal signs in the cardiovascular system. The rest of the physical examination is also normal.

Q What is the likely diagnosis?

A The acute onset, the presence of fever, and abnormal respiratory signs all suggest an acute respiratory tract infection. The grossly elevated respiratory rate, and the use of accessory muscles of respiration suggest lower respiratory tract involvement (i.e. bronchiolitis or pneumonia).

Q How should you investigate Shula?

A A chest X-ray and pulse oximetry are useful in assessing the severity of infection. A nasophayngeal aspirate (NPA), taken by passing a fine tube into the nasopharynx and applying suction (see Fig. 21.1), should be sent to the microbiology laboratory for identification of the causative pathogen.

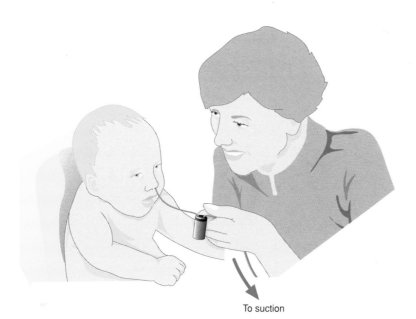

To suction

Fig. 21.1 Taking a nasopharyngeal aspirate.

Shula's chest X-ray shows evidence of hyper-inflation and increased peribronchial markings. Her oxygen saturation is 82% (normal, > 95%). You decide to admit Shula to the ward, where she can be nursed in a head-box with 30% oxygen and adequate hydration achieved via a nasogastric tube.

Q What is the most likely causative pathogen?

A There are two clues here—the age of the patient, and the time of year. Respiratory syncytial virus (RSV) infection accounts for up to 90% of cases of bronchiolitis in infancy. RSV epidemics occur annually in temperate climates and show sharp peaks of about 3 months' duration, beginning in November/December. Lower respiratory tract infection in small children may also be due to parainfluenza viruses (occur throughout the year), adenoviruses (see Case 8), influenza viruses (seasonal; see Case 17), and *Mycoplasma pneumoniae* (epidemics occur every 5 years or so; see Case 19). Recently, a novel viral pathogen has been described that may also cause symptomatic respiratory disease—human metapneumovirus (see Box 21.1).

Box 21.1 Human metapneumovirus

History—first described in 2001
Virology—belongs in same virus family as RSV (the paramyxoviridae), but in a separate genus (the metapneumovirinae)
Clinical features—symptoms and signs of viral respiratory tract infection

---

Q How will the microbiology laboratory identify the causative agent?

A The most commonly used rapid diagnostic technique is that of immunofluorescence. The principle underlying this is that cells (present in the NPA) infected with a virus will express viral-derived antigens on their surface. The presence of these antigens can be demonstrated by staining the cells with monoclonal antibodies to a variety of possible pathogens (e.g. against influenza A and B viruses, RSV, para-influenza viruses, or adenoviruses) to which a fluorescein dye has been chemically linked. Cells infected with a given organism will fluoresce under ultraviolet light if they are

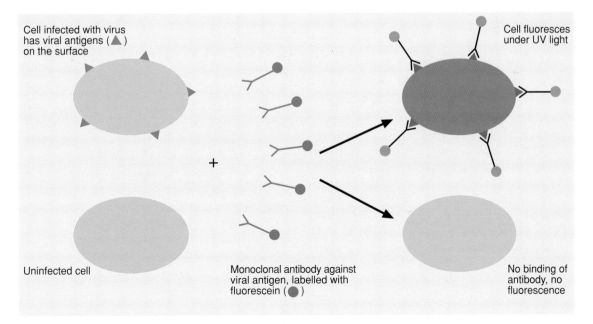

Fig. 21.2 The principle of antigen detection by immunofluorescence.

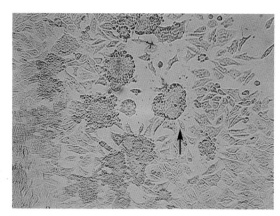

Fig. 21.3 RSV-induced cytopathic effect. Arrow shows giant cell or syncytium.

stained with the monoclonal antibody directed against that particular organism—see Fig. 21.2.

Appropriate tissue cultures will also be inoculated for virus isolation, although these may take up to 2 weeks to become positive. RSV produces a characteristic cytopathic effect in cell culture, causing formation of giant syncytial cells (see Fig. 21.3). This is how the virus acquired its name.

Q. What are the possible clinical consequences of RSV infection?

A These include:

- Most infections are asymptomatic, or result in only mild disease (75–100% of all infants are antibody-positive by the age of 2 years)
- Lower respiratory tract disease (bronchiolitis and pneumonia) display peak incidence in the first 6 months of life, resulting in hospitalization of around 1 in every 100 infants. Mortality is less than 1%—infection in infants less than 1 month old may be atypical, dominated by non-specific signs, e.g. poor feeding and lethargy. Apnoeic attacks may be the first indication of respiratory infection. RSV infection is detected in a proportion of victims of the sudden infant death syndrome
- Repeat infections occur throughout life. These present as upper respiratory tract infections in older children and adults, with cough being a marked symptom. Outbreaks of 'flu-like illness'

(see Case 17 for definition of this) due to RSV infection may occur in the elderly, e.g. in nursing homes.

Q What are the complications of RSV infection?

A These include:

- Otitis media. RSV can be recovered from middle ear aspirates either alone, or together with bacterial agents
- Severe RSV infection in infancy is associated with prolonged alterations in pulmonary function, and with further bouts of wheezing during childhood, which may be difficult to distinguish from asthma.

Q Which groups of children are at particular risk of severe disease or death from RSV infection?

A The mortality of RSV infection in infants with congenital heart disease, with underlying lung disease (including prematurity), and those who are immunosuppressed is over 25%.

The virology laboratory rings you later the same day, with a positive RSV immunofluorescence result from the NPA. You visit Shula on the paediatric oncology ward, where she is being nursed.

Q Is this the most appropriate ward for Shula to be nursed in?

A No. One hopes that in reality this would not happen! Nosocomial (i.e. spread within hospital) RSV infections are unfortunately all too common. The risk of acquiring RSV infection in this way is directly correlated with the length of hospitalization. Given the potentially devastating consequences of RSV infection in immunosuppressed hosts, great care should be taken to avoid admitting RSV-infected infants on to wards where such children may be found. The same applies to wards where infants with congenital heart defects may be present.

Q What precautions should be taken to prevent nosocomial spread of RSV?

A Spread of RSV is by inhalation of droplets, but also by direct inoculation into the pharynx of virus

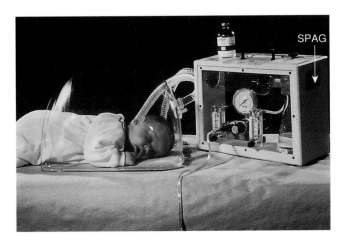

Fig. 21.4 Baby in head-box breathing in aerosolized ribavirin from a small-particle aerosol generator (SPAG).

picked up from inanimate surfaces, e.g. via nurses' hands. All known infected patients should be grouped on the same ward, or the same part of a ward, i.e. isolated. If possible, nurses should be assigned to look after either the RSV patients or the remaining patients, but not both (i.e. cohort nursing). The importance of strict hand-washing between handling of patients cannot be overemphasized.

You arrange for Shula's immediate transfer to the general paediatric ward. Shula's oxygenation improves to normal over the following 48 hours, and she is discharged home on the fourth hospital day.

Q What antiviral agent might have been used to treat Shula?

A Ribavirin is a broad-spectrum antiviral agent that interferes with the processing of viral messenger RNA. Ribavirin therapy of infants hospitalized with RSV infection results in enhanced elimination of virus excretion, symptomatic improvement, and a shorter duration of hospitalization. However, the drug has to be administered by inhalation of fine particles for at least 18 hours a day. A small-particle aerosol generator (SPAG) is thus needed, whilst the infant is nursed in a head-box (see Fig. 21.4). For an otherwise uncomplicated case, the disadvantages (cost and inconvenience) of therapy outweigh the benefits. Ribavirin does, however, reduce the mortality of RSV infection in high-risk patients (see above) and should be used in their management.

Summary: RSV lower respiratory tract infection

Clinical features
1–6 month-old child with fever, cough, and increased respiratory rate; in winter months

Diagnosis
Clinical; antigen detection in NPA

Management
Adequate hydration and oxygenation; ribavirin if severe disease

Prognosis
Full recovery usual; high mortality if underlying lung or cardiac disease or immunodeficiency

Case 22 Productive cough in Benjamin, a 14-year-old with cystic fibrosis

Benjamin, a 14-year-old youth, returns to the cystic fibrosis clinic after a 2-year absence complaining of increased cough productive of thick green sputum, breathlessness, generalized lethargy, and weight loss. Cystic fibrosis was diagnosed at 2 years of age and, apart from occasional respiratory infections, he has remained well in the intervening period. He is one of a family of four children and his 16-year-old brother also has cystic fibrosis.

Q What is the underlying defect in cystic fibrosis?

A Cystic fibrosis is the most common genetic disease among Caucasians. It is an autosomal recessive disorder and the carriage rate is approximately 1 in 20. The genetic abnormality is on the long arm of chromosome 7 in a gene coding for a chloride channel protein (cystic fibrosis transmembrane conductance regulator). This leads to altered secretions (sweat, mucus), which in turn lead to blocked ducts and retained mucosal secretions. The resulting abnormalities in mucus and other secretions of the exocrine glands result in most of the clinical complications.

Q What are the complications of cystic fibrosis?

A Cystic fibrosis is a multisystem disorder and complications include:

1. respiratory complications
   - recurrent infections
   - nasal polyps
   - haemoptysis
   - pneumothorax

2. gastrointestinal complications
   - meconium ileus at birth
   - pancreatic insufficiency
   - cirrhosis
   - diabetes mellitus

3. genitourinary complications
   - male infertility
   - amenorrhoea

At the clinic Benjamin is apyrexial but has widespread rhonchi and crepitations throughout both lung fields. His pulmonary function tests are as follows: forced vital capacity (FVC), 45%; forced expiratory volume in one second (FEV1), 50%. A chest X-ray reveals diffuse shadowing with bronchiectatic changes throughout both lung fields (Fig. 22.1). A sample of sputum is obtained for culture and he is admitted to the cystic fibrosis unit for further management.

Q What is bronchiectasis?

A This is chronic dilatation of the bronchi, which results in collections of bronchial secretions. Repeated bacterial infections follow and, occasionally, haemoptysis. The below-normal pulmonary function tests are characteristic of generalized bronchiectasis, especially during acute infections.

Q Which pathogens are likely to be grown from Benjamin's sputum?

A A number of respiratory pathogens may be isolated from the sputum of cystic fibrosis patients

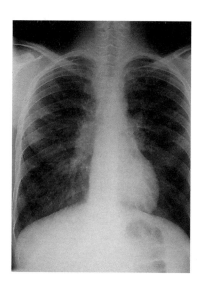

Fig. 22.1
Chest X-ray
with
bronchiectatic
changes.

Table 22.1 The major respiratory pathogens in cystic fibrosis

Respiratory pathogen	Comments
Staphylococcus aureus	Colonizes and infects before the age of 2 years. Often fatal before effective antibiotics became available
Haemophilus influenzae	Non-capsulated types and hence not protected by Hib vaccine (see Case 13). Rarely fatal
Pseudomonas aeruginosa	Colonizes in late childhood or early adulthood. Mucoid strains (due to production of extracellular polysaccharide) difficult to eradicate (see also Box 22.1)
Burkholderia cepacia	Usually multiply antibiotic-resistant
Others	Include *S. pneumoniae, M. catarrhalis, Stenotrophomonas maltophilia, Mycoplasma pneumoniae,* and *Aspergillus fumigatus,* and mycobacteria (pathogenic role of these is not certain)

(see Table 22.1). It is not unusual to recover more than one pathogen. Previous admissions to hospital for treatment of acute respiratory infections, recent antibiotics, and contact with other cystic fibrosis patients or siblings may all influence which pathogens are recovered and their antimicrobial susceptibility. Sputum culture will assist in choosing the most appropriate antibiotics, but clinical improvement despite the persistence of pathogens, especially *Pseudomonas*, following a course of antibiotics is not unusual.

Q Which antibiotic or antibiotics should be started while the results of culture are awaited?

A Most episodes of respiratory infection are bacterial in aetiology, either as a primary or a secondary (i.e. following an initial viral infection) event. Often the patient is afebrile but nonetheless appropriate, and usually intravenous (IV), antibiotics should be started promptly. The choice will be governed by the presence of the pathogens listed above and their antimicrobial susceptibility. Antibiotic cover against *P. aeruginosa* and *H. influenzae* should be instituted and an aminoglycoside (e.g. gentamicin, tobramycin, netilmicin) combined with an anti-pseudomonal penicillin (e.g. piperacillin, piperacillin/tazobactam) or a cephalosporin active against *Pseudomonas* (e.g. ceftazidime) is indicated.

It is preferable to use combination antimicrobial chemotherapy when treating *Pseudomonas* infections because of possible antibiotic synergy (enhanced activity). This is especially important if the patient has received repeated courses of antibiotics in the recent past, as isolates may be resistant to one or more agents. This combination will also be active against *Haemophilus* spp.

Benjamin was started on IV gentamicin and ceftazidime, nebulized salbutamol, and twice-daily physiotherapy. A mucoid *P. aeruginosa*

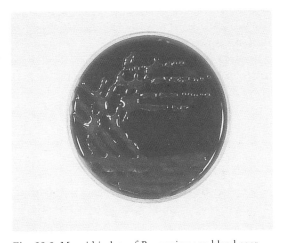

Fig. 22.2 Mucoid isolate of *P. aeruginosa* on blood agar.

(see Fig. 22.2), sensitive to gentamicin, piper-acillin/tazobactam, ceftazidime, and cipro-floxacin, was recovered from his sputum. Following a 14-day course of IV antibiotics he was considerably less breathless, his pulmonary function tests had significantly improved, he was feeling much better, and his cough was less purulent. A repeat sputum still grew the *Pseudomonas*.

Benjamin was discharged on no antibiotics as he was clinically much better and was advised about exercise and instructed on how to perform daily postural drainage to reduce the incidence of further exacerbations and help improve lung function. His pancreatic supplement, creon, was increased, levels of vitamins A and E were measured, and, because of weight loss, diabetes mellitus was excluded. Finally, he was asked to attend the cystic fibrosis clinic monthly for further follow-up.

Q Are you surprised that the pseudomonas has persisted?

A No. Antibiotics often do not eradicate pseudomonas in patients with cystic fibrosis and the clinical benefit is probably achieved by reducing the bacterial load and the inflammation.

Q Could ciprofloxacin have been used to treat the chest infection?

A Preferably not. Ciprofloxacin, a fluoroquinolone, has an important role in the management of *Pseudomonas* infections (see Box 22.1). A major advantage is that it can be administered both orally and intravenously. In cystic fibrosis it is often reserved for outpatients but is relatively contraindicated in children because of possible damage to growing cartilage and bone. This has to be weighed against the valuable contribution it can make in management, and in practice it is prescribed not infrequently in this setting. When used alone, however, resistance may emerge, especially following prolonged or repeat courses.

Q What role does nebulized colistin have in management?

> ## Box 22.1 *Pseudomonas aeruginosa*
>
> - Motile oxidase-positive Gram-negative bacillus capable of producing pigments, e.g. pyocyanin
> - Isolated from moist environments such as sinks, disinfectants. Part of the normal gastrointestinal flora
> - Causes hospital-acquired infections, e.g. urinary tract infection, bacteraemia, pneumonia, eye and skin infections
> - Is resistant to many commonly used antibiotics. Active agents include the aminoglycosides, piperacillin/azlocillin, ciprofloxacin, ceftazidime, and imipenem
> - Hospital-acquired infection may be prevented by: reversing the underlying condition, e.g. neutropenia; hand-washing (prevents cross-infection); and the correct use of disinfectants

---

A Colistin (polymyxin E) is an antibiotic active against most Gram-negative bacilli but because of its toxicity it is largely confined to topical or local use. In some centres nebulized colistin is used in chronic *Pseudomonas* carriers to reduce exacerbations, but not as part of the acute management in hospital. Parenteral colistin is occasionally used to treat infections caused by multiply-antibiotic-resistant bacteria. Nebulized tobramycin has also been shown in recent years to be effective in reducing pseudomonas colonization.

Q Should Benjamin's cystic fibrosis physician be concerned about him acquiring *Burkholderia cepacia*?

A Yes. *B. cepacia* infection may present with an acute fulminating infection, progressive deterioration in pulmonary function, or merely chronic colonization with little clinical impact. Recent molecular research has revealed that there are at least 22 different strains, some more virulent and transmissible than others. *B. cepacia* may be acquired during social contact with other patients with cystic fibrosis, e.g. at summer camps, and is almost impossible to eradicate, partly because it is susceptible to so few antibiotics.

Q How may the incidence and severity of chest infections in cystic fibrosis patients be reduced?

A This may be achieved by attention to nutrition, instruction on postural drainage, early and aggressive treatment of infections, and vaccination against the usual childhood illnesses, such as diphtheria, *H. influenzae* type b, etc. By reducing the incidence of these infections vaccination will also prevent their complications, e.g. pneumonia following whooping cough.

Q Should patients with cystic fibrosis be offered pneumococcal vaccine?

A The use of pneumococcal vaccine in cystic fibrosis is controversial because the pneumococcus is encountered relatively infrequently and, consequently, vaccination policies vary from unit to unit. On balance it is probably advisable.

Q Which other conditions predispose to the development of bronchiectasis?

A The causes of bronchiectasis may be summarized as:

1. congenital
   - cystic fibrosis (approximately 50% of all cases)
   - immotile ciliary syndrome
   - complement deficiencies
2. previous lung infections
   - adenovirus pneumonia
   - whooping cough
   - measles
   - tuberculosis (upper lobe)
   - lung abscess (upper lobe)
3. aspiration/foreign body
4. tumour

In many of these conditions the bronchiectasis may be localized and the symptoms less severe than in cystic fibrosis. The microbiology of acute infective exacerbations is similar to that of cystic fibrosis. Occasionally, a lung abscess or empyema of polymicrobial aetiology may develop that requires aspiration or drainage.

Q What factors predispose to the development of lung abscess?

A Lung abscess (i.e. a collection of pus within the lung parenchyma that may be polymicrobial in aetiology) is less common than previously because of more effective treatment for pneumonia and other suppurative lung conditions. Many abscesses are idiopathic but the remainder may arise because of:

1. necrotizing lung infection
   - pneumonia (*S. aureus*)
   - tuberculosis
2. aspiration
   - dysphagia
   - excess alcohol
   - general anaesthetic
   - cerebrovascular accident
3. dental disease/gingivitis
4. lung tumours
   - lymphoma
   - carcinoma
5. lung infarction following embolus
6. bacteraemia:
   - septic emboli settle in lungs, e.g. following infective endocarditis

---

Summary: Bronchiectasis

Presentation

Productive cough with purulent, often foul-smelling sputum, dyspnoea, and wheeze against a background of cystic fibrosis or other condition

Microbiology

H. influenzae, *S. aureus*, and *Ps. aeruginosa* are the most common pathogens but viruses and other common (*S. pneumoniae*) and less common (*B. cepacia*) bacteria must be considered

Management

Aggressive IV antimicrobial therapy to cover *Pseudomonas*, and inhaled agents also, especially during acute exacerbations; postural drainage; adequate nutrition; and vaccination against common respiratory pathogens (tuberculosis, diphtheria, etc.)

Self-assessment

1. Which of the following viruses/groups of viruses is the most common cause of croup?
   (a) Rhinoviruses
   (b) Enteroviruses
   (c) Respiratory syncytial virus
   (d) Parainfluenza viruses
   (e) Coronaviruses

2. Which one of the following antiviral agents has been shown in clinical trials to be effective in the treatment of upper respiratory tract infections due to respiratory syncytial virus?
   (a) Ribavirin
   (b) Pleconaril
   (c) Aciclovir
   (d) Amantadine
   (e) Zanamavir

3. In a patient with severe pharyngitis and generalized lymphadenopathy, which one of the following test results confirms a diagnosis of acute Epstein–Barr virus (EBV)-associated infectious mononucleosis?
   (a) EBV IgG, positive
   (b) Monospot, negative
   (c) Atypical mononuclear cells seen on blood film
   (d) EBV IgM, positive
   (e) Raised bilirubin

4. Which one of the following malignant diseases has not been associated with EBV infection?
   (a) Burkitt's lymphoma
   (b) Kaposi's sarcoma
   (c) Lymphoma in an AIDS patient
   (d) Nasopharyngeal carcinoma
   (e) Hodgkin's lymphoma

5. Which one of the following statements regarding influenza viruses is untrue?
   (a) Antigenic shift describes the process whereby new influenza viral subtypes emerge
   (b) Antigenic drift arises through spontaneous point mutations in the surface glycoproteins
   (c) Target groups for influenza vaccination in the UK include patients with pre-existing cardiac disease
   (d) Systemic manifestations of influenza virus infection (e.g. fever, myalgia) arise from the presence of virus circulating in the bloodstream
   (e) Pneumonia arising as a complication of influenza virus infection is usually due to secondary bacterial invasion

6. Which of the following groups of patients is recommended to receive influenza vaccine (may be more than one)?
   (a) Patients who have had a splenectomy
   (b) Patients with chronic respiratory disease
   (c) Patients with diabetes mellitus
   (d) Patients with renal failure
   (e) Patients with peptic ulcer disease

7. With regard to respiratory syncytial virus (RSV), which of the following statements is not correct?
   (a) Morbidity is greatest in the 1–2 year old age group
   (b) Mortality is increased in patients with immunodeficiency
   (c) Recurrent RSV infections occur throughout life
   (d) Apnoea may be the presenting feature of acute RSV infection
   (e) Infection may present as a 'flu-like illness'

8. In the diagnosis of virus infections, which of the following statements regarding immunofluorescence is *not* true?

(a) It is a rapid diagnostic technique

(b) It is dependent on the presence of live virus within the sample

(c) It can be used to distinguish between infection with influenza A and B viruses

(d) It can be used to detect bacterial as well as viral infections

(e) It is the method of choice for identification of organisms within bronchoalveolar lavage fluid

9. Which one of the following bacteria may cause an infection referred to as 'malignant otitis externa'?

(a) *Pseudomonas aeruginosa*

(b) *Staphylococcus aureus*

(c) *Clostridium perfringens*

(d) *E. coli*

(e) *Corynebacterium diphtheriae*

10. *Haemophilus influenzae* type b causes which one of the following infections in the unvaccinated child?

(a) Otitis media

(b) Sinusitis

(c) Urinary tract infection

(d) Bronchiolitis

(e) Cellulitis

11. Whooping cough is usually caused by *Bordetella pertussis* but a similar clinical syndrome may be caused by which one of the following?

(a) *Streptococcus pneumoniae*

(b) Rhinovirus

(c) Respiratory syncytial virus (RSV)

(d) *Moraxella catarrhalis*

(e) *Staphylococcus aureus*

12. Which one of the following toxins or enymes is a component of the modern acellular whooping cough vaccine?

(a) leucocidin

(b) enterotoxin

(c) endotoxin

(d) haemagglutinin

(e) extracellular polysaccharide

13. Which one of the following is not a well recognized cause of community-acquired pneumonia?

(a) *Pseudomonas aeruginosa*

(b) *Streptococcus pneumoniae*

(c) Influenza

(d) *Mycoplasma pneumoniae*

(e) *Legionella pneumophila*

14. What is the prevalence of penicillin resistance amongst strains of *Streptococcus pneumoniae* isolated in the UK?

(a) < 5%

(b) 5–10%

(c) 10–20%

(d) 20–30%

(e) > 30%

15. Which microscopic staining technique is most useful for making a diagnosis of legionellosis?

(a) Gram stain

(b) Grocot stain

(c) Ziehl–Neelsen

(d) Giemsa stain

(e) Immunofluorescence

16. Which one important biological feature of *Legionella* species is important in assisting the bacillus to survive and cause disease?

(a) Periodic mutations leading to increased virulence

(b) Presence of a capsule

(c) Survival inside protozoa

(d) Replication at temperatures <10°C

(e) Presence in many common foodstuffs such as cheese

17. Which one of the following pathogens is most likely to cause exacerbations of chronic obstructive pulmonary disease (COPD)?

(a) *Staphylococcus aureus*

(b) *Moraxella catarrhalis*

(c) *Bordetella parapertussis*

(d) *Staphylococcus saprophyticus*

(e) Cytomegalovirus (CMV)

18. Which antibiotic would be most appropriate for empirical or blind therapy of a patient with an acute exacerbation of COPD?

(a) Benzylpenicillin

(b) Gentamicin

(c) Cefotaxime

(d) Co-amoxyclav

(e) Ciprofloxacin

19. Which one of the following is an emerging respiratory pathogen in patients with cystic fibrosis?

(a) *Candida tropicalis*

(b) *Cryptosporidium parvum*

(c) *Clostridium novyi*

(d) *Stenotrophomonas maltophilia*

(e) Vancomycin-resistant *Enterococcus faecalis*

20. Nebulized antibiotics have a role to play in either the empirical treatment of exacerbations of bronchitis caused by cystic fibrosis or in suppressing the bacterial load and hence damping the inflammatory response. Which one of the following antibiotics is used for this purpose?

(a) Flucloxacillin

(b) Tobramycin

(c) Ceftazidime

(d) Ciprofloxacin

(e) Meropenem

3

CHAPTER 3

Gastrointestinal system

Gastrointestinal system

Case 23 Bertrand, a 35-year-old Frenchman with nausea, abdominal pain, and diarrhoea

Bertrand, a 35-year-old French computer programmer, is seen in the accident and emergency department at 11 a.m. on a Saturday complaining of nausea, diarrhoea, and abdominal pain. The diarrhoea woke him earlier that morning and appears to be getting worse. The abdominal pain is central in location and 'crampy' in character. He is on no medications and has never been seriously ill or required admission to hospital.

Q What further information might help in identifying the cause of his symptoms?

A Once medications have been excluded as a cause of gastrointestinal upset, the patient should be asked whether he has been abroad recently, whether other members of his household have also been unwell, and whether he can identify anything he has eaten in the last few days that might account for his illness.

Bertrand has been living in England for the past 5 years and, apart from a return trip to visit his elderly parents in Bordeaux a month ago, has not been abroad recently. His girlfriend, Michelle, with whom he shares a flat, does not have any gastrointestinal symptoms. He is uncertain about any details of what he has eaten in the last 3 days, but remarks that he attended a retirement party for a colleague at Friday lunchtime at a local hotel. On examination he is apyrexial and his pulse and blood pressure are normal. There is no abdominal tenderness or masses.

Q What is the most likely diagnosis here?

A The patient has 'gastroenteritis', probably due to food poisoning. The absence of previous gastrointestinal disease, the recent onset of symptoms, and a normal physical examination also point to this. The terms 'gastroenteritis' and 'food poisoning' are often used rather loosely, but the latter term is perhaps more likely to suggest an infective aetiology.

Q How relevant might the retirement party be?

A The provision of food for parties, receptions, weddings, etc. is often associated with problems of preparation and storage as food is being provided for larger numbers of people than is the case domestically. Details on what foods were eaten, what quantities of individual dishes were consumed, and whether any colleagues from work have been similarly affected will help in identifying the cause.

Q What are the mechanisms by which organisms cause food poisoning?

A These may be either by toxins, preformed and present in the food, or follow multiplication with or without *in vivo* toxin production and tissue invasion (see Table 23.1). For example, *Bacillus cereus* may cause two clinical forms of food poisoning: one

Table 23.1 Aetiology and pathogenesis of bacterial food poisoning

Preformed toxin	Toxin production *in vivo*	Tissue invasion
Bacillus cereus	*Clostridium perfringens*	*Campylobacter jejuni*
Staphylococcus aureus	*Bacillus cereus*	*Salmonella* spp.
Clostridium botulinum	Enterotoxigenic E. *coli*	Invasive E. *coli*
(see also Case 44)	*Vibrio* spp.	

characterized by vomiting (preformed toxin in the food) and one where diarrhoea is more prominent (toxin production *in vivo*). The different mechanisms may be reflected in the incubation period, with food poisoning mediated by toxin production having a short interval (hours) between ingestion and symptoms, as suggested in the case described here.

Q What else may cause food poisoning apart from bacteria?

A Viruses such as the noroviruses, previously referred to as 'small round structured virus', e.g Norwalk virus, and the sappoviruses, previously called caliciviruses, may cause outbreaks characterized by explosive diarrhoea (see Cases 24 and 70). Also, chemicals such as heavy metals, histamine, and neurotoxins may be ingested with food (e.g. fish) and result in gastrointestinal and other symptoms.

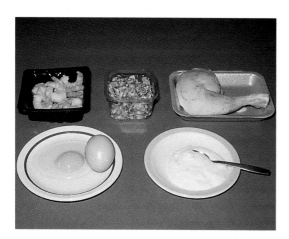

Fig. 23.1 Foods (shellfish, poultry, raw eggs, homemade mayonnaise) implicated in food poisoning.

Q Are particular foods associated with certain pathogens?

A A variety of different foods may cause food poisoning (see Fig. 23.1):

- *Clostridium perfringens* often occurs in meat or gravy, especially when reheated, when suitable anaerobic conditions occur

- foods with a high protein content, such as ham, poultry, and egg salads, are often implicated in staphylococcal food poisoning, where the organism may have come from the nose or hand of a food-handler after initial cooking or preparation

- cooked but inadequately stored rice may be responsible for *B. cereus*.

- *Salmonellae* are associated with poultry or raw or inadequately cooked eggs

- *Campylobacter jejuni*, only recognized as a human intestinal pathogen in the last 25 years, is associated with unpasteurized milk and poultry (Fig. 23.2)

- the noroviruses (small round structured viruses) cause food poisoning through contaminated shellfish or salads

Q How might one confirm which pathogen is responsible?

A Microscopy and culture of vomitus is rarely helpful in identifying the aetiology of food poisoning. A stool sample should be sent for culture and may grow *Salmonella*, *Shigella*, or *Campylobacter* spp. Most microbiology laboratories do not report the isolation of E. *coli* from all stool samples as it is part

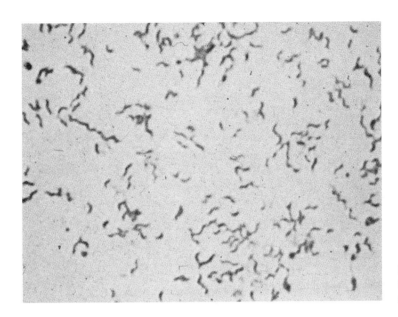

Fig. 23.2 Gram stain showing Gram-negative curved bacilli, typical of campylobacter.

of the normal flora, but in certain circumstances the presence of enterohaemorrhagic *E. coli* (EHEC) strains (see Case 25), such as *E.coli* 0157, which does cause bloody diarrhoea with renal failure as part of the haemolytic–uraemic syndrome, may be sought on culture. These strains do not ferment sorbitol, a feature that can be easily recognized in the laboratory, and they also produce a heat-labile toxin. Isolation of the organism from food is preferred when diagnosing *S. aureus* or *C. perfringens* food poisoning, as these bacteria are also part of the normal bowel flora. However, confirmation that an outbreak is due to *C. perfringens* is obtained if there is a heavy growth from the faeces of affected patients, if all the strains from multiple patients are of the same type, and if isolates from food and stools are similar.

Q What other line of investigation might help in identifying the cause?

A In the absence of remaining food from the incriminated meal, it may be possible to make a presumptive diagnosis about the cause following epidemiological investigations. This involves following up those who attended the retirement party with a questionnaire to investigate how many developed symptoms and what foods they ate. If symptoms are subsequently shown to be associated with eating, e.g. a mousse or mayonnaise, and a *Salmonella* is recovered from the stools of many of those affected (see Box 23.1), then further questioning may reveal that raw eggs were used during preparation. This type of investigation is usually coordinated by the local or

---

Box 23.1 *Salmonella* food poisoning

- Due to non-typhoidal *Salmonella* (the term typhoidal refers specifically to *S. typhi* or *S. paratyphi*; see Case 27), such as *S. enteriditis*, *S. typhimurium*, *S. dublin*, *S. agona*, etc., most of which are from animal sources

- *S. enteritidis* was responsible for much of the recent increase in salmonellosis due to contamination of egg contents

- Usually mild and self-limiting without systemic invasion, but can cause severe illness and even death in the very young (neonatal meningitis) and the very elderly (septicaemia)

- Prevention is by monitoring and sampling laying hens and eggs, slaughter of infected flocks, and advice to the public about cooking eggs and poultry adequately

public health authorities, and therefore it is essential that food poisoning is notified.

Bertrand was discharged from the accident and emergency department and subsequently improved over the next 24 hours. He was able to return to work on the Monday. It transpired that a number of Bertrand's colleagues had similar symptoms over the weekend, and the public health authorities, together with the local microbiology laboratory, undertook an investigation. There was some food remaining from the reception and, following anaerobic culture, *C. perfringens* was recovered from the roast beef, which had been eaten by 80% of those with symptoms.

Q What is the most common recognized cause of food poisoning?

A *C. jejuni*, a spiral-shaped Gram-negative bacillus, is the most common identified cause of food poisoning and may be accompanied by severe abdominal pain. This may be mistaken for an acute abdominal emergency requiring surgical investigation, with bloody diarrhoea. *Salmonella* spp. are the next most important cause.

Q How is shigellosis spread and how do *Shigella* spp. cause diarrhoea?

A Most cases of shigella in the developed world arise from person-to-person spread and *Shigella sonnei* is the species most commonly isolated. In less developed parts of the world, where classic dysentery (bloody diarrhoea) is more common, *S. dysenteriae* is relatively more common and both water and food are implicated in spread. These bacteria invade the intestinal mucosa, but most species are capable of producing an enterotoxin that is probably responsible for the watery diarrhoea seen early on in the illness.

Q How is food poisoning managed?

A Most cases are self-limiting and therefore fluid replacement is the mainstay of treatment. This is especially important where there has been severe dehydration. In these circumstances intravenous fluids such as Hartmann's solution may be necessary.

Antidiarrhoeal agents such as loperamide should be avoided if at all possible because they may affect the natural history of the disease by impairing the bowel's efforts to excrete the pathogen.

Q When, if ever, are antibiotics indicated?

A Antibiotic treatment of diarrhoea due to food poisoning or gastroenteritis is rarely indicated as there is little evidence that it will improve symptoms, and indeed it may prolong carriage or result in antibiotic-associated diarrhoea (see Case 33). Exceptions to this include:

- salmonella infection that has invaded the bloodstream, meninges, bone, etc.
- salmonella in the elderly accompanied by severe gastrointestinal symptoms
- severe shigellosis
- campylobacter infection with severe colitis or bloody stools
- salmonella, shigella, or campylobacter infection in an immunocompromised patient or a patient with relevant underlying disease, e.g. ulcerative colitis with quite severe symptoms

A quinolone such as ciprofloxacin is probably the agent of choice for the above, except for campylobacter, where erythromycin is generally recommended.

Q Which organisms causing gastrointestinal symptoms are water-borne, apart from *Shigella*?

A The distinction between food- and water-borne disease is not always clear, especially where food has been washed in contaminated water. Recognized water-borne organisms include:

- bacteria: *Campylobacter* spp.; salmonella causing enteric fever (*S. typhi*, *S. paratyphi*); *Vibrio* spp. (including *V. cholerae*); *E. coli*
- viruses: hepatitis A (see Case 28); Norwalk-like viruses (see Cases 24, 70); rotavirus (see Case 24); hepatitis E (see Case 28)
- protozoa: *Giardia lamblia*; *Cryptosporidium parvum*; *Entamoeba histolytica*

Summary: Food poisoning

Presentation

Vomiting (especially *S. aureus*, *B. cereus*), abdominal pain, and diarrhoea. Sporadic in the majority of cases, where no food is ever directly incriminated

Diagnosis

Clinical diagnosis having excluded other possibilities such as appendicitis. Stool for culture and other appropriate tests with epidemiological investigations if part of an outbreak

Management

Fluid replacement. Antibiotics rarely required

Case 24 Damian, a 13-month-old baby with vomiting and diarrhoea

Damian, a 13 month-old baby, is brought to see you by his mother in the week before Christmas. For the past 2 days, Damian has been vomiting, and this morning he has already soiled four nappies with profuse watery diarrhoea. He has not eaten anything unusual over the last 4 days. He attends a day-care nursery when his mother is working. He has reached all his developmental milestones at an appropriate age, and has received full courses of dipththeria–pertussis–tetanus (DPT), polio, and *Haemophilus influenzae* type b (Hib) vaccines. On examination, Damian is febrile (38.5°C), and assessment of skin turgor suggests that he is moderately dehydrated.

Q What is the diagnosis?

A Damian has acute gastroenteritis. The acute onset, the presence of fever, and lack of any relevant past medical history make infection the most likely cause. Viruses are more frequent than bacterial pathogens as causes of infantile gastroenteritis in temperate climates.

Box 24.1 **Noroviruses (aka Norwalk virus, Norwalk-like agents, SRSVs) and caliciviruses (see also Case 70)**

- Genome analysis suggests that all these viruses are related to each other; hence the current classification of the norovirus genus within the calicivirus family

- These agents are particularly associated with outbreaks of gastroenteritis that affect people of all ages, e.g. winter vomiting disease

- Spread by food (especially shellfish) and water

- Aerosols, generated by forceful vomiting, also important in transmission

- Symptomatic disease is usually short-lived, e.g. 48 hours

Q Name four groups of viruses that cause gastroenteritis.

A These include:

1. Rotaviruses—the most common cause in young children

2. Enteric adenoviruses (serotypes 40 and 41; see Case 8)

3. Noroviruses (previously known as small round structured viruses (SRSVs) or Norwalk-like viruses). These viruses belong to the family of viruses known as caliciviruses. (See Box 24.1 and also Case 70)

4. Astroviruses, so-called because of their star-like morphology. Astrovirus gastroenteritis is usually mild and rarely necessitates hospitalization

Coronaviruses, enteroviruses, and small round viruses (SRVs; also known as small featureless viruses) are also found in human stools, but their role as causative agents of diarrhoea has not been proven.

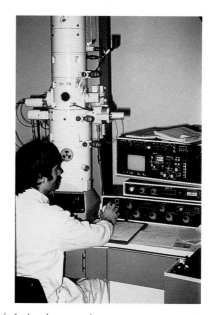

Fig. 24. 1 An electron microscope.

Q How should you confirm your diagnosis in Damian?

A A sample of stool should be sent as soon as possible to the virology laboratory for electron microscopy (EM; see Fig. 24.1). None of the above-mentioned viruses will grow in the tissue culture cell lines maintained in a routine diagnostic laboratory, so virus culture is not possible. However, all are excreted in extremely large amounts (> 10^6 particles per ml) in infected stools and vomitus during the early phase of acute gastroenteritis, and therefore they can be visualized with an EM. Virus excretion does, however, fall off rapidly with time—hence the need for specimens taken as soon as possible, and certainly within 48 hours of onset.

Each virus is recognized by its characteristic morphology (see Fig. 24.2). A bacterial cause (e.g. *Salmonella*) of Damian's illness must also be excluded by appropriate culture of his stool.

Electron microscopy is a rapid diagnostic technique (a positive result can be available within 3 hours) and is also comprehensive, i.e. it will detect whatever virus is there, provided the virus is present in sufficient quantity. However, it is expensive and alternatives are being developed, including antigen detection by enzyme-linked immunosorbent assay (ELISA) and latex particle agglutination. These are rapid and cheaper techniques, but will only detect specific viruses, e.g. a rotavirus. More modern approaches to diagnosis, such as genome amplification by polymerase chain reaction

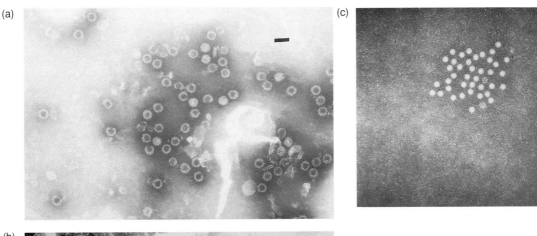

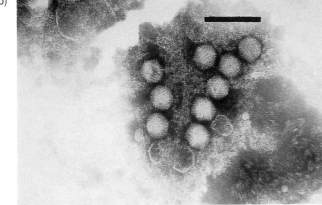

Fig. 24.2 (a) Rotaviruses (scale bar, 100 nm); (b) adenoviruses (scale bar, 200 nm); (c) noroviruses.

(PCR) assay, are being developed, especially for the Norwalk group of viruses, but are only available in larger centres or research laboratories.

Q What are the short-term complications of viral gastroenteritis?

A Excessive fluid loss may result in dehydration and electrolyte imbalance, most commonly a metabolic acidosis.

You decide to refer Damian to the local hospital, because of his profuse diarrhoea, and signs of dehydration. A stool sample is sent to the laboratory, where a rotavirus is seen by EM. On the ward, an initial attempt at oral rehydration is made, but abandoned after persistent vomiting, and an intravenous (IV) drip is set up. After 48 hours of IV fluid replacement, Damian's stool output declines and over the next 48 hours oral feeding is gradually re-established.

Q Should Damian be nursed on an open ward?

A Preferably not. There is a significant risk of nosocomial spread of rotavirus infection, and ward staff must be aware of this. Adherence to strict hand-washing protocols is the single most useful measure to reduce the risk of spread. Patients should ideally be nursed in single rooms but this is not always practicable or possible.

Q Could you describe this as a typical case of rotavirus gastroenteritis?

A Yes. The features of rotavirus infection are listed in Table 24.1.

Q Which patients are at risk of chronic rotavirus infection?

A Immunosuppressed children or adults may suffer from chronic diarrhoea (> 3 months). Management is difficult, but there are reports of successful treatment of this condition with human immunoglobulin containing antibodies to rotavirus.

Table 24.1 Features of rotavirus infections in temperate climates

More common in autumn/winter

Peak incidence between 6 and 24 months of age; severe disease unusual after the age of 3 years

Transmission mainly by faecal–oral route

Severity varies from a 24-hour illness to overwhelming gastroenteritis, with occasional deaths

Vomiting, a prominent feature, may precede diarrhoea by 48 hours

Fever > 38.5°C almost universal

Watery diarrhoea on average persists for 5–7 days. Blood or pus in stools suggests concurrent bacterial infection

Q How does rotavirus infection differ in less developed countries?

A Rotaviruses are the most common single cause of diarrhoeal illness worldwide, with an estimated annual incidence of 125 million cases, and 8–900 000 deaths most of which occur in poorer countries. No specific antiviral agents are available, and management is dependent largely on oral rehydration with solutions containing glucose and electrolytes. Breast-feeding significantly reduces the chances of diarrhoeal illness, presumably via passive immunization.

Q Is rotavirus infection preventable?

A Not at present. Much effort has been expended in the development of rotavirus vaccines. One particular vaccine, containing a rhesus–human reassortant virus, showed very promising results in large-scale clinical trials, and was licensed in the USA in 1998. Unfortunately, however, this vaccine had to be withdrawn because of reports of an increased incidence of intussusception following vaccine administration. It is to be hoped that an effective and safe vaccine will be developed soon.

Summary: Rotavirus gastroenteritis

Presentation

Vomiting, profuse watery diarrhoea, usually in a small child

Diagnosis

Examination of faecal sample by electron microscopy (will also allow diagnosis of other causes of gastroenteritis, e.g. adenoviruses (children), calici- and noro-viruses (cause outbreaks in adults), astroviruses)

Management

Supportive; fluid replacement

Case 25 Fraser, a 37-year-old business executive with abdominal pain, diarrhoea, and flatulence

Fraser, a 37-year-old business executive, complains of central abdominal pain, moderate to severe diarrhoea, and flatulence for 4 days. He has no relevant previous medical history, is on no medications, and neither his wife nor his two children have any gastrointestinal symptoms. Physical examination is unremarkable. On further questioning it transpires that Fraser has spent a week in Central America, returning 2 days ago.

Q What else would it be useful to know about his recent trip abroad?

A It is certainly likely that his symptoms relate to his trip abroad, but details of where he was in Central America, whether his trip was confined to cities, what foods or liquids he consumed, and whether he took any drugs, such as antibiotics, before, during, or after returning home are very relevant.

Fraser's trip was to Nicaragua and he spent most of the time in cities, but there were a few field trips. He avoided drinking anything except bottled liquids where at all possible, and most of the food he ate was freshly cooked. He did not take any medication before travelling, although he remarked that a number of his colleagues who had been on the trip with him had been on medication since returning.

Q What is the general term for this condition and how common is it?

A Fraser has probably acquired traveller's diarrhoea, the most common medical condition among people travelling to tropical or subtropical parts of the world. It occurs in about 20–50% of travellers.

Q What are the causes?

A About 70% of episodes are due to an infective agent of one kind or another (see Table 25.1). However, a proportion may be due to overindulgence in alcohol or food, and some cases may be accounted for by chemical poisoning, e.g. scombrotoxin. Bacterial pathogens account for about 70% of infective cases.

Q What initial investigations should be made?

A A sample of faeces should be sent for culture. In addition, microscopy for ova, trophozoites (in fresh liquid faeces), and parasite cysts should be requested, and full clinical details plus information on where the patient has been, and whether he has been on antibiotics, should be included on the request form, so that less common parasitic causes in particular will be considered.

Table 25.1 Common causes of traveller's diarrhoea

Bacteria	Parasites	Viruses
Escherichia coli	*Giardia lamblia*	Noro-viruses
Salmonella spp.	*Cryptosporidium parvum*	Rotavirus
Campylobacter jejuni	*Entamoeba histolytica*	
Shigella spp.	*Cyclospora cayetanensis*	
Vibrio cholerae and other spp.		

Table 25.2 Important features of *Giardia lamblia*

Organism

- Flagellated enteric protozoan
- Trophozoite is free-living; encystation occurs in intestine

Transmission

- Faecally contaminated water
- Person-to-person spread, e.g. day-care nurseries
- Sexual, i.e. homosexual

Pathogenesis

- Disruption of brush border of the small intestine
- Disaccharidase deficiencies

Clinical disease

- Asymptomatic
- Self-limiting diarrhoea (25–50%)
- Chronic diarrhoea and malabsorption

Diagnosis

- Faeces for trophozoites (early stages of disease) or cysts following ether concentration
- Duodenal aspirate for microscopy

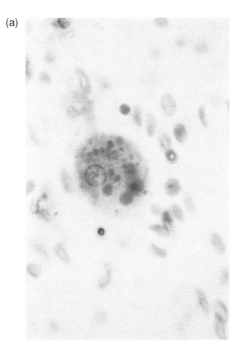

(a)

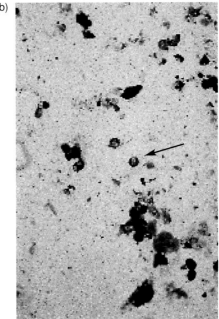

(b)

Cysts of *Giardia lamblia* (see Table 25.2 and Fig. 25.1) are seen under light microscopy in two consecutive stool samples. Culture for bacterial pathogens, including *Vibro* spp., is negative. Fraser is put on appropriate treatment and makes an uneventful recovery.

Q What is the appropriate therapy for giardiasis?

A Rehydration and oral metronidazole for 10 days.

Q What should the patient be told before taking metronidazole?

A Metronidazole may cause a disulfiram-like reaction, with flushing and hypotension following alcohol ingestion, and therefore alcohol should be avoided during treatment. Prolonged use of

Fig. 25.1 Protozoan causes of traveller's diarrhoea. (a) *Entamoeba histolytica* (trophozoites); (b) *Cryptosporidia* (cysts) see arrow; (c) *Giardia lamblia* (cysts).

(c)

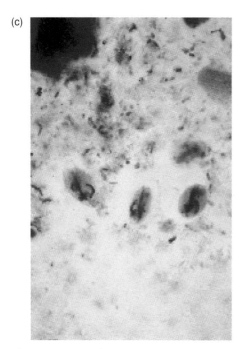

Fig. 25.1 (c) *Cont'd.*

metronidazole may result in peripheral neuropathy and, although it has been used frequently during pregnancy for the treatment of vaginal discharge, it should be avoided if possible, especially during the first trimester. Metronidazole is also the treatment of choice for amoebiasis caused by *Entamoeba histolytica* (Box 25.1; see also Case 30) but is ineffective against cryptosporidiosis (Box 25.2).

Q Is giardia the most common cause of traveller's diarrhoea?

Box 25.1 *Entamoeba histolytica*

Clinical illness

Diarrhoea and abdominal pain, dysentery (bloody diarrhoea), toxic megacolon, extraintestinal spread (liver abscess, lung, brain)

Diagnosis

Stool for cysts (trophozoites seen in fresh specimens only), colonoscopy, serology, and CT/MRI scans if invasive

---

Box 25.2 *Cryptosporidium parvum*

Clinical illness

Self-limiting diarrhoeal illness in immunocompetent host; severe watery diarrhoea in HIV patients with, occasionally, cholecystitis. No antimicrobial therapy effective

Diagnosis

Modified Ziehl–Neelsen stain on stool sample

A No. Enterotoxigenic strains of *E. coli* are more common and account for approximately 50% of cases. Diarrhoea-producing *E. coli* may be subdivided into:

- *enteropathogenic*—strongly adherent to intestinal epithelial cells. Cause infantile gastroenteritis in the tropics and sometimes in hospitals

- *enterotoxigenic*—produce either a heat-labile or heat-stable toxin, together with adhesive factors. Major cause of traveller's diarrhoea

- *enteroinvasive*—cause an illness similar to shigella dysentery in patients of all ages

- *cytotoxin-producing*—*E. coli* 0157 is the most common serotype and the toxin is closely related to the shiga toxin of *Shigella dysenteriae*. Causes a variety of diarrhoeal diseases, including colitis and the haemolytic uraemic syndrome and may be acquired from food (see Case 23).

Q How may traveller's diarrhoea be avoided?

A Improved food hygiene practices in warmer climates may in time reduce the incidence, but in the meantime travellers should eat only freshly prepared foods that are served hot and fruit or vegetables that can be peeled. Salads in particular should be avoided. Hot tea or coffee, recently boiled drinks, or bottled beverages are safe but tap water and ice cubes should be avoided if at all possible. Travellers to a cholera-endemic area may receive whole-cell cholera vaccine (of questionable efficacy) before travelling (see Case 31). It is not clear what precise role prophylactic antibiotics (mainly to prevent infection caused by *E. coli*) have in preventing this condition, but if used they should be started on arrival and continued for 2–3 days after returning. Travellers for whom prophylaxis should be considered are:

- those with inflammatory bowel disease
- patients with diabetes mellitus
- the elderly
- patients with AIDS
- those travelling to the tropics for a brief but very important visit

The potential side-effects of the agents listed below, plus their loss as a therapeutic option due to resistance, are arguments against routine prophylaxis. The agents most commonly prescribed are:

- co-trimoxazole: resistance increasingly emerging
- doxycycline: less frequently used now. To be avoided in children or during pregnancy
- quinolones, e.g. ciprofloxacin, etc., if antibiotic resistance prevalent
- bismuth compounds: used more frequently by travellers from North America

Q What are the principles of management of traveller's diarrhoea?

A The key features are:

- fluid and electrolyte replacement
- antimotility drugs such as loperamide but used with caution
- a short course of ciprofloxacin or co-trimoxazole (if symptoms persist and giardiasis or amoebiasis, for which metronidazole is recommended, are excluded).

Summary: **Traveller's diarrhoea**

Presentation

Diarrhoea and abdominal pain shortly after arriving or returning from a visit to a tropical or subtropical area

Diagnosis

One or more stool samples, preferably fresh, for culture and microscopic examination for ova, cysts, etc. Important to inform the laboratory of areas visited to ensure all potential pathogens are looked for

Management

Likelihood of contracting diarrhoea when travelling may be reduced by careful attention to foods consumed and, occasionally, prophylactic antibiotics. Treatment involves fluid replacement, loperamide, and either ciprofloxacin or co-trimoxazole if bacterial; metronidazole for giardiasis and amoebiasis

Case 26 Bob, a 55-year-old retired coal miner with abdominal pain

Bob is a 55-year-old retired coal miner who is referred to the accident and emergency department by his family doctor with a 10-day history of increasing crampy abdominal pain, vomiting, and constipation. The abdominal pain has become severe in the preceding 24 hours. On examination Bob has a temperature of 39.5°C, is tender in the right lower quadrant with rebound tenderness, and has absent abdominal bowel sounds.

Q What is the diagnosis?

A The history and physical findings are suggestive of peritonitis, most likely due to a perforated viscus. Although peritonitis *per se* does not automatically mean infection, it is likely that spillage of bowel contents into the peritoneum will result in infection. This might be caused by a perforated appendix (the patient is a little old for this), diverticulitis, large-bowel neoplasm, inflammatory bowel disease, or a perforated peptic ulcer.

Q What microbes may be causing the peritonitis?

A This depends on the site of perforation. The number of commensal organisms increases as one descends through the gastrointestinal tract (see Table 26.1). Anaerobes such as *Bacteroides* spp.,

Prevotella spp., and *Clostridium* spp. become the dominant bacterial flora in the large bowel. Potential pathogens such as *Escherichia coli*, *Proteus mirabilis*, and *Pseudomonas aeruginosa* are less numerous, but become more so following instrumentation or broad-spectrum antibiotic therapy.

Shortly after admission Bob is taken to theatre for a laparotomy, which reveals a tumour and a perforated descending colon with a walled-off abscess and localized peritonitis. The tumour is resected but the procedure is technically difficult and there is spillage of pus into the peritoneum. An anterior resection with defunctioning colostomy is performed. A swab of the pus is obtained for culture and Bob, who is allergic to penicillin, is started on intravenous antibiotics.

Q Was a swab the best specimen to send for culture?

A No. Unless there is insufficient material to collect or it is difficult to aspirate, actual pus or tissue is always preferable to a swab, especially when trying to isolate anaerobes. In addition, a Gram stain of the pus may give an early idea of the likely pathogens. Pus may be collected and forwarded to

Table 26.1 Normal flora of the gastrointestinal tract

Site	Number of organisms (cfu/g)*	Common microbes	Comment
Stomach	$<10^3$	Lactobacilli, streptococci, yeasts	Numbers increase with age, achlorhydria
Small bowel	$10^3–10^9$	As above plus clostridia, enterobacteriaceae, enterococci	Increase distally. Antibiotics affect relative numbers
Large bowel	$10^8–10^{12}$	As above plus protozoa (*Chilomastix*, *Trichomonas*), yeasts	Anaerobes outnumber facultative organisms by 1000–10 000:1

* cfu/g, Colony-forming units per gram.

the laboratory in a sterile container or a syringe sealed with a rubber plug.

Q What antibiotic or antibiotics are indicated here and, ideally, when should they be started?

A The details of Bob's condition suggested intraabdominal sepsis and therefore antibiotics should have been administered before laparotomy. This will also ensure that Bob is protected when the first incision is made, or if pus or the contents of a viscus is spilled into the peritoneum, resulting in possible bacteraemia.

Metronidazole will cover anaerobes, including *Bacteroides fragilis*, which are often resistant to penicillin. If there is a history of penicillin allergy every effort should be made to confirm this, as otherwise the patient will be deprived of some of the best antibiotics available. A genuine history of allergy may be indicated by a history of a skin rash, anaphylaxis, or angioneurotic oedema. Diarrhoea or a fainting attack following an intramuscular injection do not represent allergy. Gentamicin, or a cephalosporin such as cefuroxime or cefotaxime, should be given here as these will cover most coliforms. Gentamicin and metronidazole with or without benzylpenicillin or ampicillin still remain a good combination in the absence of a history of penicillin allergy. The β-lactam/β-lactamase inhibitor combination, piperacillin/tazobactam, is also useful as second-line treatment as it is effective against many antibiotic-resistant bacteria and has a broad spectrum of activity, i.e. it is active against aerobic Gram-negative bacilli including *Pseudomonas aeruginosa*, enterococci, and anaerobes. There is approximately a 10% chance of cross-allergy to cephalosporins, but this should be balanced against the severity of the patient's condition and the nature of the original allergic reaction. Erythromycin has poor activity against Gram-negative bacilli and results in thrombophlebitis when given intravenously.

Q How does the use of antibiotics as part of surgical chemoprophylaxis differ from that of treatment?

A Chemoprophylaxis implies the use of antibiotics to prevent infection arising from the surgical pro-

---

> ### Box 26.1 **Principles of surgical antimicrobial prophylaxis**
>
> *Identify patients at risk*, e.g. large-bowel resection, amputation of ischaemic limb, prosthetic joint implantation
> *Match antibiotics with pathogens*, e.g.
>
> - cefuroxime + metronidazole: abdominal surgery
> - co-amoxyclav: gynaecological surgery
> - flucloxacillin: joint implant
>
> *First dose before incision*: at induction or with premedication but *not* days before surgery, during, or after operation
> *Discontinue after surgery*: at most two doses if the procedure takes longer than 3 hours. Administering more doses than this has no prophylactic benefit. Treatment as opposed to prophylaxis may require different antibiotics

---

cedure, rather than to treat established infection. In particular, the timing of the first dose and duration are critical in chemoprophylaxis (see Box 26.1).

Bob is transferred to the intensive care unit (ICU) after surgery for ventilation and monitoring. He develops the adult respiratory distress syndrome (ARDS), acute renal failure (serum creatine 250 μg/ml), and requires positive pressure ventilation to maintain satisfactory blood gases and inotropes, i.e. he has multiorgan failure. Blood cultures subsequently grow *E. coli*, resistant to cephradine and ampicillin but sensitive to gentamicin, cefuroxime, and cefotaxime, and *B. fragilis* (Fig. 26.1). The swab taken at laparotomy also grows the same two organisms plus enterococci. Gentamicin is added to the metronidazole, and cefotaxime (a third-generation cephalosporin) is started postoperatively.

Q What is the significance of the enterococci isolated from the swab?

A Although enterococci are part of the normal bowel flora and frequently recovered from intra-

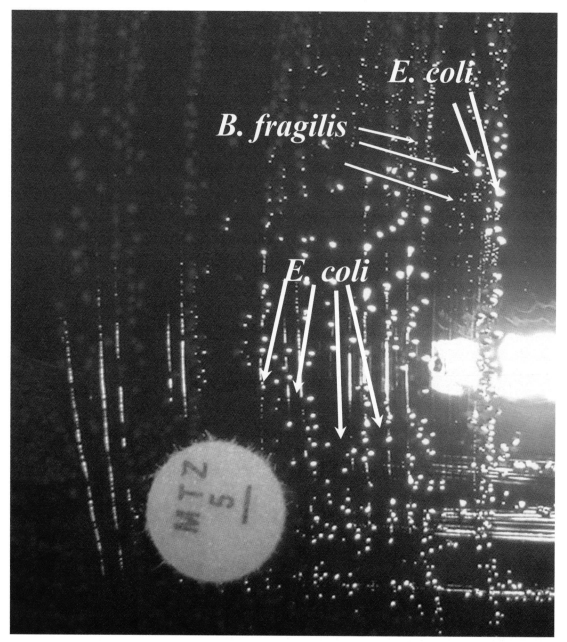

Fig. 26.1 Mixed growth of *E. coli* and *B. fragilis* (does not grow near metronidazole disc) on blood agar isolated from blood cultures and swab.

abdominal and wound specimens, they are usually less pathogenic than anaerobes or coliforms such as *E. coli* unless they cause intravascular line infection or bacteraemia.

Q Was it wise to add gentamicin in light of the poor renal function?

A The aminoglycosides (e.g. gentamicin, tobramicin, netilmicin, amikacin) are among the most

Box 26.2 Serum aminoglycoside assays

1 Should be carried out in *all* patients who receive more than three doses. Toxic:therapeutic ratio is low and there is considerable variation in pharmacokinetics between patients

2 Imperative in the elderly, neonates, patients with declining renal function, or patients on other nephrotoxic agents

3 First set of levels should be done around the second to fourth dose and include a pre-dose, i.e. just before a dose (trough) and post-dose level, i.e. 1 hour after an IV dose (peak). Alternatively, for once-daily dosing, instead of taking a sample 1 hour after administration, a sample can be taken 8 hours after the dose with no pre-dose sample required. Blood samples should not be taken through the intravascular line in which the aminoglycoside is given

4 Should be repeated every 3–4 days at least and more frequently if initial levels are toxic, if the patient is extremely ill, or if renal function declines

5 Acceptable levels for once-daily administration are:
- gentamicin: trough, < 1 µg/ml; peak, >10 µg/ml or 1.5–6 µg/ml if taken 8 hours after the dose
- tobramycin and netilmicin: as for gentamicin
- amikacin: trough, < 5 µg/ml; peak, > 50 µg/ml

active agents against Gram-negative bacteria. Their use is not contraindicated in deteriorating renal function or failure but the dose and dosage interval need to be modified and frequent, if not daily, serum assays carried out (see Box 26.2). Aminoglycosides are now administered in a single daily dose as this results in higher peak serum concentrations, is less expensive, saves time, and may even reduce toxic side-effects. The exception to this is in the treatment of infective endocarditis (see Case 49). The addition of gentamicin to cefotaxime (*E. coli* sensitive to both) is justified because of the uncontrolled Gram-negative sepsis with multi-organ damage.

Five days after admission to the ICU Bob remains pyrexial, has a white cell count of $24 \times 10^9/l$, and requires inotropic support. Computerized tomography (CT) reveals a residual paracolic abscess, which is drained using a percutaneous catheter under radiological control (see Fig. 26.2), and a drain is left *in situ*. 20 ml of sterile pus (Fig. 26.3) is aspirated initially. Pus in decreasing amounts continues to drain for 4 days. Bob's pyrexia settles and his general condition improves over the next week. He remains on intravenous antibiotics for 14 days, but is eventually discharged from the unit despite developing a number of superinfections.

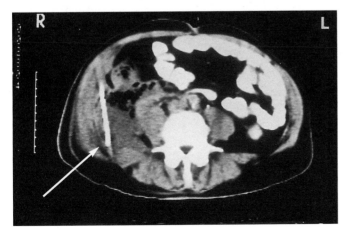

Fig. 26.2 CT scan demonstrating right-sided abdominal abscess with drain *in situ* (see arrow).

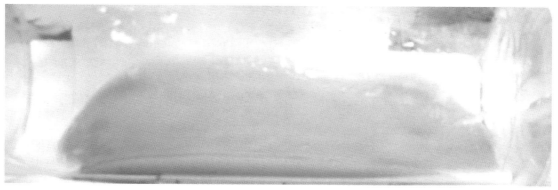

Fig. 26.3 Pus aspirated from abdomen; more likely to yield pathogens than a swab, especially if obtained before the start of antibiotics.

Q What is a superinfection?

A A 'superinfection' is a new infection that arises as a complication of antimicrobial therapy to treat an existing infection. Examples include:

- oral thrush: occurs in immunosuppressed patients or patients on corticosteroids who have recently been on broad-spectrum antibiotics such as ampicillin or cephalosporins

- antibiotic-associated diarrhoea: most commonly due to enterotoxin produced by *Clostridium difficile* (see Case 33)

- enterococcal urinary tract infection (UTI): *Enterococcus faecalis* and *E. faecium* are low-grade pathogens but symptomatic infection may occur in a catheterized patient (see Case 34) on antibiotics with little anti-enterococcal activity, used to treat another infection, e.g. ciprofloxacin, cephalosporins.

Summary: Peritonitis

Presentation
May be localized or generalized but usually presents with an 'acute abdomen'

Diagnosis
Usually clinical and confirmed at surgery. Ultrasound is helpful in localizing intraabdominal abscesses and the drainage of pus. Blood cultures should also be taken as bacteraemia may occur

Management
Surgery is usually required to correct the underlying disease, e.g. removal of perforated tumour, and for drainage. Broad-spectrum antibiotics (to cover Gram-negative bacilli and anaerobes) also indicated and admission to ICU if evidence of organ failure

Case 27 Belinda, a 25-year-old non-Caucasian with malaise, myalgia, and fever

Belinda, a 25-year-old non-Caucasian woman, is referred to the accident and emergency department of a local hospital by her GP. She has been unwell for a week and complains of malaise, headache, myalgia, and some minor upper respiratory symptoms. Belinda is on no medications, has no relevant previous medical history, and her husband and two children are well. Apart from a temperature of 38°C, physical examination is unremarkable.

Q What aspects of Belinda's background require clarification?

A Some infections, e.g. tuberculosis, are more common in certain ethnic groups or immigrants from the underdeveloped world, even when they have lived for some years in the developed world. Other infections, e.g. malaria (see Case 50) and enteric fever, may be contracted during visits to see relatives. Consequently, it is essential to ask about family history, whether there has been recent travel, and, if so, what areas were visited and whether the patient was immunized before travel.

Further questioning reveals that Belinda was born in Bombay but that she and her family moved to Britain when she was 5 years of age. Family history is unremarkable. She had visited her grandmother in India 2–3 weeks previously and had returned 6 days before presentation. Neither her husband nor her children had accompanied her. Apart from the routine vaccinations received as a child, she had not been vaccinated before travel. Belinda did, however, take mefloquine prophylaxis for malaria.

Q What organ system apart from the respiratory tract should you ask about?

A It is possible that she has a minor viral-type illness contracted since her return but travel-associated illnesses must be excluded, in particular those affecting the gastrointestinal system. A history of diarrhoea, vomiting, and abdominal pain may suggest traveller's diarrhoea (see Case 25).

On further questioning the respiratory symptoms are considered minor, but she admits to a short bout of nausea and diarrhoea shortly after arriving in India. This settled quickly and she is now if anything a little constipated.

Q What might the combination of pyrexia, evidence of a systemic illness (malaise, myalgia), and a history of recent gastrointestinal upset suggest?

A Enteric fever. Enteric or typhoid fever is an illness caused by infection with *Salmonella typhi* or *S. paratyphi* (paratyphoid fever) and may be contracted by people resident in temperate climates following travel abroad to tropical or subtropical areas. The clinical features are:

- pyrexial illness in a returned traveller
- malaise, headache, anorexia, myalgia, mild respiratory symptoms such as a cough
- diarrhoea or constipation, but *neither* may be present
- fever with relatively slow pulse
- rose spots—maculopapular lesions that blanch on pressure—are a late manifestation and are present in < 20% of cases
- abdominal tenderness and hepatosplenomegaly may be present

Q How may the diagnosis be confirmed and what should be included in the differential diagnosis?

A The diagnosis is made when there are clinical features such as those described above, together with isolation of the bacterium from appropriate sites such as blood, faeces, and urine (see Fig. 27.1). Laboratory abnormalities that may point towards enteric fever include leucopenia due to neutropenia, disseminated intravascular coagulation with

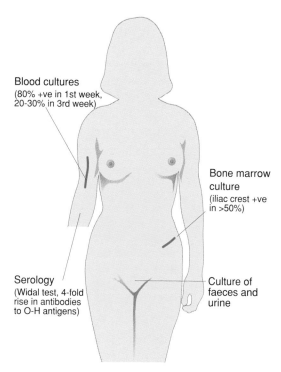

Blood cultures
(80% +ve in 1st week,
20-30% in 3rd week)

Bone marrow
culture
(iliac crest +ve
in >50%)

Serology
(Widal test, 4-fold
rise in antibodies
to O-H antigens)

Culture of
faeces and
urine

Fig. 27.1 Investigation of a patient with suspected
enteric fever.

low platelets, and elevated hepatic enzymes such as
SGOT (serum glutamic-oxaloacetic transaminase).
The differential diagnosis includes malaria,
intraabdominal pathology such as appendicitis or a
paracolic abscess, amoebic colitis, brucellosis, and
even respiratory tract infection where respiratory
symptoms are more prominent. Notwithstanding
the malaria prophylaxis (see Case 50) she could still
have malaria, especially if prophylaxis was not
started before travel and continued for 2 weeks following return as usually recommended.

Q What other laboratory test is often requested
when making a diagnosis of enteric fever?

A The Widal test.

Q What is the basis of this test?

A This test determines the presence of antibodies
to H (flagellar) and O (cell wall) salmonella antigens. The results, however, are not always easy to
interpret and there may be some cross-reactions

with non-enteric salmonellae. The Widal test is
often not especially helpful in diagnosing infection
caused by *S. paratyphi* because it is affected by vaccination against typhoid fever; there may also be
false-positive results in patients with connective
tissue diseases. Therefore, although included as one
of the investigations for the diagnosis of typhoid
fever, it is frequently not very helpful in the individual patient. It may, however, have a role in epidemiological surveys.

Q What are the complications of enteric fever?

A These include:

• toxaemia with hepatic, renal, and bone marrow
dysfunction

• gastrointestinal perforation (single or multiple)
and haemorrhage

• metastatic infection such as osteomyelitis,
endocarditis

• persistent infection resulting in relapse or
chronic carriage (see Table 27.1)

**Table 27.1 Epidemiology and spread
of enteric fever**

Spread

The bacterium enters the body via the mouth and
humans are the only reservoir. Person-to-person
spread is possible with poor standards of hygiene,
but less likely than with other gastrointestinal
pathogens, e.g. *Shigella*

Chronic carrier

Arises from inadequate treatment. Bacterium may
persist in the gallbladder

Water-borne

Important source in underdeveloped world and
spread occurs where sewage contaminates drinking
water supplies

Food-borne

• Food washed or prepared with contaminated
water

• Food-handler with poor standards of hygiene
who is a chronic carrier

An early diagnosis with prompt and aggressive treatment instituted in hospital is important in avoiding the complications that account for fatalities.

Q What is the treatment of enteric fever?

A Antimicrobial chemotherapy is essential as this is a systemic condition with life-threatening complications. The agent chosen should be active against the infecting strain as confirmed by sensitivity testing. Chloramphenicol was traditionally the agent of choice, as most isolates are sensitive, but ciprofloxacin is now increasingly used because it is as effective and does not have the bone marrow side-effects of chloramphenicol. It should, however, be used with caution in children, as it can adversely affect growing cartilage and bone. Alternative but less effective antibiotics include ampicillin and co-trimoxazole. Management must also include treatment of complications, such as fluid replacement for dehydration, blood transfusion following haemorrhage, surgery for perforation, and organ support if required.

Belinda is admitted to hospital, initially for observation and investigation. Blood and faeces cultures taken on admission grow a non-lactose fermenter (Fig. 27.2), subsequently identified as *S. typhi*, sensitive to ampicillin,

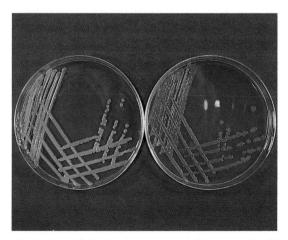

Fig. 27.2 *E. coli* (lactose fermenter) on left, compared with salmonella species (non-lactose fermenter) on right on MacConkey agar.

chloramphenicol, and ciprofloxacin. She is started on ciprofloxacin intravenously, which is subsequently changed to oral administration. Investigations to exclude typhoid fever in her husband and children are negative.

Q Why is ciprofloxacin more effective than ampicillin?

A Ciprofloxacin and chloramphenicol achieve relatively high intracellular concentrations and this, together with good penetration into the intestinal mucosa, probably explains the superior efficacy of these agents compared to ampicillin or co-trimoxazole, despite equivalent susceptibility of the organism in vitro.

Q How can enteric fever be prevented?

A Prevention in the developing world is achieved by the separation of drinking water supplies from sewage, and greater attention to the preparation of food. Travellers from the developed world to endemic areas should be careful about what they eat, especially when eating out (see Case 25). A whole-cell heat-killed vaccine consisting of *S. typhi* is available which should be given as a primary course of two doses 4–6 weeks apart. There is also an oral typhoid vaccine consisting of a live attenuated strain, which appears to be as efficacious as the parenteral vaccine. In addition there are now Vi capsular polysaccharide and Vi conjugate vaccines. Vaccination is recommended for travellers to areas of the world where enteric fever is prevalent such as Africa, Asia, and Central and South America. It is also offered to laboratory workers handling specimens that may contain the typhoid bacillus. Vaccination is not recommended for contacts, carriers, or as part of the management of an outbreak.

Q What are the characteristics of enteric *S. typhi* and *S. paratyphi* and non-enteric salmonellae?

A Both enteric and non-enteric salmonellae share many similar features that distinguish them from other members of the *Enterobacteriaceae* and that are important in distinguishing them from other bacteria in the laboratory (see Box 27.1).

Box 27.1 Genus *Salmonella*

- Lactose-negative coliforms, of which there are > 200 species

- Ferment glucose and mannitol, which distinguishes them from other non-lactose fermenters in stool specimens

- Kauffmann–White scheme classifies salmonellae to species on the basis of somatic (cell wall), flagellar, and capsular antigens

- enteric (*S. typhi* and *S. paratyphi*) and non-enteric (the remainder)

The non-enteric salmonellae are animal in origin and are a major cause of food poisoning (see Case 23). They may be contracted from poultry (chickens, turkeys), cows, pigs, and, to a lesser extent, birds and domestic pets. Infection is usually by ingestion of contaminated food such as eggs (*S. enteritidis*) or meat (*S. typhimurium*) and the symptoms are similar to those of other causes of food poisoning. Unlike infection caused by the enteric salmonellae, most cases are self-limiting, sporadic, and do not require antimicrobial chemotherapy. The incidence is highest in the period from July to November in the UK. Cross-infection may occur occasionally in institutions if hygiene standards are poor. Some species, such as *S. virchow* and *S. cholerasuis*, may be more virulent and are associated with bacteraemia, meningitis, and osteomyelitis. When this occurs aggressive antimicrobial chemotherapy is required.

Before discharge from hospital, Belinda remarks in conversation that she helps her brother a couple of days a week in a sandwich bar.

Q What precautions need to be taken to prevent spread in this setting?

A Six consecutive negative specimens of faeces are required before it is considered safe for her to go back to work, because of the serious consequences of prolonged carriage with subsequent transmission to the general public.

Q How do these precautions differ in a food-handler who has contracted salmonella food poisoning?

A A food-handler who has contracted non-enteric salmonellosis such as food poisoning may return to work when symptoms have resolved if he or she can be relied upon to practise good personal hygiene, especially hand-washing, even if the faeces are still positive. Clearance specimens (negative faeces) are therefore not necessary, but if good personal hygiene cannot be guaranteed negative specimens usually are required.

Summary: Enteric fever

Presentation

Pyrexial illness with non-specific gastrointestinal symptoms in a traveller returned from an endemic area. Physical examination often unremarkable

Diagnosis

Culture of blood and faeces for *S. typhi* or *S. paratyphi*. Urine and bone marrow may also be positive. Serology often not diagnostic, especially if vaccinated in the past

Management

Careful attention to food hygiene and pre-exposure vaccination when travelling will prevent acquisition. Ciprofloxacin or chloramphenicol are the antibiotics of choice

Case 28 Anorexia, malaise, and nausea in Eddie, 25 years old

Eddie, a 25-year-old solicitor, presents with a 5-day history of anorexia, malaise, fever, and nausea. He has been persuaded to visit his GP by his friends, who have told him his eyes have become yellow (see Fig. 28.1), and he has also noticed some abdominal discomfort on the right-hand side. On closer questioning he admits to smoking 15 cigarettes a day, but has not been able to face one since he began to feel ill. He has noticed that over the past couple of days that his urine has become very dark, which he attributes to not having taken in much fluid. He has not noticed any change in the colour or consistency of his stools. Prior to this illness he has been fit and healthy, with no past medical history of note. He is not on any regular medication.

Q What is the likely diagnosis?

A Eddie is clearly jaundiced. Although there are a large number of causes of jaundice, the non-specific prodromal illness with fever is highly suggestive of an acute infective—most probably viral—hepatitis. Other possibilities include acute alcoholic hepatitis and drug-induced hepatitis, either of which may mimic acute viral hepatitis. Many patients with acute hepatitis give a history of tobacco and alcohol intolerance. The right upper

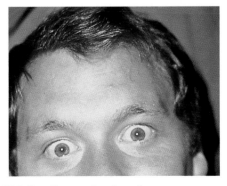

Fig. 28.1 Jaundice seen in sclera of eyes.

quadrant pain is due to acute enlargement of the liver, stretching the innervated liver capsule. Occasional patients, especially those with hepatitis B virus infection, may give a history of a rash and/or a polyarthritis prior to the onset of jaundice, features that arise from immune complex formation between virus and antibody.

Q What are the possible causative agents of acute infective hepatitis?

A A large number of infectious agents can cause acute hepatitis, including hepatitis A, B, C, D, and E viruses, Epstein–Barr virus (see Case 15), cytomegalovirus (see Case 56), yellow fever virus (see Case 68), and leptospira (see Case 53).

Q Are the hepatitis viruses A–E all closely related variants of the same type?

A No. The only thing these viruses have in common is that they are all hepatotropic (i.e. they demonstrate an ability to infect hepatocytes). The five hepatitis viruses each belong to different virus families, possessing entirely different properties (see Table 28.1).

Q How are the hepatitis viruses spread?

A There are a number of different routes, and the viruses differ in the extent to which they are spread by these routes.

Hepatitis A and E viruses (HAV, HEV) are enterically spread, i.e. via the faecal–oral route. These viruses are excreted in faeces. Ingestion of contaminated food or water then results in transmission. Whilst any food can act as a vehicle for transmission, certain foods carry an increased risk, e.g. shellfish, as these are able to concentrate virus if grown in contaminated water. Gross contamination, e.g. faecal contamination of water supplies through inadequate sewage disposal, may result in thousands of individuals being exposed. Such huge epidemics have been well described for HEV. On a smaller scale, if a food-handler with acute infection does not observe scrupulous hand hygiene, then

Table 28.1 Salient features of hepatitis A–E viruses

Hepatitis A virus

RNA genome; belongs to picornavirus family

Spread	Faecal–oral transmission
Risk groups	Those who eat/drink contaminated food, e.g. shellfish, and water
	Travellers to areas of high endemicity with low hygiene standards
	Carers or contacts (e.g. within families) of cases of acute HAV infection
Incubation period	2–6 weeks
Diagnosis	The presence of IgM anti-HAV
Outcome	Asymptomatic seroconversion; acute hepatitis; fulminant hepatitis (less common than with HBV). No chronic carriage
Vaccine	Killed whole-virus vaccine—for frequent travellers, sewage workers

Hepatitis B virus

DNA genome; belongs to hepadnavirus family

Spread	Vertical (i.e. mother-to-baby)
	Sexual
	Contact with contaminated blood or blood products
Risk groups	Newborns of carrier mothers
	Sexual partners of carriers
	Sexually promiscuous, both heterosexual and male homosexuals
	Injecting drug users who share needles
	Patients receiving or exposed to blood/blood products, e.g. haemophiliacs, haemodialysis patients, blood transfusion recipients
	Health-care workers exposed to potentially contaminated blood/blood products
	Members of population groups known to have high carriage rates
Incubation period	6 weeks–6 months
Diagnosis	HBsAg indicates current infection; IgM anti-HBc confirms recent infection
Outcome	Asymptomatic seroconversion; acute hepatitis; fulminant hepatitis. Chronic carriage may lead to cirrhosis, hepatocellular carcinoma
Vaccine	Subunit HBsAg—for risk groups (see Table 28.2)

Hepatitis C virus

RNA genome; belongs to flavivirus family

Spread	Contact with contaminated blood or blood products
	Vertical. Note: much less common than with HBV
	Sexual—controversial. Very inefficient compared to HBV
	Other 'natural' routes of transmission unidentified

Table 28.1 *cont'd*	
Risk groups	Injecting drug users who share needles
	Blood/blood product recipients
	Health-care workers exposed to contaminated blood/products, e.g. through needlestick injuries
Incubation period	Up to 3 months
Diagnosis	Anti-HCV indicates past infection; HCV RNA confirms current infection
Outcome	As for HBV. Fulminant hepatitis unusual
Vaccine	None as yet

Hepatitis D virus

Incomplete RNA genome; as yet unclassified family; deltavirus genus. Requires HBV as a helper virus

Spread	As for HBV
Risk groups	As for HBV. In the UK, most HDV-infected patients are injecting drug users
Diagnosis	Detection of delta antigen, anti-delta antibodies
Outcome	Acute hepatitis; fulminant hepatitis (increased risk in HBV/HDV co-infection); chronic carriage leading to cirrhosis, hepatocellular carcinoma
Vaccine	HBV vaccine. Anti-HBs protects against HDV infection

Hepatitis E virus

RNA genome, was classified as a calicivirus, but now some uncertainty over this

Spread	Faecal–oral
Risk groups	Travellers to areas where HEV is highly endemic, e.g. Indian subcontinent, South America, Russia
Incubation period	Up to 12 weeks; occasional prolonged incubation reported
Diagnosis	IgM anti-HEV indicates acute infection
Outcome	As for HAV but mortality higher in pregnant women
Vaccine	None as yet

virus of faecal origin may arrive in soon-to-be consumed food. Intrahousehold spread of HAV is a fairly common event.

Hepatitis B, C, and D viruses (HBV, HCV, HDV) are, in contrast, blood-borne viruses. Thus, they can all be transmitted via the parenteral route. This is most obviously achieved by means of transfusion of a contaminated unit of blood, although in the UK and many other countries blood donors are screened to try and prevent this happening (see Case 29). More subtle parenteral transmission occurs through sharing of needles between individuals who inject drugs for recreational use or through needlestick injuries (see Case 57). Inapparent exposure to blood can occur through sharing toothbrushes or razors, or via bites and scratches. Horizontal transmission of HBV between children, presumably through the latter route, is an important means of spread in some countries.

Blood-borne pathogens may gain access to all body fluids and compartments via the bloodstream, thus raising other possible routes of transmission. HBV is certainly present in seminal fluid and female genital tract secretions, and HBV is a sexually transmitted infection (STI)—indeed, this is how much of acute HBV infection in the UK arises. Certain sexual practices may increase the risk of transmission, e.g. if there is also blood exposure through abrasions. HCV, however, is much less efficiently transmitted sexually than is HBV, and should not be regarded as an STI.

For all blood-borne pathogens, there is the possibility of mother-to-baby, or vertical, transmission. This may arise from exposure of the baby to virally infected maternal blood, or through passage through an infected birth canal, or even postnatally through contaminated breast milk. Vertical transmission is by far the most important route of transmission of HBV worldwide.

Q What further clinical details should be elicited from Eddie in order to pinpoint the most likely cause of his hepatitis?

A He should be asked about recent travel (and any prophylactic measures taken before travel), recent contact with jaundiced individuals, sexual history (and any recent changes in sexual partners), whether he has ever injected drugs, and, if so, whether he shared needles, and transfusion history. As part of the differential diagnosis, he should also be asked about medication and alcohol intake.

Eddie is not on any form of medication and his alcohol intake amounts to an average of 3–4 pints of beer per week. He gives no history of travel abroad in the last 6 months. He does not eat shellfish. He has not been in contact with anyone else who is jaundiced. He denies ever having injected drugs and has never received a blood transfusion. He reveals that he is a homosexual, and he acquired a new sexual partner about 4 months ago. On examination he is febrile (38.0°C), jaundiced, and his liver is

tender and palpable 2 cm below the intercostal margin, but he has no stigmata of chronic liver disease and there are no other clinical signs.

Q How should Eddie be investigated further?

A The most likely diagnosis is now acute HBV infection, most probably acquired from his new sexual partner, although HAV infection from an unknown source is also a possibility. Apart from the standard investigations (full blood count, liver function tests), blood for hepatitis serology should also be sent to the microbiology laboratory All samples from Eddie should be clearly labelled as 'risk of infection' to alert porters and laboratory staff to the potential dangers of handling such material and to ensure safe transport. Note that the diagnosis of viral hepatitis relies on the detection of the viruses or antibodies to the viruses using serological or molecular techniques. None of the hepatitis viruses can be grown in routine tissue culture, so it is *not* useful to send a faecal sample to the laboratory.

Q What tests would you expect the laboratory to perform initially, to identify: (1) HAV infection; (2) HBV infection; (3) HCV infection?

A The tests are slightly different for each of these viruses, and therefore are potentially confusing.

- Hepatitis A. Detection of IgM anti-HAV antibodies. IgM antibodies are markers of recent infection, and their presence confirms the diagnosis with a single test
- Hepatitis B and C viruses. Detection of the viruses (or parts of them), as opposed to antibodies to the viruses, in a peripheral blood sample

The initial screening test for HBV infection is to look for presence of the hepatitis B surface antigen (HBsAg; see below). This antigen is synthesized in excess by infected hepatocytes, and is present in the peripheral blood in all patients currently infected with HBV. Thus, a negative HBsAg result effectively excludes this diagnosis.

Serum can be tested for anti-HCV antibodies, but (1) available kits do not distinguish between IgG and IgM antibodies, and (2) anti-HCV is not always present at the time of clinical presentation. Therefore, tests for acute HCV infection involve genome detection assays (i.e. HCV RNA), which are expensive. Diagnosis of chronic HCV infection is discussed in Case 29.

The following preliminary report is received from the microbiology laboratory: hepatitis A IgG detected; hepatitis A IgM *not* detected.

Q What are the significant differences between IgM and IgG antibodies?

A IgM antibodies are only present for a short period following infection, whereas IgG antibodies persist for many years, if not for life. Thus the presence of virus-specific IgM in a serum sample is a definitive indication that the patient has recently been infected with that virus, whereas the presence of virus-specific IgG only indicates that the patient has been infected with that virus at some unspecified time during his or her life (see also Fig. 59.2 in Case 59). One other important difference, not relevant in this particular case, is that IgM,

being a large pentameric molecule, is unable to cross the placenta, whereas IgG can.

Q How would you interpret the above results?

A The IgG anti-HAV indicates that Eddie has at some stage been infected with HAV, but the absence of IgM anti-HAV means that the infection was some time ago, and is not the cause of his current jaundice.

Q What diagnostic assays are available for characterizing HBV infection?

A A schematic diagram of HBV is given in Fig. 28.2. Various component parts (i.e. antigens) of the virus can be detected in the laboratory. Similarly, antibodies to these antigens can also be detected. The antigen–antibody systems can be summarized as:

Antigen	Abbreviation	Antibody
Hepatitis B core antigen	HBcAg	Anti-HBc
Hepatitis B e antigen	HBeAg	Anti-HBe
Hepatitis B surface antigen	HBsAg	Anti-HBs

'e' is short for 'extractable. HBeAg is, in fact, derived from the same gene as the core antigen.

Q What are the possible consequences of acute HBV infection? How do these differ from those of acute HAV infection?

A These are shown in diagrammatic form in Fig. 28.3. Statistically speaking, the most likely outcome is asymptomatic seroconversion, i.e. there is not sufficient liver damage to cause symptoms. Alternatively, the patient may be acutely jaundiced (like Eddie). About 1% of acute HBV infections are said to be fulminant, i.e. the amount of liver damage is so great that the patient goes into liver failure. This carries a high mortality, the best treatment being liver transplantation. Finally, some patients with acute HBV infection will fail to clear the virus from their livers, and will become chronically infected (chronic carriers). Chronic carriage may result in inflammatory liver disease, leading

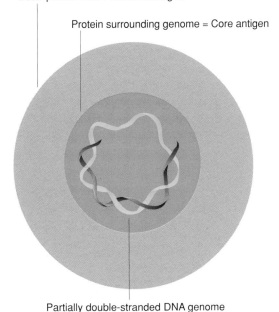

Outer protein coat = Surface antigen

Protein surrounding genome = Core antigen

Partially double-stranded DNA genome

Fig. 28.2 Schematic diagram of hepatitis B virus.

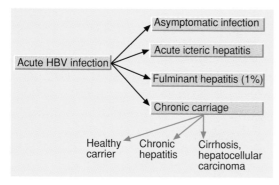

Fig. 28.3 Outcome(s) of infection with hepatitis B virus.

over a prolonged period of time (e.g. 20 years) to cirrhosis and a considerably (over 300-fold) increased risk of development of primary liver cell cancer. The risk of chronic carriage is not related to the severity of the acute infection but to the age at acute infection: 5–10% of otherwise immuno-competent adults will become chronic carriers following acute infection, whereas over 95% of infected neonates become carriers. Patients who are immunosuppressed are also at greater risk of becoming chronic carriers. e.g. HIV-infected patients, transplant recipients.

The potential outcomes for HAV infection differ in that fulminant hepatitis is less common, and there are no chronic sequelae of HAV infection (or HEV, for that matter). Thus, recovery from HAV is associated with viral clearance and lifelong immunity to further infection.

You receive the following result from the virology laboratory on Eddie's serum: hepatitis B surface antigen (HBsAg), present.

Q How do you interpret this result?

A The presence of HBsAg indicates active viral replication in the liver, i.e. current HBV infection.

Q Can you be sure, then, that Eddie's jaundice is due to acute HBV infection?

A No. The HBsAg result gives no information about *when* the infection took place. It is possible that this is acute HBV infection—but it is also possible that Eddie is a chronic carrier of HBV, and that his current jaundice may therefore be unrelated.

Q What assay will the laboratory perform to determine whether this is acute or chronic HBV infection?

A As explained above, the best serological marker of recent infection with a virus is the presence of IgM class antibodies to the virus. In the case of HBV, the standard diagnostic assay is to look for the presence of IgM anti-HBc. The significance and usefulness of the other markers of HBV infection are discussed below.

A further report from the laboratory reads: HBsAg, positive; IgM anti-HBc, positive; indicates recent infection with hepatitis B virus.

Q What steps should be taken in the further management of Eddie?

A These include:

1. He should be observed carefully during the acute stage of his illness. If there is any indication of fulminant hepatitis (e.g. impairment of conscious level, liver flap) he should be referred to hospital for specialist care

2. He, and all those responsible for caring for him, should be aware that he is an infection risk. His blood and body fluids will contain HBV. Care should be taken to avoid needlestick accidents (this should be standard practice whether or not a patient has HBV infection). He should be advised not to share razors or toothbrushes as the amount of blood present on these may be sufficient to transmit infection

3. After Eddie has recovered from his acute illness, he should be followed up to determine whether he is one of the 10% of patients who become chronic carriers. Chronic carriage is defined as the persistence of HBsAg for longer than 6 months

4. Eddie's sexual partner should also be tested for HBsAg. If positive, he should also be followed up to determine whether he is a chronic carrier

or not. If negative, he should be offered appropriate prophylaxis (see below)

5. Both Eddie and his partner should be counselled about HIV infection (see Case 38)

Eddie recovers from his episode of jaundice, although it is 4 months before he is fit enough to return to work. Follow-up testing demonstrates the disappearance of HBsAg from his serum after 12 weeks, and the appearance of anti-HBs after 16 weeks, confirming elimination of the virus. His partner gives a history of jaundice 1 year previously and, on testing of serum samples taken 6 months apart, is shown to be HBsAg-positive, confirming that he is a chronic carrier. The laboratory report also indicates that his serum is HBeAg-positive.

Q What is the purpose of testing for HBeAg and anti-HBe?

A Not all HBV carriers are equal. They are not all equally infectious, and they are not all equally at risk of serious chronic liver disease. The HBeAg/ anti-HBe system has been used for many years to distinguish between different groups of HBV carriers.

HBeAg is derived from the same viral gene as the core antigen, and is a surrogate marker of the extent of HBV replication occurring in the liver, i.e. the more virus turnover in the liver, the more likely an HBeAg positive result. HBeAg carriers, sometimes referred to as 'supercarriers', are highly infectious (e.g. through a needlestick injury) and also at most risk of serious liver disease. On an annual basis, a small percentage of such carriers will lose their HBeAg from serum, indicating a significant decrease in virus production within the liver (the pathogenesis of this is not completely understood). At this stage, their serum may contain equal amounts of HBeAg and anti-HBe, which will render both markers undetectable as they will associate into immune complexes. Some time later the anti-HBe will be in excess, and the serum will be HBeAg-negative, anti-HBe-positive. Anti-HBe-positive patients are much less infectious (e.g. transfusion of unit of blood needed to transmit infection) and have a reduced risk

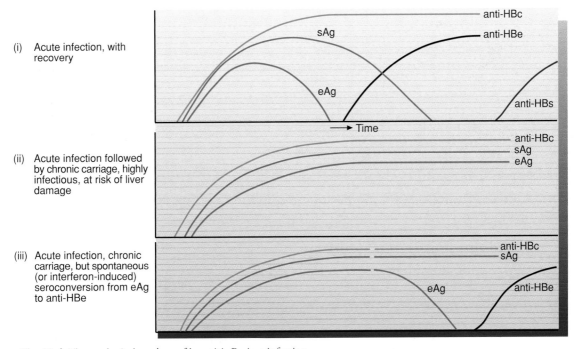

(i) Acute infection, with recovery

(ii) Acute infection followed by chronic carriage, highly infectious, at risk of liver damage

(iii) Acute infection, chronic carriage, but spontaneous (or interferon-induced) seroconversion from eAg to anti-HBe

Fig. 28.4 The serological markers of hepatitis B virus infection.

of long-term liver disease. The 'e' status of all carriers should be determined, as it gives prognostic information and also informs as to the infectiousness of the patient.

Note that HBeAg and anti-HBe are only surrogate markers of what is going on in the liver of HBsAg carriers. A more exact measure is the presence and quantity of HBV DNA in serum, but assays for this are not available in most routine diagnostic laboratories.

Figure 28.4 shows in diagrammatic form the serological results obtained from various categories of patients infected with HBV.

Further investigation of Eddie's partner reveals moderately deranged liver function tests, with a raised alanine aminotransferase. A liver biopsy reveals chronic active hepatitis.

Q Is there anything further that could be done for him?

A Yes. He is a candidate for alpha-interferon (IFN) therapy. This immunomodulatory agent works by enhancing the elimination of HBV-infected hepatocytes by the host's own immune system. Patients who respond to IFN become HBeAg-negative and then anti-HBe-positive. Loss of HBsAg and complete elimination of the virus may take some years. However, seroconversion from HBeAg to anti-HBe positivity is a successful clinical end-point, as the risk of progressive hepatitis is now much reduced and the patient is very much less infectious. Not all patients respond to IFN. Response rates are reduced in carriers who have been infected since birth and in immunosuppressed patients (e.g. HIV-infected).

Q Are there any alternative forms of therapy for chronic HBV infection?

A Yes. The replication cycle of HBV, which is extremely unusual, includes a step whereby viral RNA is reverse transcribed into DNA. This is carried out by the viral polymerase enzyme. Recognition of this process has led to the use of reverse transcriptase inhibitors, originally developed for the treatment of HIV infection (see Case 38), in clinical trials for chronic HBV carriers. The

most studied drug in this class is lamivudine. In addition, promising results have been reported using adefovir, a nucleotide phosphonate analogue (see Appendix 3) that is a broad-spectrum viral DNA polymerase inhibitor.

Q Is HBV infection preventable by immunization?

A Yes, by both passive and active immunization.

1. Passive immunization
   - Hyperimmune hepatitis B immunoglobulin (HBIg, contains high-titre anti-HBs)
   - For newborns of HBeAg-positive carrier mothers (see Case 60)
   - For non-responders to vaccine who suffer exposure, e.g. needlestick injury (see Case 57)

2. Active immunization
   - Hepatitis B vaccine—recombinant HBsAg (i.e. a subunit vaccine)
   - No risk of inadvertent transmission of HBV
   - Three intramuscular injections at 0, 1, and 6 months
   - Check anti-HBs levels 4–6 weeks after end of course: >10 mIU/ml are regarded as protective, although responses > 100 mIU/ml are desirable
   - Non-responders (up to 10% of recipients) are not protected
   - World Health Organization (WHO) policy is for HBV vaccination to be universal. However, current UK policy is for selective vaccination, i.e. only for those at risk of HBV infection (see Table 28.2)

Table 28.2 Risk groups recommended for HBV vaccination

Babies of HBV carrier mothers (see Case 60)

Parenteral drug misusers

Individuals who change sexual partners frequently

Sexual and close family contacts of a case or carrier

Patients with chronic renal failure (see Case 56)

Health-care workers (because of risk of occupational exposure)

Summary: Acute viral hepatitis

Presentation

Non-specific prodrome, fever, malaise, nausea, and alcohol and nicotine intolerance, followed by jaundice

Causative agents

Hepatitis viruses A–E; occasionally EBV, CMV

Diagnosis

IgM anti-HAV; HBsAg, IgM anti-HBc; anti-HCV, HCV RNA

Spread

Faecal–oral route (HAV, HEV); vertical, sexual, blood contact (HBV, HCV, HDV)

Complications

Fulminant hepatitis; chronic hepatitis leading to cirrhosis and liver cell cancer (HBV, HCV, and HDV only)

Treatment of HBV

Supportive; interferon-alpha; lamivudine; adefovir; liver transplantation (fulminant hepatitis, end-stage chronic hepatitis)

Prevention

Reduction in risk activities, e.g. sharing needles; safe sex; vaccination (against HAV, HBV) for selected at-risk groups; screening of blood supply (HBV, HCV)

Case 29 Tim, a 43-year-old business manager, is keen to donate blood

Tim, a 43 year-old IT business manager, goes to the local blood centre, keen to donate blood. He reads the leaflet supplied to him concerning who should and who should not, donate blood, decides that he is eligible, and a unit of blood is duly withdrawn from an antecubital vein. One week later, he is surprised to receive a letter from the blood transfusion service, telling him that one of his blood tests has given an abnormal result, and asking him to return to the centre for an appointment with a counsellor.

Q What tests will have been performed on Tim's blood?

A A full blood count to check his haemoglobin and several assays to ensure that his blood will not transmit a blood-borne infection—specifically human immunodeficiency virus (HIV), human T cell lymphotropic virus (HTLV; see Case 66), hepatitis B and C viruses (HBV, HCV), and syphilis—to the recipient of his donation. For the virus infections, the precise tests include anti-HIV, anti-HTLV, hepatitis B surface antigen, and anti-HCV.

Tim attends for counselling, and is told that his blood sample was anti-HCV-positive. His blood therefore cannot be used. Tim is astounded, and doesn't understand how he could have caught HCV infection.

Q What does the test result 'anti-HCV-positive' indicate?

A The presence of antibodies to HCV in Tim's blood means that at some time he has been infected with HCV. This result does not tell us whether he is still infected with the virus.

Q What questions should Tim be asked in order to shed light on how he may have become infected?

A As always, this kind of question requires an understanding of the routes of spread of the virus under consideration (see Table 28.1, Case 28).

HCV is present in the peripheral blood of chronically infected patients, and therefore the important questions to ask about risk factors are the following.

- Has Tim ever injected drugs?
- Has he ever received a transfusion of blood or blood products and, if so, when and in what country?
- Has he any tattoos or ear- or body-piercing?
- Has he had courses of acupuncture?

After some reflection, Tim remembers that he did experiment with injecting 'speed' when at University in the late 1970s, but he insists he only did this twice. He had a road traffic accident in 1998 in the UK that resulted in him receiving a transfusion, although he doesn't recall how many units were transfused. He has one tattoo, performed in a licensed parlour in 1994.

Q What is the most likely source of Tim's exposure to HCV?

A By far the most likely time of infection was in the late 1970s, when using injectable drugs. The epicentre of the current epidemic of HCV infection is amongst drug users—roughly 75% of all HCV-infected individuals in the UK give a positive history of injecting drugs. Tim may regard it as unlucky to acquire infection when only injecting on a small number of occasions, but unfortunately that may happen. The history of blood transfusion may raise eyebrows, but all donated blood in the UK has been screened for HCV (as indeed, Tim's was!) since late 1991, so a transfusion in London in 1998 is unlikely to be the source of infection. The tattoo may also be regarded with suspicion, but there are good epidemiological data that a history of tattoo performed by a professional tattooist is not a significant risk for HCV infection. This is reassuring evidence that messages about needle sterility have been acted on. Of course, 'home-brew' or 'amateur' tattoos will not necessarily be as safe.

Whether HCV can be transmitted sexually is controversial. It is impossible to state with certainty that it cannot be transmitted in this way, but this appears to be a very inefficient route for HCV, certainly in comparison with HBV, which is definitely a sexually transmitted infection. HCV can also be passed from

You must not give blood if:

- You think you need a test for HIV/AIDS or hepatitis.

You must never give blood if:

- You are HIV positive.

- You are a hepatitis B carrier.

- You are a hepatitis C carrier.

- You are a man who has **ever** had oral or anal sex with another man, even if you used a condom or other protective.

- You have **ever** received money or drugs for sex

- You have **ever** injected, or been injected with, drugs; even a long time ago or only once. This includes body-building drugs. **You may be able to give if a doctor prescribed the drugs. Please ask.**

You must not give blood for at least 12 months after sex (even if you used a condom or other protective) with:

- A partner who is, or you think may be:
  - HIV positive.
  - A hepatitis B carrier.
  - A hepatitis C carrier.

- (If you are a woman) a man who has **ever** had oral or anal sex with another man, even if they used a condom or other protective.

- A partner who has **ever** received money or drugs for sex.

- A partner who has **ever** injected, or been injected with, drugs; even a long time ago or only once. This includes body-building drugs. **You may be able to give if a doctor prescribed the drugs. Please ask.**

- A partner who has, or you think may have been, sexually active in parts of the world where HIV/AIDS is very common. This includes most countries in Africa. **There are exceptions, so please ask.**
Please read the next page

Fig. 29.1
Extract from blood donor leaflet.

mother to baby (i.e. vertical transmission), but again, this is very much less common (e.g. 5%) than with HBV-infected mothers (see Case 60).

Q In view of his history, should Tim have donated blood?

A No. The leaflet given to all potential blood donors (see Fig. 29.1) specifically asks those who have ever injected drugs to self-defer from donation. Tim's 'excuse' will be that he had no perception of himself as 'a druggie', having only injected a couple of times many years ago, and therefore he did not believe that that advice applied to him.

Q What are the chances that someone who is anti-HCV-positive is also a chronic carrier of HCV infection?

A Of 100 anti-HCV positive individuals, around 80 will be chronically infected. In comparison, only 5–10% of HBV-infected adults become chronic carriers; for HIV, we do not recognize a phenomenon of viral clearance—thus 100% of anti-HIV positive patients are believed to be chronically infected.

Q What further test should be performed to determine whether Tim is one of the lucky 20% who have cleared the virus?

A The most sensitive tests for HCV detection are genome (i.e. RNA) detection tests, e.g. by reverse transcriptase polymerase chain reaction (RT/PCR) or other genome amplification assays. Recently, a test for HCV core antigen (i.e. viral-derived protein) has been developed, and shows much promise as a cheaper, and more easily performed, alternative.

The following results are obtained from a repeat serum sample from Tim: anti-HCV, positive; HCV RNA (RT/PCR assay), positive. He is referred to the local hospital for further investigation.

Q What further tests should be performed?

A The results above confirm that Tim is chronically infected with HCV. This puts him at risk of progressive chronic inflammatory liver disease, leading ultimately to cirrhosis, and an increased

risk of primary hepatocellular carcinoma. Investigations should now focus on whether or not he has evidence of liver disease. Standard liver function tests (LFTs) would be a good place to start.

When seen in the clinic, Tim reports that he is in good health. He is on no medication, and drinks, on average, 10 pints of beer and 6–8 glasses of wine a week. The following results are obtained from the clinical chemistry laboratory:

bilirubin	7 mmol/l (normal, up to 17)
alanine aminotransferase (ALT)	32 IU/ml (normal, up to 50)
gamma-glutamyl transferase (GGT)	24 IU/ml (normal, up to 70)
alkaline phosphatase (AP)	43 IU/ml (normal, 40–120)

Q How should you interpret the above results?

A The liver function tests are all within the normal range.

Q In view of Tim's good health, and the normal LFT panel, is it necessary to consider any further investigations?

A Yes. Unfortunately, a single set of LFTs is not a reliable way of assessing the degree of liver damage in chronic HCV infection. The ALT is the best marker of disease activity (being an enzyme released by dead or damaged liver cells), but the natural history of chronic hepatitis C is one of flares and remissions over time so that, even in patients with severe underlying liver damage, it is possible that LFTs may be normal on occasion. There is as yet no serum marker that provides a reliable guide to the severity of underlying liver pathology.

Tim's apparent feeling of well-being is also not sufficient to rule out underlying liver pathology. Chronic HCV hepatitis is largely a clinically silent disease, until eventually the liver damage is so advanced that patients present with symptoms and signs of end-stage liver disease.

Q What factors influence the rate of progression of liver damage in chronic HCV infection?

A Increased age at infection is associated with faster disease progression. Most importantly, alcohol, a liver toxin, is a significant co-factor for disease progression. Regardless of anything else in Tim's management, he should be strongly advised to reduce his alcohol intake. Whether or not there is a 'safe' level of alcohol consumption in carriers of HCV infection is controversial. Ideally, Tim should stop altogether.

Q What further investigation should be discussed with Tim?

A The only way to be sure about the severity of liver damage in an HCV-infected patient is to perform a liver biopsy.

Tim undergoes a percutaneous liver biopsy. The pathology report reads: 'Microscopy: An adequate liver biopsy showing normal architecture. There is a moderate chronic inflammatory infiltrate in the portal tracts but no interface or lobular inflammation. No fatty change, fibrosis, or excess iron seen.'

Q Is there any treatment for chronic hepatitis C infection?

A Yes. Optimal current therapy consists of a combination of pegylated alpha-interferon (PEG-IFN) plus ribavirin. PEG-IFN is essentially a slow-release preparation of IFN given by once-weekly intramuscular injection, which results in evenly sustained serum levels of the drug.

Q What factors influence the response to antiviral therapy in chronic HCV infection?

A A number of large-scale clinical trials have identified several such factors. The likelihood of sustained clearance of infection is greater in:

- females
- patients under the age of 40
- patients without fibrosis evident on liver biopsy
- patients infected with non-genotype 1 virus
- patients with a low viral load

Q What is meant by the genotype of HCV?

A HCV 'isolates' are classified into genotypes and subtypes according to their degree of genome homology. Currently, six different genotypes of HCV have been well characterized. The pathogenicity of the different genotypes appears to be much the same, i.e. genotype does not influence degree of liver damage to any great extent. However, the response to current therapy is clearly different—patients with type 1 virus are much less likely to clear infection.

Q What are the disadvantages of antiviral therapy for chronic HCV infection?

A It has to be prolonged—6 months for non-genotype 1, 12 months for genotype 1 infection. It has side-effects, e.g. headaches, myalgia, 'flu-like illness', and depression from the IFN and haemolysis from

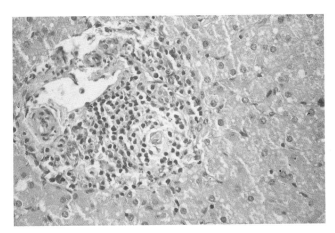

Fig. 29.2 Histology showing chronic inflammatory cell infiltrate in a portal tract.

the ribavirin. It is expensive. It is not always successful ('cure rates' are around 40% for genotype 1, 80% for non-1). At present, it is recommended only for patients with moderate to severe disease as indicated histologically (see Fig. 29.2).

Q Can HCV infection be prevented?

A There is no vaccine for HCV at present nor is there any preparation of antibodies that has been shown to be effective as passive immunization. Measures to reduce the spread of HCV infection include screening blood and tissue donors and public health measures to reduce injecting drug abuse *per se* and the sharing of needles amongst injecting drug users.

Q Does the screening of blood donors by anti-HCV and anti-HIV testing mean that there is no risk of acquiring HCV or HIV infection from a blood transfusion in the UK?

A Unfortunately no, although the risk in the UK is low, about 1 in a million. Infection with a virus is followed at an interval, known as the window period, by appearance of antibodies to that virus. For both HCV and HIV, the window period may be quite prolonged, e.g. up to 3 months. Thus, there is a risk that a blood donor will donate blood whilst in this period. If this happens, the donor checks out as being anti-HCV- or anti-HIV-negative, but the blood from that donor contains high titres of the virus and will transmit infection if transfused into a recipient.

Q Is there anything that can be done to reduce this risk?

A Yes. An alternative way of screening blood donors for HCV and HIV would be to use a test that identifies the virus itself in peripheral blood, rather than antibodies to the virus. Such a test could be an antigen or a genome detection test. Genome detection tests are more sensitive. The feasibility of nucleic acid testing (referred to as NAT) of blood donors is being explored in the UK, specifically for HCV. However, it should be borne in mind that the cost of NAT is considerable, and the risks of acquiring HCV from a blood transfusion are far smaller than many other serious potential adverse events arising from blood transfusion (e.g. bacterial infection, being given the wrong blood).

Summary: Chronic hepatitis C virus infection

Diagnosis

By detection of anti-HCV. Often performed as screening test, e.g. in blood donors, or in individuals who give a history of having injecting drugs

Further investigation

HCV RNA testing to determine whether infection is chronic; liver function tests; liver biopsy

Treatment

Pegylated interferon-alpha plus ribavirin combination therapy. Response rate dependent on age, sex, degree of liver fibrosis, viral genotype, and viral load

Case 30 Upper abdominal pain in Gareth, a 46-year-old sheep farmer

Gareth, a 46-year-old sheep farmer, complains of upper abdominal pain of increasing severity that has been present for about 1 month. Nausea, anorexia, and a general lassitude have recently affected his work. On examination Gareth is apyrexial and anicteric, with a pulse rate of 80/min. In the right upper abdominal quadrant there is a smooth and well circumscribed mass, which appears to be hepatic in origin.

Q What specific investigations are likely to be useful in determining the cause of this hepatic mass?

A The differential diagnosis includes neoplasia (primary hepatic, although relatively rare, and secondary), haemangioma, gall bladder disease, or an abscess. Also, one should not forget tuberculosis as a possible diagnosis in a patient who has been unwell for some weeks or months, even in the absence of a fever. Non-pulmonary tuberculosis can present in a variety of different and occult ways (see Case 52). Ultrasound, which is usually available and is non-invasive, should outline the nature of the mass and indicate whether it is cystic, solid, or fluid-filled. Computerized tomography (CT) or magnetic resonance imaging (MRI) scans may be required to confirm this.

Ultrasound showed a double-walled cystic lesion in the right lobe of the liver (see Fig. 30.1). The full blood count revealed an eosinophil count of 1.2×10^9/L.

Q What is the likely diagnosis?

A The appearance of this mass and the background history of sheep farming (herbivorous animals), together with a peripheral eosinophilia, is compatible with hydatid disease caused by the tapeworm *Echinococcus granulosus* (see Fig. 30.2).

Q The radiologist who performed the ultrasound examination offers to aspirate the contents of this cyst to confirm the diagnosis. The attending physician refuses. Why?

A Rupture of the cyst and spillage of the contents is a possible complication of this procedure, and severe systemic symptoms such as rigors and high fever may follow. Serological investigation for antibodies to *E. granulosus* using enzyme immunoassay (often only available in reference centres) should confirm the diagnosis. The Casoni skin sensitivity test rarely adds further to the diagnosis.

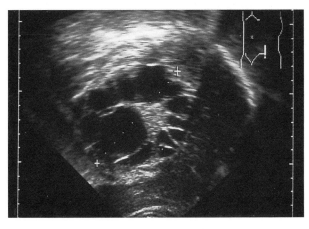

Fig. 30.1 Ultrasound of right lobe of liver showing double-walled cystic lesion (between the +s).

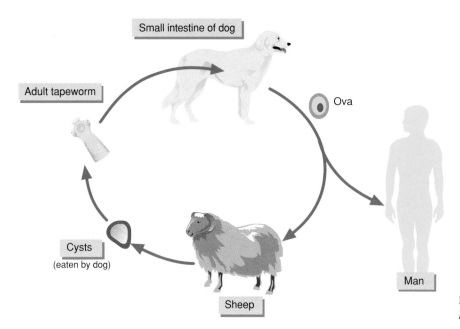

Fig. 30.2 Life cycle of *Echinococcus granulosus*.

Q Is surgical removal required?

A Unless the cyst is very large such that there are pressure effects or the patient is unresponsive to chemotherapy, surgical removal is not indicated. Most patients respond to albendazole or mebendazole which is administered for 6 weeks or more.

Q What other microbes cause liver abscesses?

A Most liver abscesses are pyogenic and caused by bacteria such as *Streptococcus anginosus* (see Cases 5 and 43), *Staphylococcus aureus*, and *Bacteroides* spp. and coliforms such as *Escherichia coli* originating from the large bowel (see Case 26). Fungal infections of the liver may also involve the spleen, and are usually found only in the severely immunocompromised, such as bone marrow transplant patients. *Entamoeba histolytica* (Fig. 30.3) liver involvement following amoebic colitis may occur in patients or travellers from endemic areas (see Box 30.1).

Box 30.1 Amoebic liver abscess

Clinical features

- Younger age group than those with pyogenic abscesses and usually a history of recent travel abroad
- Diarrhoea or colitis in 30–40%
- Point tenderness may be present

Investigations

- Eosinophilia in 80%
- Amoebae may be seen in biopsy of edge of abscess; rarely seen in aspirated fluid
- Rise in antibodies

Treatment

- Metronidazole and diloxanide furoate

Résumé for undergraduate students

The differential diagnosis of a mass in the liver is an important clinical scenario in medicine and infection is one of the causes of such a mass. Whilst a pyogenic abscess is the most common and likely infective cause, amoebic or hydatid infections should not be forgotten.

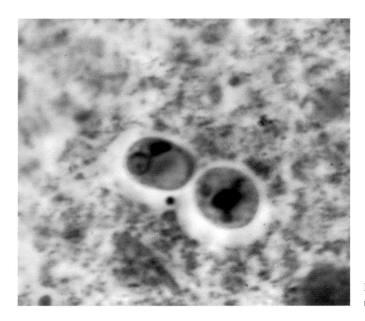

Fig. 30.3 Cysts of *Entamoeba histolytica* on microscopy of stool specimen.

Summary: Hydatid disease

Presentation
Abdominal mass/liver abscess; occupation may be relevant

Diagnosis
Ultrasound but not aspiration! Serology

Management
Albendazole, mebendazole; surgery occasionally

Case 31 Continuous non-bloody diarrhoea in Paul, a 35-year-old aid worker

Paul, a 35-year-old male aid worker who has spent the previous 6 months working in a refugee camp, becomes ill on taking a long flight from Lima, Peru to London. He complains of almost continuous non-bloody diarrhoea for the preceding 18–24 hours, nausea, and severe fatigue. On arrival in the airport health centre in London, he is apyrexial, dehydrated, drowsy, and has postural hypotension.

Q What additional information would be helpful in coming to a provisional diagnosis?

A The presence of abdominal pain and the passage of blood per rectum is very suggestive of a colitis or enteritis due to *Salmonella*, *Campylobacter*, or *Shigella* (dysentery). A history of similar symptoms from fellow passengers or aircraft crew might indicate an outbreak of toxin-mediated food poisoning caused by *Staphylococcus aureus*, *Bacillus cereus*, or *Clostridium perfringens* and a food history might point to the source and likely cause (see Case 23). Further information from the patient is required concerning the nature of his work in the refugee camp, the social conditions there, and whether colleagues have had similar symptoms.

Further questioning of Paul indicates that there has been minimal if any abdominal pain, and that he is now passing liquid non-bloody stools every 30–40 minutes. Before he left Lima he had been engaged for the last 2 weeks in fieldwork in the foothills of the Andes, where conditions had been primitive and water in short supply.

Q What is the likely diagnosis?

A The profuse watery diarrhoea without abdominal pain leading to marked dehydration is consistent with cholera (aetiological agent *Vibrio cholerae*; see Table 31.1). Cholera has been endemic in many parts of the world for some years, and spreads along trade and travel routes rather than by human carriage. Risk factors include drinking untreated or unboiled water and attendance at social events where food washed in untreated water may be consumed.

Q How does *V. cholerae* induce diarrhoea?

A The bacterium does not gain access to the bloodstream and never enters any tissue of the body. It replicates only in the small intestine following attachment, where it finds suitable conditions. There it elaborates an enterotoxin that acts

---

Table 31.1 *Vibrio cholerae*

- Motile Gram-negative curved bacillus
- Requires specific media but grows luxuriantly in alkaline medium, which is used to isolate it from stool specimens
- Causes diarrhoea by the production of an enterotoxin, whereas other *Vibrio* spp. such as *V. parahaemolyticus* are invasive
- Classic biotype replaced by El Tor in the 1960s and different serotypes, e.g. *Ogawa*, *Inaba* distinguished by somatic (O) antigens

---

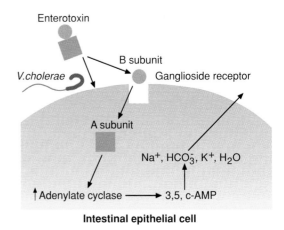

Intestinal epithelial cell

Fig. 31.1 Mechanism of action of cholera enterotoxin.

by stimulating adenylate cyclase (see Fig. 31.1), not unlike some of the toxins elaborated by *Escherichia coli* or *Salmonella*. The toxin's effects on water and electrolyte metabolism result in an alkaline environment, which in turn provides ideal growth conditions for the bacterium.

Q What is the management of cholera?

A Fluid replacement is the key to effective management and in severe cases this should be by the intravenous route. Lactated Ringer's solution or saline with added glucose and potassium may be used, with regular assessment of electrolytes, blood glucose, and acid balance. Antibiotics are believed to shorten the duration of diarrhoea but are not always necessary. Tetracyclines are the agents of choice, with co-trimoxazole, chloramphenicol, and quinolones as alternatives.

Q How may cholera be prevented?

A Improved sanitation, especially the separation of sewage from drinking water, reduces endemic disease. Untreated water and contaminated food (e.g. shellfish) or food washed in water should be avoided. Cholera, whether microbiologically confirmed or otherwise, should be notified and stool specimens forwarded to the laboratory accompanied by appropriate travel and other details, as culture for cholera is not routine in most UK laboratories. A phenol- and heat-inactivated parenteral vaccine is available but is only 50% protective, effective for no more than 3 months, and is not pro-

tective against *V. cholerae* 0139. It is indicated for travellers to endemic areas but is not useful for the control of outbreaks. An orally administered live recombinant vaccine is also available and is more efficacious than the inactivated vaccine but again does not protect against *V. cholerae* 0139.

Résumé for undergraduate students

Cholera is rare in temperate climates and confined to the returned traveller with diarrhoea. However, it is a major cause of morbidity and mortality in many other parts of the world and the pathogenic mechanism via adenylate cyclase is one of the best described for diarrhoea.

Summary: **Cholera**

Presentation
Continuous watery diarrhoea in a resident of an endemic or epidemic area or a returned traveller

Diagnosis
Culture of faeces on selective media (should be requested as not routine); urea and electrolytes to assess degree of dehydration

Management
Fluid replacement (e.g. saline with glucose and potassium); antibiotics (i.e. tetracyclines) sometimes necessary

Case 32 Winston, 68 years old, with nausea and vomiting

Winston, 68 years old, is admitted to hospital complaining of nausea and vomiting, colicky abdominal pain, and diarrhoea that has been present for a number of days. He has not been abroad recently, but up to his retirement 3 years ago he worked for the United Nations, travelling back and forth to South-east Asia. He lives with his wife, Edith, who is well. He suffered a myocardial infarction 8 years previously and chronic lymphocytic leukaemia was diagnosed 4 years ago, but he has since remained well on no medication. His physical examination is unremarkable.

Q What microbiological investigations should be instigated?

A Stool samples for culture should be sent to the microbiology laboratory for the diagnosis of gastro-enteritis caused by *Campylobacter*, *Shigella*, *Salmonella*, etc. and for microscopy to detect ova and parasites. Blood cultures should also be taken because his chronic leukaemia renders him immunosuppressed. If any food is incriminated this should also be analysed. Consideration should be given to non-infectious causes such as diverticulitis, inflammatory bowel disease, and bowel neoplasia, and appropriate investigations undertaken, e.g. ultrasound, colono-scopy, especially if the symptoms do not settle.

Forty-eight hours after admission, Winston develops rigors, a temperature of 39.5°C, and becomes cold, clammy, and hypotensive. He is immediately transferred to the intensive therapy unit (ITU) for resuscitation. Blood cultures subsequently grow *Escherichia coli*. Urine culture is sterile. The laboratory also reports seeing larvae in the second sample of faeces submitted.

Q What might these larvae be?

A Rhabditiform larvae of *Strongyloides stercoralis* were seen following concentration of faeces. This roundworm is endemic in the tropics but may be seen in temperate climates in institutions, where continuous self-infection may occur. Alternatively, it may be diagnosed in patients who have spent some time in the tropics (the organism is acquired from soil and is endemic in indigenous popu-lations) even some years previously, as in the case described here. In the immunosuppressed patient (e.g. those with leukaemia, lymphoma, or on corti-costeroids) there may be an interval of some years between the original infestation and presentation. The diagnosis is usually made by seeing larvae in the stool or by detecting a rise in antibodies by enzyme immunoassay (only available in reference laboratories).

Q Is there a connection between the strongyloidi-asis and the Gram-negative bacteraemia?

A Yes. Acute presentation as described here may also be accompanied by bacteraemia induced by gastrointestinal upset in the immunosuppressed host, and this may be fatal.

Q How is strongyloidiasis contracted and what are the common clinical presentations?

A Filariform larvae penetrate the skin, especially the soles of the feet, enter the bloodstream, migrate to the lungs, and eventually settle in the small intes-tine where they mature. This sequence takes about 2–3 weeks. The larvae may remain in the intestine for some years and, where personal standards of hygiene are poor, repeated autoinfection may occur. Patients with strongyloidiasis may present with:

- asymptomatic infestation (diagnosed on screen-ing)
- nausea, vomiting, diarrhoea, abdominal pain
- a malabsorption-type syndrome
- creeping skin eruptions occurring over many years
- pneumonitis with eosinophilia
- infestation accompanied by bacteraemia

Box 32.1 **Other helminths (worms) and the diseases they cause**	
Helminth	*Diseases/complications*
Nematodes (roundworms)	
Ascaris lumbricoides	Intestinal obstruction
Onchocerca volvulus	River blindness (onchocerciasis)
Wucheria bancrofti	Elephantiasis
Enterobius vermicularis (thread or pinworm)	Perianal irritation
Toxocara canis	Asthma, epilepsy, ocular lesions
Cestodes (tapeworms)	
Taenia solium (pigs)	Epilepsy from cystercisosis may occur
Echinococcus granulosus (dogs)	Hydatid disease with cysts (see Case 30)
Trematodes (flukes)	
Schistosoma spp.	Cystitis (bilharzias, see Case 39), gastrointestinal bleeding
Fasciola hepatica	Cholangitis, cholecystitis

Winston is successfully resuscitated in the ITU with intravenous fluids but does not require ventilation. The bacteraemia is treated with intravenous cefotaxime (see Case 47). Winston is also started on thiabendazole (or ivermectin), which is given for 3 days to treat the strongyloides, and follow-up stool samples are clear of larvae.

Q What is the most common roundworm infestation in the UK?

A *Ascaris lumbricoides* is probably the most common worm (helminth) encountered in temperate climates (see Box 32.1), and infestation is usually seen in children 3–8 years of age, who present with failure to thrive, bowel obstruction, or eosinophilia accompanied by respiratory symptoms. Piperazine is the treatment of choice.

Résumé for undergraduate students

Strongyloidiasis is a relatively uncommon infection in temperate climates but it is of some impor-

tance in the returned traveller or the immunocompromised host who may develop overwhelming infection. This and other helminth infestations are responsible for a wide variety of diseases and they should be included in the differential diagnosis of a variety of conditions affecting a number of systems.

Summary: Strongyloidiasis

Presentation
Usually acquired in the tropics, with symptoms of diarrhoea and abdominal pain. Occasionally overwhelming infection

Diagnosis
Larvae seen in faeces under microscopy; eosinophilia in blood count; and rise in antibodies

Treatment
Thiabendazole or ivermectin

Case 33 Maria's diarrhoea after discharge to nursing home

Maria Smith is a 78-year-old woman who is recovering from a partial colectomy in a community hospital. Three days after transfer from the local general hospital, her general practitioner has been called to see her because she has a low-grade fever (38.5°C) and some diarrhoea. She is tolerating oral fluids but is still somewhat weak.

Q Is there any other information you would like in attempting to make a diagnosis?

A Apart from details as to whether she has any other symptoms such as vomiting or dysuria, you would like to know details of any medications she may be on, especially those that may cause diarrhoea such as laxatives and digoxin, and whether or not she has recently been on nasogastric feeds, a not uncommon cause of diarrhoea in hospital. In addition, you need to know when and what antibiotics she was on at the time of her surgery.

Apart from a thiazide diuretic and occasional nonsteroidal anti-inflammatory drugs, Joan is on no other medications. She completed a course of co-amoxyclav on the day of discharge from hospital.

Q What investigations are indicated?

A A full blood count and urea and electrolytes will indicate whether there is a leucocytosis (suggestive of infection) and indicate if she is dehydrated. Blood cultures should also be taken even if she does not appear overtly septic, as in the elderly a high fever is not always present. A sample of faeces should also be sent to the laboratory.

Q What should the faeces be processed for?

A Normally, most routine laboratories will look for *Salmonella*, *Shigella*, and *Campylobacter* as these are the common causes of gastroenteritis in food poisoning. However, in the setting of a patient who

has recently been on antibiotics, analysis for *Clostridium difficile* toxins should also be requested.

Maria is given some fluids intravenously to augment her oral intake. Her investigations are normal apart from the presence of *C. difficile* toxin in the faeces.

Q Is the isolation of *C. difficile* sufficient to confirm a diagnosis of antibiotic-associated diarrhoea due to this organism.

A No. *C. difficile* commonly colonizes the bowel and only the demonstration of toxin production is sufficient evidence that the symptoms are due to this organism. Colonoscopy, which is not always indicated, may also be diagnostic of pseudomembranous colitis, which is most likely due to *C. difficile* (Fig. 33.1).

Q Is there any specific treatment for *C. difficile* diarrhoea?

A Discontinuation of antibiotics and oral or intravenous rehydration are often all that is required but, in the more ill patient, oral metronidazole is indicated. Metronidazole is preferred to oral vancomycin as it is cheaper and the frequent use of oral vancomycin encourages the emergence of vancomycin-resistant enterococci.

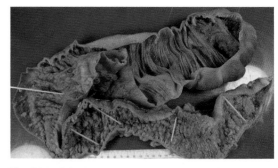

Fig. 33.1 Colonic mucosa (on post-mortem) characteristic of pseudomembranous colitis caused by *C. difficile*.

Q Is there any other measure that should be taken here and why?

A Maria should be moved to a side room to prevent the nosocomial spread of *C. difficile*. Patients with diarrhoea due to infective causes represent a risk to other patients, especially if the diarrhoea is frequent or explosive. As *C. difficile* can form spores and therefore persist for long periods in the environment, it is particularly important to ensure that the clinical area surrounding Maria is adequately clean and decontaminated with appropriate disinfectants.

Q What major complications may follow *C. difficile* infection?

A Toxic megacolon with perforation and overwhelming sepsis do sometimes occur as a complication of pseudomembranoues colitis (Fig. 33.2), especially if the diagnosis is delayed. Occasionally,

total colectomy is required as part of the management in such circumstances.

Q Is *C. difficile* confined to hospitals and nursing homes?

A No. Any patient who has received antibiotics, either for prophylaxis or treatment, is at risk of developing *C. difficile*-associated diarrhoea, but most cases seem to present in hospital. It may be that in the community, where patients are generally less ill, the disease is milder.

Q Which antibiotics are likely to cause *C. difficile* diarrhoea?

A Almost all antibiotics are capable of causing *C. difficile* diarrhoea but broad-spectrum agents that disrupt the normal bowel flora are especially likely (Table 33.1). Clindamycin, which was the first antibiotic described, is less commonly used in Europe than in the USA.

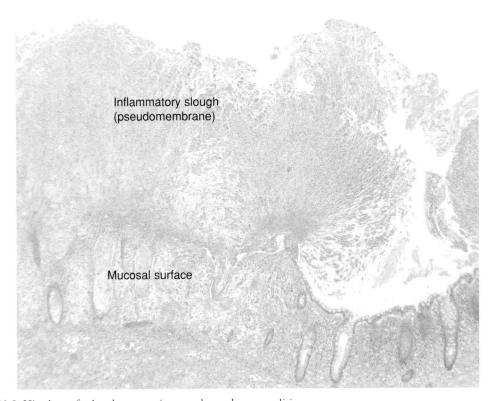

Inflammatory slough (pseudomembrane)

Mucosal surface

Fig. 33.2 Histology of colon demonstrating pseudomembranous colitis.

Table 33.1 Antibiotics commonly implicated in *C. difficile* diarrhoea

Clindamycin
Ampicillin/amoxycillin
Co-amoxyclav
Cefuroxime/cefotaxime
Others, e.g. tetracyclines, rifampicin, etc.

Q What strategies do you know of to prevent *C. difficile* diarrhoea?

A The intelligent and appropriate use of antibiotics is essential and includes the following.

- Only give antibiotics if really necessary: sometimes it is appropriate to carry out investigations and await results before starting antibiotics

- Use narrow-spectrum agents such as benzylpenicillin (if appropriate) and keep courses short. In hospital, most courses can be as short as 5–7 days

- Certain antibiotics are more prone to cause *C. difficile* diarrhoea than others, especially cephalosporins, and these should be avoided if possible (see Table 33.1).

- Also, symptomatic patients should be isolated and the patient's environment adequately decontaminated, especially if there is visible soiling; hand-washing, as ever, is essential between contacts with patients.

Summary: *C. difficile*-associated diarrhoea

Presentation

Diarrhoea in any patient on or recently on antibiotics, especially broad-spectrum agents

Diagnosis

Detection of *C. difficile* cytotoxin in stool or from isolate.

Management

Stop antibiotics (if possible) or change to narrow-spectrum agents; rehydrate, orally or intravenously; oral metronidazole

Complications

Perforation; megacolon

Self-assessment

1. Which one of the following viruses is not associated with acute diarrhoeal illness?

(a) Rotaviruses

(b) Enteroviruses

(c) Adenoviruses

(d) Caliciviruses

(e) Noroviruses

2. Which one of the following is not characteristic of disease caused by noroviruses?

(a) Can be diagnosed by electron microscopy of stools

(b) Vomiting

(c) Occurs commonly in both children and adults

(d) Jaundice

(e) An illness that lasts 24–48 hours

3. Match the following serological profiles with the most appropriate interpretation.

(a) IgG anti-HBcAg positive, HBsAg negative

(i) Highly infectious carrier of HBV

(b) IgG anti-HBcAg negative, anti-HBs positive

(ii) Responder to HBV vaccine

(c) IgM anti-HBcAg positive, HBsAg positive

(iii) Past HBV infection, cleared

(d) IgG anti-HBcAg positive, HBsAg positive

(iv) Past HBV infection, not cleared

(e) HBsAg positive, HBeAg positive

(v) Recent HBV infection

4. Which one of the following viruses is not transmitted by the enteric route?

(a) Hepatitis A virus

(b) Hepatitis C virus

(c) Hepatitis E virus

(d) Poliovirus

(e) Adenovirus 41

5. Which one of the following indicates a poor prognosis for the likelihood of response to therapy for chronic HCV infection?

(a) No fibrosis evident on liver biopsy

(b) Female sex

(c) Age 35 years

(d) Low viral load

(e) HCV genotype 1

6. Which one of the following statements regarding viral hepatitis is not true?

(a) The mortality from HEV infection is higher than that from HAV infection

(b) Fulminant hepatitis is more likely with HBV than with HCV infection

(c) The majority of individuals infected with HCV become chronic carriers

(d) HAV infection can be prevented by use of a subunit vaccine

(e) Individuals given HBV vaccine who fail to generate an anti-HBs response are not protected from HBV infection

7. Which one of the following species of salmonella is not a recognized cause of salmonella food poisoning in the UK?

(a) *Salmonella typhimurium*

(b) *Salmonella derby*

(c) *Salmonella enteridis*

(d) *Salmonella dublin*

(e) *Salmonella paratyphi*

8. In investigating an outbreak of food poisoning after a wedding banquet, what information is likely to be of greatest use in determining the likely source?

(a) The occupation of the guests

(b) The proportion of symptomatic and asymptomatic guests that ate each foodstuff

(c) The ambient temperature on the day of the wedding

(d) A list of all medications that the guests were on

(e) The cost per head of the meal from the caterers

9. Which one of the following is not an appropriate indication for the use of metronidazole?

(a) Anaerobic bacterial vaginosis

(b) Vaginal thrush

(c) Giardiasis

(d) Amoebiasis

(e) Surgical prophylaxis

10. What proportion of cases of traveller's diarrhoea is caused by enterotoxigenic *E. coli*?

(a) 10%

(b) 30%

(c) 50%

(d) 80%

(e) 90%

11. What are the predominant normal flora of the large intestine?

(a) Staphylococci

(b) Enterococci

(c) Anaerobic Gram-negative bacilli

(d) Coliforms such as *E. coli*

(e) Candida

12. Which one of the following statements about aminoglycosides, e.g. gentamicin, is correct?

(a) They have a wide therapeutic index

(b) They penetrate well into the cerebrospinal fluid (CSF)

(c) They are potent agents against aerobic Gram-negative bacilli

(d) Once-daily dosing has removed the need for routine assays of blood levels

(e) Tobramycin is significantly less toxic than gentamicin

13. Which one of the following investigations is most appropriate in confirming a diagnosis of enteric fever?

(a) Elevated C reactive protein (CRP)

(b) White cell count indicating a leucopenia

(c) Positive Widal test

(d) Positive skin test

(e) Blood cultures

14. Which antibiotic is most appropriate in the treatment of enteric fever caused by *Salmonella typhi*?

(a) Ampicillin

(b) Gentamicin

(c) Ciprofloxacin

(d) Vancomycin

(e) Flucloxacillin

15. Which one of the following is a well recognized cause of liver abscess?

(a) *Pseudomonas aeruginosa*

(b) *Giardia lamblia*

(c) *Entamoeba histolytica*

(d) *Coxiella burnetti*

(e) Beta-haemolytic streptococci, group B (*Strep. agalactiae*)

16. Which haematological feature is associated with parasitological infections or infestations?

(a) Leucopenia

(b) Lymphocytosis

(c) Atypical lymphocytes present on the blood film

(d) Thrombocytopenia

(e) Eosinophilia

17. Which laboratory feature is characteristic of *Vibrio cholerae*?

(a) Grows well in alkaline media

(b) Urease production

(c) Grows well on chocolate blood agar

(d) Lipase production

(e) Non-motile

18. What role do antibiotics have in the management of cholera?

(a) They prevent spread

(b) They shorten the duration of diarrhoea

(c) They treat subclinical bacteraemia or bloodstream infection

(d) They reduce the likelihood of prolonged faecal carriage

(e) They reduce the production of cholera enterotoxin

19. Through which pathogenic mechanism does *Clostridium difficile* cause diarrhoea?

(a) Mucosal tissue invasion

(b) Overgrowth of the bacterium in the bowel lumen

(c) Production of enterotoxin

(d) Subclinical bacteraemia or bloodstream infection with distal effects on the colon

(e) Stimulation of pancreatic enzymes

20. Which one of the following antibiotics is least likely to lead to antibiotic-associated diarrhoea caused by *C. difficile*?

(a) Piperacillin–tazobactam

(b) Moxifloxacin

(c) Benzylpenicillin

(d) Meropenem

(e) Ampicillin

4

CHAPTER 4

Genitourinary system

SECTION 4
Genitourinary system

Case 34 Gillian, a 23-year-old receptionist with frequency, dysuria, and haematuria

Gillian, a 23-year-old receptionist, has a 2-day history of frequency, dysuria, and slight haematuria. She also complains of suprapubic pain but there is no vaginal discharge. Six weeks previously her GP had prescribed ampicillin for 5 days for a similar episode, and the symptoms had gradually resolved. There is no other relevant previous history and physical examination is unremarkable.

Q What is the likely diagnosis and why?

A The symptoms as described above in a young woman are very suggestive of lower urinary tract infection (UTI) and, in particular, cystitis, i.e. infection of the bladder. A urethritis or cervicitis due to *Neisseria gonorrhoeae* or other sexually transmitted diseases would be characterized more by dysuria during the early part of micturition, and a discharge (see Case 36). Enquiries about changes in

(a)

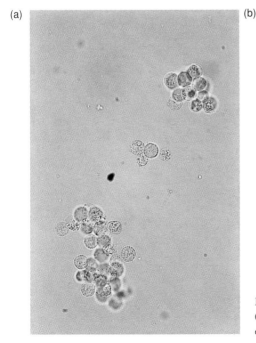

(b)

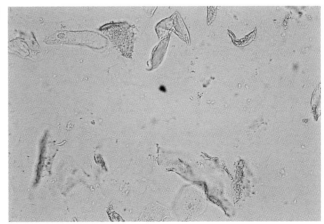

Fig. 34.1 Microscopy of: (a) infected urine with numerous 'pus' cells; (b) contaminated or poorly taken urine, i.e. not a true MSU, as indicated by squamous epithelial cells.

sexual habits or partners, however, should always be made with this type of presentation.

Q What are the possible complications of this infection?

A Symptoms such as frequency, dysuria, and haematuria are indicative of lower renal tract involvement. Infection of the kidney or renal pelvis is more likely to be accompanied by fever, vomiting, rigors, and perhaps abdominal or flank pain. Loin or renal angle tenderness is typical of pyelonephritis, which may be accompanied by bacteraemia.

Gillian's family doctor obtains a midstream urine specimen (MSU), which is cloudy, and sends it to the local microbiology laboratory for microscopy and culture before starting Gillian on trimethoprim for 5 days. The microscopy report on the urine is as follows: >100 white cells/mm^3; <10 red cells/mm^3; small numbers of epithelial cells seen (see Fig. 34.1).

Q What is the interpretation of the above microscopy report?

A Normally, urine has <5 white or pus cells/mm^3 and a count of 10–30/mm^3 may indicate early or partly treated infection. Large numbers of pus cells (>100/mm^3) are diagnostic of infected urine, although this may not occur if the patient is incapable of mounting a normal inflammatory response, as with neutropenia. The epithelial cells represent possible vulval or vaginal contamination and, consequently, culture may grow more than one organism or insignificant numbers of harmless skin flora. A Gram stain is not usually done for urine specimens as it does not add to the above or indicate the most appropriate therapy.

Q What pathogens most frequently cause urinary tract infection?

A Gram-negative bacilli such as *Escherichia coli* are the most common cause, as outlined in Table 34.1.

Culture of the urine grew a pure growth of >10^5/ml of *Staphylococcus saprophyticus* (Fig. 34.2) that, on sensitivity testing, was resistant to ampicillin, nitrofurantoin, cephradine, and nalidixic acid, but sensitive to trimethoprim (see Table 34.2). The patient's symptoms completely resolved after 2–3 days of the 5-day course of trimethoprim.

Q Could the isolation of a *Staphylococcus* here not represent skin contamination as indicated by the microscopy?

A No. The presence in pure growth of a recognized urinary pathogen, *S. saprophyticus*, is diagnostic here. *S. saprophyticus* is a coagulase-negative staphylococcus that is distinguished in the laboratory by intrinsic resistance to novobiocin, a rarely used antibiotic. It is second in importance to *Escherichia coli* as a cause of cystitis in young women (see Table 34.1). It is almost exclusively confined to women during the reproductive years, and there

Table 34.1 Aetiology of urinary tract infection (UTI)

Organism	Frequency (%)	Comment
Escherichia coli	> 50	Most common cause by far
Proteus spp.	10–15	Often associated with renal stones
Klebsiella spp.	10	Hospital/catheter-associated
Enterococci	8–10	Usually low-grade pathogens
S. saprophyticus	5–8	Confined to young women
S. epidermidis/aureus	2–6	Hospital/catheter-associated or bacteraemia (*S. aureus*)
Pseudomonas aeruginosa	4	Recurrent UTI or underlying pathology

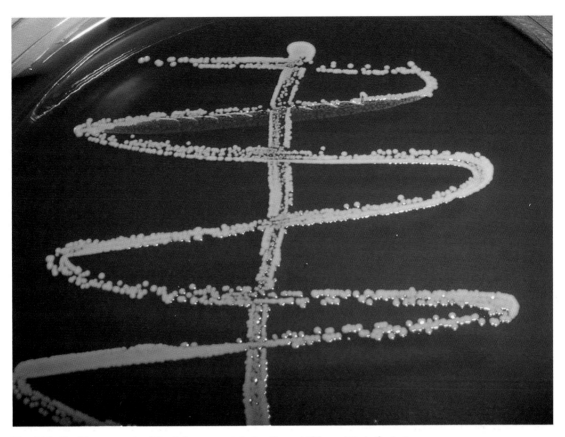

Fig. 34.2 Significant growth of *Staphylococcus saprophyticus* (i.e. > 10^5 bacteria/ml of urine).

Table 34.2 Commonly prescribed oral antibiotics to treat UTI

Antibiotic	Comment
Ampicillin	Most hospital and up to 50% of community isolates resistant. Should not therefore be used as empirical or 'blind' treatment
Trimethoprim*	Very useful agent to treat UTI in hospital and the community
Nalidixic acid	Early quinolone, urinary antiseptic. Poor against staphylococci and streptococci. Less frequently used now
Nitrofurantoin*	Useful agent and a urinary antiseptic. Inactive against *Proteus*
Co-amoxyclav	Effective against many ampicillin-resistant isolates
Cephalexin	As for co-amoxyclav
Cephradine	As for co-amoxyclav
Ciprofloxacin/levofloxacin	Second-line agent to treat complicated UTIs or more resistant organisms
Norfloxacin*	

* Preferred agents for antimicrobial prophylaxis before instrumentation or lithotripsy, or in recurrent infections or those associated with coitus.

appears to be a seasonal peak incidence in late summer and early autumn. Like most urinary pathogens it is acquired from the rectum and, although not sexually acquired *per se*, is associated with recent sexual intercourse or menstruation. Like many coagulase-negative staphylococci, such as *S. epidermidis*, *S. saprophyticus* is often resistant to β-lactam agents such as ampicillin and cephradine (Table 34.2).

Q Does Gillian warrant further investigation?

A No. Although urinary tract infection may occur as a result of underlying disease of the genitourinary tract, it is not uncommon in females and the recent episode described here probably represents relapse of an earlier infection, partially treated with ampicillin. High concentrations of many antibiotics are achieved in the urine as this is their route of excretion and, although the *S. saprophyticus* was resistant to ampicillin *in vitro*, some inhibition of growth is likely to have occurred; this, together with increased oral fluid intake leading to a dilution effect, ensured a temporary resolution in symptoms. The presentation and outcome described do not suggest complicated UTI, and consequently none of the factors necessary to merit further investigation are met (see Box 34.1).

Box 34.1 Indications for radiological investigations

Adults (intravenous urography (IVU) or ultrasound (US))

- First infection in men
- Recurrent infection or persistent symptoms
- Frank or persistent haematuria
- Unexpected pathogen
- Suspected renal abscess (US)

Children (US)

- All children require ultrasound investigation
- < 2 years: if US normal, cystoscopy and scintigraphy; if abnormal, IVU, micturating cystourethrography
- 2–10 years; if US normal, no further investigations; if abnormal, IVU and micturating cystourethrography

---

Q Do the symptoms and the microbiology results fulfil the criteria for the 'urethral syndrome'?

A No. This patient had a significant bacteriuria with a well recognized cause of urinary infection and there is nothing especially unusual about this episode. The features of the 'urethral syndrome' are outlined in Box 34.2.

Box 34.2 Urethral syndrome

Definition

Symptoms of dysuria and frequency in women during the reproductive years, without significant bacteriuria (i.e. < 10^5 bacteria/ml)

Possible causes

- Less common urinary pathogens, e.g. *Chlamydia trachomatis*, *Neisseria gonorrhoeae*, *Gardnerella vaginalis*, herpes simplex
- Conventional bacteria but with counts as low as 10^2/ml
- Fastidious bacteria such as lactobacilli, diphtheroids
- Non-infective, e.g. psychological factors, trauma from intercourse

---

Summary: Urinary tract infection

Presentation

Frequency, dysuria, and haematuria indicate lower tract infection. Fever, vomiting, rigors, and flank pain are more suggestive of upper renal tract involvement

Diagnosis

An MSU should reveal pyuria and a bacterial colony count of >10^5/ml. Lower counts may be seen in partly treated infection or less common causes, as seen in the urethral syndrome

Management

Increased fluid intake and an oral antibiotic or urinary antiseptic such as trimethoprim or nitrofurantoin. Ultrasound or intravenous pyelogram should be considered in children, men, and following recurrent episodes in women

Case 35 Joan's cloudy bag (This postgraduate case contains some undergraduate material.)

A 55-year-old woman, Joan, has chronic renal failure secondary to pyelonephritis and is on continuous ambulatory peritoneal dialysis (CAPD). She has noticed that the bag containing the dialysate has become cloudy in the past few days. She has also experienced some mild abdominal discomfort, but is apyrexial. She has no other abdominal or gastrointestinal symptoms.

Q What is the likely diagnosis?

A The dialysate bag is normally clear, but a cloudy bag in a patient on CAPD with or without abdominal symptoms is characteristic of CAPD peritonitis. CAPD has been widely used since the mid-1980s as a form of renal replacement, and is based upon hyperosmolar ultrafiltration across the peritoneal membrane. This is achieved by insertion of a Tenckhoff catheter (see Fig. 35.1), which is permanent and allows the continuous instillation of 1–2 l of dialysis fluid for 4–8 hours. Compared with haemodialysis it is more economical, does not require vascular access, entails fewer electrolyte restrictions, is less likely to be associated with elevated blood pressure, and ensures greater mobility for the patient.

Q How frequent is CAPD peritonitis and how does it arise?

A The rate of infection is around 1–1.5 episodes per patient per year, which is about half of what it was during the early years. This is a relatively low incidence, considering that there is permanent access to the peritoneal cavity and that this sealed system is broken about 1500 times a year. Infection may arise from the exit site, the tunnel through which the catheter passes (see Fig. 35.2), the peritoneum itself, or via the haematogenous route. The latter two sources are relatively infrequent.

Q How may the diagnosis be confirmed?

A A sample of fluid should be sent to the laboratory for microscopy and culture or, if this cannot be done immediately, the fluid should be refrigerated. A cloudy bag usually contains >100 pus cells/mm^3, predominantly polymorph neutrophils. The Gram stain is relatively insensitive in detecting microorganisms and consequently culture is essential to confirm an aetiological diagnosis. Samples of fluid are incubated aerobically and anaerobically after centrifugation and enrichment to maximize the yield from culture.

Pending the results of culture and sensitivity testing, Joan's renal physician prescribes intraperitoneal cefuroxime and vancomycin

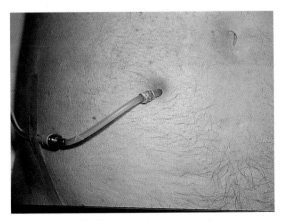

Fig. 35.1 Tenckhoff catheter inserted into the abdomen.

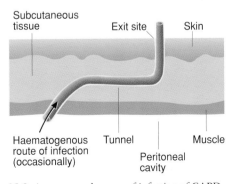

Subcutaneous tissue

Exit site   Skin

Haematogenous route of infection (occasionally)   Tunnel

Peritoneal cavity   Muscle

Fig. 35.2 Anatomy and source of infection of CAPD.

(administered in the dialysis fluid), and follow-up is arranged. In the peritoneal fluid 250 white cells/mm^3 are seen and *Staphylococcus epidermidis* (the most common aetiological agent), sensitive to vancomycin but resistant to cefuroxime, is isolated. The cefuroxime is discontinued and over the next few days the bag becomes less cloudy and her symptoms resolve.

Q What local factors contribute to staphylococcal peritonitis?

A Considerably fewer bacteria are required to cause CAPD than surgical peritonitis. The presence of the catheter results in the formation of a biofilm on the surface, composed of extracellular slime that protects organisms from the body's host defences such as mononuclear cells and that inhibits penetration by antibiotics. The low pH and relatively high osmolarity of CAPD fluid will also suppress the activity of these cells in the dialysate.

Q What is the success rate for the treatment of CAPD peritonitis with first-line antimicrobial agents?

A The conventional approach to the management of uncomplicated CAPD peritonitis before the results of culture are available is usually intraperitoneal vancomycin plus an aminoglycoside but, if symptoms are more severe, a loading dose of an intravenous antibiotic is administered. This approach is successful in approximately 80% of cases. Antibiotic treatment should be modified following antimicrobial sensitivity results, and it is possible to subsequently administer the aminoglycoside to alternate bags rather than to each bag.

Occasionally, it is necessary to remove the Tenckhoff catheter if infection persists or relapses, if there is an associated tunnel infection, or if infection is caused by fungi or *Pseudomonas*, both of which are difficult to eradicate. The newer quinolone antibiotics have been used recently because they may be administered orally and achieve excellent intraperitoneal levels.

Six months later, after making a full recovery from the first episode, Joan becomes seriously ill with vomiting, severe abdominal pain, cloudy dialysate, and a temperature. This time she is admitted to hospital and *Escherichia coli* and *Bacteroides fragilis* are isolated from her dialysis fluid.

Q What is the significance of these two organisms compared with *S. epidermidis*?

A Skin organisms such as *S. epidermidis* are most frequently implicated in CAPD peritonitis (see Table 35.1). Coliforms and other gut flora are less common, but when they occur they often reflect

Table 35.1 **Organisms most frequently implicated in CAPD peritonitis**

Organism	Frequency (%)	Comment
Coagulase-negative staphylococci	45	*S. epidermidis* in 80%
Staphylococcus aureus	15	Associated with tunnel infections
Streptococci	12	Include enterococci
Escherichia coli	8	Consider bowel perforation
Other coliforms	5	Consider bowel perforation
Pseudomonas aeruginosa	4	Tunnel infection and abscesses
Diphtheroids	2	Relapse common
Fungi	2	*Candida albicans* most frequent
Miscellaneous	7	

intraabdominal pathology, such as a perforated viscus. Consequently, investigation and management should be as for surgical peritonitis (see Case 26) and include abdominal X-rays, ultrasound, surgical consultation, and possibly a laparotomy.

Following investigation, diverticulitis with localized abscess formation is diagnosed, which requires removal of the catheter, surgical resection, and drainage. Following a course of intravenous gentamicin, ampicillin, and metronidazole, Joan makes a full recovery but, because of distortion to the peritoneum arising from the surgical peritonitis, she is unable to go back on peritoneal dialysis and is haemodialysed instead until she can undergo renal transplantation.

Q What measures may be taken to minimize CAPD infection?

A Strategies to prevent infection very much depend on the patient and the attention that he or she gives to the procedure of changing bags. It also involves:

- insertion of the Tenckhoff catheter by an experienced surgical team who carry out the procedure regularly
- training of patients in the cleaning and dressing of the exit site and the application of occlusive dressings. Patient motivation is all-important
- eradication of nasal carriage with mupirocin where *S. aureus* infection recurs

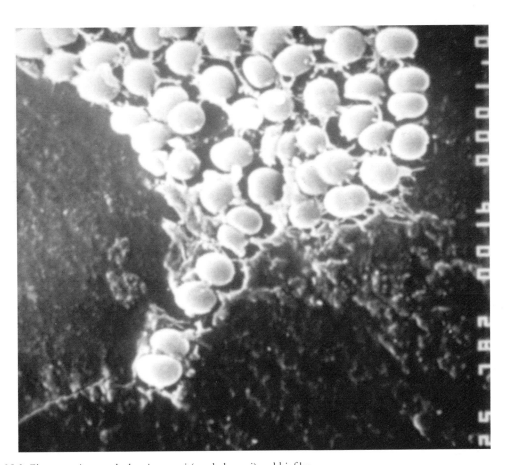

Fig. 35.3 Electron micrograph showing cocci (staphylococci) and biofilm.

- development of improved catheter materials that inhibit the adhesion of bacteria and the formation of biofilms, and the incorporation of antimicrobial agents in the catheter

- there may be a place in some cases for the use of filters, routine alcohol rinses, or prophylactic antibiotics.

Q When are coagulase-negative staphylococci, especially *S. epidermidis*, important as pathogens?

A These skin bacteria are likely to cause infection whenever foreign bodies are inserted into the bloodstream or a body cavity. These include intra-vascular catheters (peripheral, arterial, and central) and prosthetic joints (see Box 35.1). The ubiquitous distribution of these bacteria, their resistance to multiple antibiotics, the production of extra-cellular slime resulting in biofilm formation (see Fig. 35.3), and problems with typing that hamper our understanding of their epidemiology make the prevention and treatment of infection especially difficult.

Q What are the risk factors for intravascular catheter infections?

A These include:

- inexperience or poor technique by the operator

- insertion of central rather than peripheral catheters

- insertion during an emergency, e.g. cardiac arrest

- duration of catheterization, especially if longer than 3–4 days

Many intravascular devices become infected during insertion, but infection may also arise from contaminated infusates (rare now but implicated previously in outbreaks of *Citrobacter* spp. bacteraemia) and contamination of hubs or giving-set junctions.

Résumé for undergraduate students

Peritonitis associated with CAPD is confined to patients with end stage renal disease requiring renal replacement therapy. The most common cause is coagulase-negative staphylococci, also the commonest cause of device-related infections, which are associated with biofilm formation. Many device-related infections require the removal of the device as antibiotic therapy alone is often unsuccessful.

Box 35.1 Important infections caused by coagulase-negative staphylococci

- Bacteraemia: common organism (see Case 47)

- Endocarditis: 5% of native and 40% of prosthetic valve infection

- CSF shunt: 50% of infections. Diphtheroids increasing in importance

- Prosthetic joint: 30% of infections; usually introduced at time of surgery

- Vascular grafts: 60% of infections, e.g. aortofemoral

- Urinary tract infection: *S. saprophyticus* in young women (see Case 34)

Summary: CAPD peritonitis

Presentation
Cloudy bag or dialysate. Frank abdominal pain less a feature than with surgical peritonitis

Diagnosis
>100 pus cells/mm^3 and bacteria grown from fluid after centrifugation or enrichment. *S. epidermidis* the most common cause

Management
Intraperitoneal antibiotics. Removal of catheter rarely required

Case 36 Elizabeth, a 28-year-old prostitute, attends the clinic for a check-up

Elizabeth, 28 years old, attends the genito-urinary medicine clinic for a check-up. She has recently started work in a 'massage parlour', and it is the policy of the owner to ensure all 'girls' attend for regular assessment. She has no relevant past medical history and is not on any regular medication apart from the oral contraceptive pill. Her last menstruation was 2 weeks ago. She has noticed a whitish vaginal discharge, not very profuse, over the past couple of days, but no other symptoms related to the genitourinary tract, in particular, no dysuria or vaginal irritation. On examination, the vaginal walls do not look inflamed, although there is a small amount of purulent material visible. On passing a speculum, a mucopurulent discharge is seen coming from the cervix.

Q What is your provisional diagnosis?

A Elizabeth has a mucopurulent cervicitis. The vaginal discharge has presumably arisen from the cervix. The absence of vaginal irritation or signs of vaginal wall inflammation support this hypothesis.

Q What organisms may cause this condition?

A Mucopurulent cervicitis may arise from infection with *Neisseria gonorrhoeae* (see Box 36.1) or *Chlamydia trachomatis* strains D–K (see below). Herpes simplex virus may also infect the cervix, resulting in a profuse mucopurulent discharge, especially during a primary attack of genital herpes (see Case 37), but the absence of visible ulceration makes this diagnosis less likely.

Q What investigations should you perform?

A A cervical smear should be Gram-stained. Gonococci may be seen as intracellular Gram-negative diplococci (see Fig. 36.1). A swab for culture for *N. gonorrhoeae* should preferably be plated out on appropriate media in the genitourinary medicine (GUM) clinic (the organism is fragile and may not survive prolonged storage prior to plating out).

A further cervical swab, together with a urethral swab, for chlamydia diagnosis should also be taken.

Q How will the laboratory attempt to confirm infection with *C. trachomatis*?

A Although chlamydia are classified as bacteria, they do not grow on inanimate media. Isolation can be attempted in cell culture, where the replicating organisms produce large inclusion-bodies, the presence of which can be demonstrated by appropriate staining, but this is time-consuming and labour-intensive and has largely been superseded by other, more rapid, diagnostic approaches. Antigen detection by enzyme-linked immunosorbent assay (ELISA) or by staining with fluorescently labelled monoclonal anti-chlamydia antibodies are two popular alternatives. Ideal samples for these techniques

---

Box 36.1 *Neisseria gonorrhoeae*

- Gram-negative intracellular diplococcus
- Males: usually symptomatic, with involvement of urethra (profuse purulent discharge + dysuria), anus and rectum, pharynx (from oral sex), prostate, epididymis, and testes
- Females: often asymptomatic, with involvement of endocervix, urethra, rectum, pharynx. May cause pelvic inflammatory disease (see Box 36.4)
- Neonates: ophthalmia neonatorum—a severe purulent conjunctivitis shortly after birth, due to acquistion of infection on passge through an infected birth canal (see Case 61)
- Bacteraemia may occur (more common in females), with involvement of skin and joints
- Diagnosis by smear and culture (see Fig. 36.1)
- Antibiotic treatment: depends on knowledge of local resistance patterns as penicillin resistance is no longer uncommon, and not always due to β-lactamase production. Examples include single high dose of amoxicillin plus probenecid; single dose of a quinolone (e.g. ciprofloxacin)

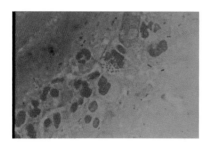

Fig. 36.1 Intracellular Gram-negative diplococci.

are an endocervical swab (females) or a urethral swab (males). However, as in many other areas of diagnostic microbiology, molecular techniques involving genome amplification are becoming the norm for diagnosis. Their exquisite sensitivity means that chlamydial DNA can be detected in urine, which is a much easier (and less painful!) specimen for the patient to provide.

Q Should you offer Elizabeth any other tests?

A All new female patients attending a GUM clinic, regardless of sexual proclivity, should be offered:

- serological screening for syphilis (see Box 36.2)
- cervical smear for cytology if due or clinically indicated
- cervical smear and culture for *N. gonorrhoeae* and swab for *C. trachomatis* detection
- vaginal smear, culture, or wet prep as clinically indicated (see below)
- throat and/or rectal cultures for *N. gonorrhoeae* dependent on sexual history
- urinalysis
- tests for HIV and hepatitis B virus infection if clinically indicated

Q What investigations are routine for new male patients attending the GUM clinic?

A New male patients should be offered:

- syphilis screening
- microscopy and urinalysis of initial voided urine

- urethral smear and culture for *N. gonorrhoeae* and swab for *C. trachomatis* detection if symptomatic or at high risk for these infections
- tests for HIV and hepatitis B virus infection if clinically indicated

---

Box 36.2 Syphilis

Causative agent

- *Treponema pallidum*, a spirochaete

Stages of disease

- Primary: painless, indurated ulcer ('hard' chancre) usually in genital area
- Secondary: 6–8 weeks later; fever, headache, widespread rash, generalized lymphadenopathy, ± mucosal mouth ulcers and wart-like lesions (condylomata lata) in moist warm sites
- Latent: may then ensue, and last several years
- Tertiary: includes granulomatous lesions or gummata at various sites (e.g. skin, bones, joints)
- Quaternary: involves the cardiovascular (e.g. aortic aneurysm) and central nervous systems (tabes dorsalis, general paralysis of the insane)
- Congenital syphilis: in offspring of infected mothers

Diagnosis

- Screening is via the detection of specific treponemal antibodies using standard ELISA formats. The presence of specific IgM indicates recent infection. Alternatively, there are a number of non-specific screening tests based on cardiolipin or reagin (e.g. WR, VDRL, RPR), which would require confirmation with specific treponemal tests (e.g. TPPA, FTA)
- Dark-ground microscopy may demonstrate organism in exudate from chancre, mucous ulcers, condylomata lata, but not in later stages of disease

Treatment

- High-dose penicillin (or doxycycline or erythromycin), with appropriate serological follow-up to confirm cure

For patients of either sex, HIV serology may be offered if appropriate after pre-test counselling and consent (see Case 38). Similarly, those at risk of HBV infection should be offered HBV serology and, if negative for both HBsAg and anti-HBcAg (see Case 28), a course of vaccination.

Patients such as Elizabeth, who are at continued risk of acquisition of sexually transmitted diseases, will require screening at regular intervals for all of the above.

Q What treatment should you offer Elizabeth at this stage?

A If the cervical smear is positive for Gram-negative diplococci, you should treat her for gonorrhoea (see Box 36.1) and also for a presumptive chlamydial infection (e.g. with a 7-day course of doxycycline (not if pregnant) or single dose of azithromycin), as the two infections can often co-exist. If the smear is negative, you should treat the presumptive chlamydial infection only.

Q What are the other principles of management of a patient with a sexually transmitted disease (STD)?

A These include:

1. *Contact tracing.* Treating the patient with antibiotics is only half the battle. In simple terms, 'it takes two to tango'! Identification and tracing of all contacts of patients with an STD is a vital function of the clinic. Contacts should be advised to attend the clinic in person, when appropriate counselling, testing, and treatment can be offered.

2. *Prevention of infection.* The most effective method is the use of barrier methods of contraception (i.e. condoms and diaphragm), the use of which should be encouraged.

3. *Education.* It is important that any patient with an STD should appreciate that they are potentially infectious and that they should therefore abstain from sexual intercourse until their infection has been appropriately treated. In addition, teenage children should be made

aware of STDs and how to avoid them by appropriate teaching in the school setting.

Elizabeth's cervical smear, examined in the clinic, shows many polymorphs, but no organisms are seen. You prescribe a 1-week course of doxycycline, and counsel Elizabeth about the risks of spreading her infection, advising her to abstain from sexual intercourse for 7 days. You ask her to return to the clinic in 2 weeks time. The cervical swab from Elizabeth is reported as 'chlamydia antigen, positive'. At her return visit to the clinic, speculum examination reveals a normal cervix.

Q Are any further actions warranted?

A Yes. You should make a posttreatment assessment of compliance with the antibiotics, and of the success or otherwise of the contact tracing. The risk of re-infection from an untreated partner should be stressed.

Q What clinical syndromes are associated with genital *C. trachomatis* infection?

A These include:

- Non-specific urethritis (NSU; see Box 36.3)
- Prostatitis or epididymitis
- Mucopurulent cervicitis (this case)
- Pelvic inflammatory disease (see Box 36.4)
- Reiter's syndrome (triad of arthritis, conjunctivitis, NSU, usually in HLA B27-positive individuals; see Case 69)
- FitzHugh–Curtis syndrome (right upper quadrant pain due to perihepatitis). High titres of antibodies to *C. trachomatis* may be diagnostic
- Trachoma inclusion conjunctivitis (infection of neonate acquired on passage through infected birthcanal; see Case 61)
- Infertility (in females; there may not be a history of symptomatic infection)

Elizabeth returns to the clinic at regular intervals for routine checks. At one such visit, she complains of a thin, smelly vaginal discharge.

Q What are the common causes of a vaginal discharge?

A Candidosis, trichomoniasis, and 'bacterial vaginosis' (see Boxes 36.5–36.7).

Box 36.3 Non-specific urethritis (NSU)

- Previously known as non-gonococcal urethritis (NGU); most common STD in UK
- Urethral symptoms (dysuria, mucopurulent discharge); usually only in males
- Causative organisms include *C. trachomatis* (30–60%), certain strains of ureaplasma and mycoplasma, e.g. *M. genitalium* (20%), and possibly *Trichomonas vaginalis*
- May coexist with gonococcal urethritis
- In asymptomatic patients, presence of polymorphs (> 5 per high power field) in urethral smear or initial-voided urine may indicate urethritis
- Treatment: a tetracycline or erythromycin. Relapse may occur

---

Box 36.4 Pelvic inflammatory disease (PID)

- Presentation: lower abdominal pain and tenderness (± peritonism), dyspareunia, pelvic pain and tenderness (± mass *per vaginam*), mucopurulent cervicitis, and fever
- Differential diagnosis: appendicitis, ectopic pregnancy, tubo-ovarian abscess, urinary tract infection
- Causative organisms: *N. gonorrhoeae, C. trachomatis*, coliforms, and streptococci; anaerobes
- Management: varies from outpatient antibiotics to cover chlamydia and anaerobes (e.g. a tetracycline, and metronidazole) to urgent admission to hospital for laparotomy and drainage. Partner should be investigated and treated accordingly

---

Box 36.5 Vaginal candidosis

- Causative agent: *Candida albicans* (a yeast). May be part of normal flora of gastrointestinal tract, and thus not necessarily a sexually transmitted disease
- Predisposing factors include diabetes mellitus, oral contraceptives, pregnancy, broad-spectrum antibiotics, steroid therapy
- Presents with profuse white vaginal discharge and vaginal itching. Diffuse erythema extending to vulva seen on examination
- Diagnosis by clinical history and presentation, vaginal smear (budding yeasts and pseudomycelium seen), and/or swab of exudate cultured on Sabouraud's medium
- Treatment with topical clotrimazole, miconazole, or oral fluconazole or itraconazole
- Attacks may recur. Consider treatment of sexual partner, if he is symptomatic

---

Box 36.6 Trichomoniasis

- Causative agent: *Trichomonas vaginalis*, a protozoan
- Presents with thin yellowish discharge with an offensive smell ± irritation, dysuria. Punctate erythema and abundant discharge seen on examination
- Diagnosis by microscopy of vaginal wet preparation. Difficult to culture
- Treatment with metronidazole or tinidazole for both patient and partner

Box 36.7 Bacterial vaginosis (also known as non-specific vaginitis; this is not a sexually transmitted disease)

- Causative agents: a heterogeneous mix of anaerobes, *Gardnerella vaginalis*, mycoplasmas
- Presents with scanty but offensive smelling discharge
- Diagnosis: vaginal pH > 5 (normal < 4.5), positive amine test, vaginal smear shows 'clue' cells—epithelial cells coated with Gram-variable bacteria—and absence of lactobacilli
- Treatment: metronidazole
- Recurrence of symptoms is common

Summary: Sexually transmitted diseases

Presentation

May be asymptomatic (especially in females); vaginal, cervical, or penile discharge; frequency and dysuria; pelvic pain, dyspareunia; genital ulceration

Diagnosis

Urethral and cervical smears; vaginal, urethral, cervical swabs for appropriate culture; vaginal wet prep; serology; urinalysis

Management

Antibiotic therapy where appropriate; contact tracing; education and encouragement of safe sex practices; regular screening of the sexually promiscuous (e.g. prostitutes)

Case 37 Sharon, a 24-year-old personnel manager with a blistering genital rash

Sharon, a 24-year-old personnel manager, attends the genitourinary medicine (GUM) clinic in great distress. She has developed several painful blisters in and around her vagina over the past 72 hours. She complains that passing urine is excruciatingly painful, and she is also finding it difficult to walk. On examination, Sharon is febrile (38°C) and looks generally unwell. Painful inguinal lymphadenopathy is noted bilaterally. The appearance of the external genitalia is shown in Fig. 37.1. A mucopurulent cervical discharge is seen on speculum examination, and there are ulcers visible on the cervix (Fig. 37.2).

Q What is the diagnosis?

A Sharon has an extensive blistering rash. Ulcers can be seen, where the roofs of the blisters have been eroded. These lesions are typical of herpes simplex virus (HSV) infection. The systemic manifestations (fever, malaise), bilateral lymphadenopathy, and widespread distribution of the lesions, including spread on to the adjacent skin of the thigh, are typical of a primary attack (the classification of HSV infections is discussed in Case 4).

Q How would you confirm your diagnosis?

A By sending vesicle fluid or a swab of an ulcer base to the virology laboratory for virus isolation. HSV grows readily in cell culture in 24–48 hours. Alternatively, electron microscopy of vesicle fluid will demonstrate the presence of herpesvirus particles or direct immunofluorescence can be performed by staining cells from the ulcer base with appropriately labelled monoclonal antibodies.

Q What complications may arise from an attack of primary genital herpes?

A These include:

- lesions near to urethra/urethral meatus may lead to acute urinary retention

- sacral nerve root involvement may also lead to urinary and/or faecal retention

- spread to lumbosacral meninges leading to meningitis

- local extension to cervix (cervicitis) and, rarely, uterus and Fallopian tubes, leading to pelvic inflammatory disease

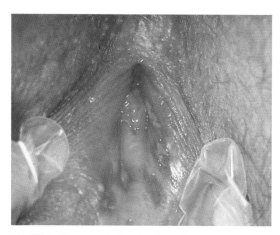

Fig. 37.1 Ulcerative lesions in the vagina.

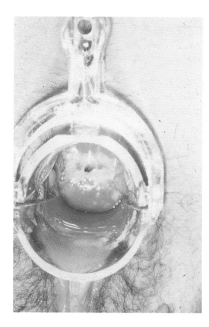

Fig. 37.2 Cervix with ulcers and discharge.

Q How should you manage this patient?

A Primary genital herpes is a clear indication for antiviral therapy—without treatment, this severe, debilitating illness may continue for 2–3 weeks. Whilst oral therapy on an outpatient basis may suffice for many patients, the extent of Sharon's attack warrants admission to hospital.

You admit Sharon to hospital and initiate intravenous aciclovir therapy. Within 48 hours, her fever subsides, she feels much better, and no new lesions have appeared. However, when you next visit her on the ward, her husband of 5 years, Jason, demands to see you, wanting to know how his wife acquired her infection. He has never had genital herpes, and therefore he believes that she must be having an extramarital affair. Sharon steadfastly denies this—and you are convinced she is telling the truth.

Q How then, might Sharon have acquired the infection?

A There are two possibilities. Firstly, Jason may suffer from cold sores, i.e. recurrent orolabial herpes. These lesions contain high titres of infectious virus, which can be passed to the genital area of a sexual partner either by orogenital sex, or by direct inoculation via contaminated fingers. Although orolabial herpes is usually due to infection with HSV-1, and genital herpes due to HSV-2, both viruses can infect at either site, and primary genital infection with HSV-1 is clinically indistinguishable from that due to HSV-2.

Secondly, despite the absence of previous symptoms, Jason may nevertheless have acquired genital herpes, possibly many years ago, with an asymptomatic primary infection. Virus will have spread to his sacral ganglia, where for the most part it will exist in a latent state, but may reactivate from time to time. Such recurrent attacks, which are also likely to be subclinical, will give rise to infectious virus on his external genitalia, leading to transmission to his wife.

Genital HSV infection is an emotionally charged subject, and the emergence of disease in one part-

---

Box 37.1 Epidemiology of HSV-2 infection

- Seroepidemiological studies indicate that 15–25% of the adult population has evidence of HSV-2 infection
- Less than 25% of anti-HSV-2 positive individuals give a history of symptomatic genital herpes (see also Case 63)
- Asymptomatic shedding from anti-HSV-2-positive individuals without a positive history is usually of low titre, and transient (e.g. 24 hours only). Recent evidence suggests a transmission rate of 10% per year to uninfected partners.

---

ner of an apparently monogamous couple, such as described here, inevitably raises suspicions. Jason may not take kindly to being told that he does, after all, have HSV infection, and may also find the suggestion that he has passed this on to his partner after 5 years of monogamy faintly ludicrous. It may be as well to re-iterate the salient data on which this conclusion is based (see Box 37.1).

Jason and Sharon accept your explanations and, after 72 hours of intravenous therapy, Sharon is discharged with a further 7 days of oral valaciclovir. On her return to clinic 2 weeks later, although physically well, she bursts into tears, and after much coaxing, explains that she is afraid her life will be blighted by painful recurrent attacks of genital herpes.

Q What are the risks of recurrent disease?

A These are:

- Having acquired the virus, she will indeed carry it for the rest of her life (prompt antiviral therapy does *not* prevent HSV latency)
- She may suffer recurrences, but it is impossible to predict their frequency, which may vary from none to one every 3–4 weeks, even in immunocompetent individuals. The basis for this variability in the virus–host relationship is not understood

Q Are recurrent attacks likely to be as severe as the primary attack?

A No. Recurrences are less severe; systemic manifestations are rare; the number of lesions will be dramatically less; the lesions will be localized (usually unilateral, no spread to adjacent skin, cervical lesions in 5% cases only); the average time to healing is 6–7 days.

Despite your reassurances about the milder nature of recurrent disease, Sharon is still worried in case she falls into the category of having very frequent recurrences.

Q Is there any management strategy that can improve the lot of such individuals with frequent recurrences?

A Yes, prophylactic antiviral therapy (i.e. aciclovir or derivatives). Continuous low-dose therapy for months at a time dramatically reduces the frequency of attacks. Breakthrough attacks may occur, but are usually mild and infrequent. Unfortunately, attacks return on cessation of therapy, at the same frequency as before. Many patients in the USA have now been on such regimens for a number of years, without ill effects.

Q Is there a potential drawback to such a strategy?

A An initial worry was that continuous therapy would lead to the emergence of drug-resistant mutants. Although such mutants have been described, their occurrence is rare in an immunocompetent host, and most are of reduced pathogenic potential and therefore not a clinical problem. The one setting where fully virulent mutants may emerge is in immunosuppressed patients (e.g. those with HIV infection).

Sharon's final anxiety concerns the effect her genital herpes may have should she become pregnant, but I reassure her on that point (see Case 63).

Q Many patients attending GUM clinics have much less florid disease than Sharon, e.g. solitary ulcers. What is the differential diagnosis of genital ulceration?

A The common causes of ulceration confined to the genital area are genital herpes, chemical burns from disinfectants, trauma (including excoriation of marked acute candidal vulvitis), pyogenic infection, and fixed drug eruption

Other causes include:

- syphilis (primary chancre, see Case 36)
- chancroid, granuloma inguinale, and lymphogranuloma venereum (see Boxes 37.2–37.4) are seen almost exclusively among travellers
- genital ulceration as part of systemic diseases, such as Behcet's disease, or erythema multiforme (HSV infection may act as a trigger for the latter)

Any of these conditions may closely mimic another, although intact vesicles are almost exclusive to HSV infection. Single lesions, which may appear trivial to the patient (e.g. 1 mm in diameter), are often due to genital herpes and should not be

---

Box 37.2 Chancroid

- Causative organism: *Haemophilus ducreyi*
- 'Soft chancre': single or multiple papules on the genitalia that ulcerate
- Lack of induration distinct from 'hard chancre' of syphilis
- Inguinal adenopathy prominent; may break down to form an abscess or discharging sinus in groin
- Diagnosis: Gram-negative bacilli in smears
- Treatment is with tetracycline

Box 37.3 Granuloma inguinale

- Causative organism: *Klebsiella granulomatis* (formerly known as *Donovania granulomatis*)
- Papules on genitalia or groins. Subsequently ulcerate and become secondarily infected
- Diagnosis: biopsy appearance of Donovan bodies (intracellular bacilli) in macrophages
- Treatment is with tetracycline

<table>
<tr><td>

Box 37.4 **Lymphogranuloma venereum**

- Causative organism: *Chlamydia trachomatis*, strains L_{1-3}
- Small genital ulcer; may go unnoticed
- Presentation with painful enlarged inguinal nodes, leading to multiple abscesses that may rupture
- Diagnosis: serology or intradermal skin test with Frei's LGV antigen
- Treatment is with tetracycline

</td></tr>
</table>

ignored. The approach to diagnosis of such a lesion is the same as discussed earlier—a swab of the ulcer should be sent to the laboratory for virus isolation or direct immunofluorescence. Using these techniques, it is also possible to type the virus to determine whether it is HSV-1 or -2.

Q Is typing of virus clinically useful?

A Most laboratories do not type HSV. However, typing may be useful in tracing routes of spread of infection, e.g. in suspected child sexual abuse, where the child may have acquired genital herpes by direct inoculation of virus from his/her own oro-labial source (likely to be type 1) rather than from the genital area of the abuser (likely to be type 2).

Typing of virus also has some limited prognostic value—genital type 2 infection is more likely to recur than genital type 1 infection, whereas the reverse is true of orolabial infection.

Summary: Genital herpes simplex infection

Presentation

- *Primary*—extensive painful genital ulceration; inguinal adenopathy; fever
- *Recurrence*—asymptomatic; if lesions, then usually few in number, localized, not indurated; no adenopathy or systemic response

Diagnosis

Clinical; swab in viral transport medium for virus isolation; demonstration of virus in vesicle fluid/ulcer base by electron microscopy, antigen detection

Management

Aciclovir for primary attack and prophylaxis if frequent or severe recurrences; barrier methods of contraception to prevent spread

Case 38 Jane, 27 years old, requests an AIDS test

Jane, a 27 year-old accountant previously fit and well, arrives in your surgery in a state of great agitation. Immediately after sitting down, she asks you for an acquired immunodeficiency syndrome (AIDS) 'test'. It quickly becomes clear that Jane is worried that she may be infected with the human immunodeficiency virus (HIV). Before ordering an appropriate diagnostic test, you need to ascertain whether Jane has any risk factors for acquisition of HIV infection.

Q What are the routes of transmission of HIV?

A There are three possible means by which HIV is spread between individuals:

- sexual
- vertical (i.e. mother to baby)
- exposure to infected blood or blood products, e.g. transfusion of blood, administration of factor VIII, sharing of needles between injecting drug users, needlestick injuries

There is no evidence to suggest that HIV can be transmitted via droplet spread or by insects.

Q To which family of viruses does HIV belong?

A The retroviruses.

Q Why are retroviruses so called?

A Retroviruses have an RNA genome, but can convert this into a DNA copy by virtue of the virally encoded enzyme reverse transcriptase. One of the central tenets of molecular biology is that genetic information flows unidirectionally from DNA to RNA to protein. Thus, the apparent 'backward' step of making RNA into DNA led to the adoption of the term 'retroviruses' to describe this family of viruses. Eukaryotic cells do not have a reverse transcriptase, and thus this enzyme is an ideal target for anti-retroviral drugs.

You ask Jane why she is worried about HIV infection. It transpires that she has just returned from a holiday abroad with several friends. During this trip, she had unprotected sexual intercourse with a casual acquaintance, whom she has just learned is an injecting drug user. Intercourse took place on one occasion only, this being 5 days ago. On direct questioning, Jane denies any other risk factors for HIV infection. Apart from her understandable anxiety, she has no other symptoms and examination reveals no abnormalities.

Q What is the basis of the standard laboratory test for HIV infection?

A Laboratory diagnosis of HIV infection is usually made by demonstrating the presence of antibodies to the virus in patients' sera, not by detection of the virus or viral antigens. Note that there is no such thing as an 'AIDS test'.

Q Jane is obviously distraught. Are you able to confirm whether or not she has not contracted HIV infection?

A Unfortunately, no. There is a lag time (known as the 'window period') between infection with HIV and the production of antibodies. This varies, but the vast majority of HIV-infected patients will be antibody-positive 3 months after acquisition of infection. A test on Jane's serum now would be negative, and you could not exclude the possibility of HIV infection until a sample taken 3 months after the potential exposure is also shown to be negative.

You explain this dilemma to Jane, and ask her to return to see you in 3 months time for an anti-HIV test. In fact she returns 4 weeks later, complaining of a sore throat and non-specific malaise. On examination, you note a fine macular rash on her trunk and moderate cervical and axillary lymphadenopathy.

Q What is your differential diagnosis, and what investigations should you order?

Table 38.1 HIV-seroconverting illness

- Onset. 1–6 weeks after exposure
- Symptoms. Fever, sweats, myalgia, anorexia, nausea, diarrhoea, sore throat, rash
- Signs. Lymphadenopathy, rash, non-exudative pharyngitis. More rarely—oral ulcers, enlarged liver, spleen
- Differential diagnosis. Infectious mononucleosis (see Case 15); other viral infections, e.g. influenza, viral hepatitis, measles, primary HSV infection; secondary syphilis (see Case 36)

A Jane now has a glandular-fever like illness. While the most common cause of this syndrome is acute Epstein–Barr virus (EBV) infection (see Case 15), there is also the possibility that this may be due to acute HIV infection—the acute retroviral syndrome or HIV-seroconverting illness. This is reported in 40–70% of patients with HIV infection. The features of this syndrome are listed in Table 38.1.

Q How should you investigate Jane?

A A full blood count and film would be useful. In HIV-seroconverting illness, this would typically show a reduced total lymphocyte count, with the presence of atypical mononuclear cells. It would be important to exclude EBV infection—a heterophile antibody test should be negative. Tests for other infections, listed in the differential diagnosis in Table 38.1, would be appropriate in patients with particular features associated with those infections.

All specimens sent to the laboratory should be clearly indicated as 'high risk'. If Jane is suffering from acute HIV infection, her blood will be infectious, and it is important that laboratory staff are aware of this potential risk.

Q How would you prove the diagnosis of HIV infection?

A The routine anti-HIV tests are usually negative at the time of an HIV-seroconverting illness, becoming positive about 2–6 weeks after onset of symptoms. One method of making a definitive diagnosis at this stage would be to demonstrate the presence of HIV RNA in serum using a genome amplification technique, but this is not always available.

A full blood count from Jane reveals a moderate lymphopenia, with atypical mononuclear cells seen. The monospot is negative. At Jane's insistence, you request an anti-HIV test, the result of which is negative. Jane makes an uneventful recovery from her illness, and returns 4 weeks later, for a repeat anti-HIV test. The result of this test is positive.

Q Is there anything further you should do before accepting the diagnosis of HIV infection?

A Yes, because of the seriousness of the diagnosis, you should order a repeat anti-HIV test. Even though your patient has a defined risk exposure, and her illness 4 weeks previously is entirely consistent with an acute HIV infection, the diagnosis of HIV infection should *always* be confirmed by sending a second serum sample from the patient for testing. In any laboratory, there is the possibility of error (e.g. mislabelling of tubes, inserting the wrong sample in the test, assigning a result to the wrong patient), and there are well-documented instances where such errors have led to the erroneous labelling of a patient as being anti-HIV positive.

Q What is the risk of acquisition of HIV infection through unprotected intercourse with a known HIV-positive partner?

A It is difficult to quote a precise risk, although it is considerably less than for some other sexually transmitted diseases (e.g. gonorrhoea, syphilis). Factors that affect the likelihood of transmission include the stage of HIV infection in the donor (progression of HIV infection to AIDS is associated with higher titres of virus in peripheral blood and genital secretions) and the presence of genital ulceration in either partner. Although it will be no comfort to her, Jane may consider herself very unlucky to have acquired infection after a single sexual exposure.

After much anguish, Jane eventually comes to terms with her diagnosis.

Q Which cells are infected by HIV, and why?

A The cellular receptor for HIV is a molecule known as CD4. This is normally only present on certain cells of the immune system—a subset of T lymphocytes and cells of the monocyte/macrophage lineage. Thus, HIV infects these cells, and the damage to these cells caused by the virus is reflected in a gradual loss of immune function.

Q What is the natural history of HIV infection?

A The defining characteristic of HIV infection is the inexorable decline in immune function over time. The consequences for the HIV-infected individual will therefore be the development of diseases associated with immunodeficiency.

Q What is AIDS?

A AIDS is a very carefully defined diagnosis, made on clinical and laboratory grounds. In order to fulfil the criteria for a diagnosis of AIDS, an HIV-infected patient must either have evidence of one of a number of specific illnesses—therefore known as AIDS-defining conditions—or have a CD4 count of less than $200/mm^3$. The AIDS-defining illnesses (discussed in more detail in Case 51) are ones that are indicative of serious underlying cellular immunodeficiency, e.g. *Pneumocystis carinii* pneumonia or Kaposi's sarcoma. The addition of a low CD4 count in the definition of AIDS was made in its most recent revision, and reflects the fact that patients with <200 CD4 cells/mm^3 are in imminent danger of acquiring an AIDS-defining illness.

Note that HIV infection is a necessary, but not sufficient, cause of AIDS. HIV-infected individuals may exhibit a range of clinical consequences from asymptomatic infection through to the severe debilitating and life-threatening immunodeficiency state known as AIDS. Before the advent of antiretroviral therapy, the mean incubation period between infection with HIV and the development of AIDS was 8–12 years.

Q How are the various stages of HIV infection classified?

A In recognition of the different stages of HIV infection, and in order to facilitate comparison of patient groups in different studies, the Centres for Disease Control in Atlanta, Georgia, have devised classification systems for HIV infection, which have been revised on several occasions.

The current system categorizes HIV-infected patients on the basis of two parameters—their clinical status and their peripheral blood CD4 count—see Table 38.2. In clinical category A, persistent generalized lymphadenopathy (PGL) is defined as two or more extrainguinal sites of lymphadenopathy for a minimum of 3 months for which no other cause can be found. Typical symptomatic, but non-AIDS-defining illnesses included in category B are oral candidiasis, recurrent oral/genital herpes, herpes zoster, and oral hairy leucoplakia (OHL; see Fig. 38.1 and Box 38.1). The occurrence of these diseases is indicative of a declining host immune function. Category C contains the very precise list of 'AIDS-defining' illnesses, which are indicative of severe immunodeficiency. As a CD4 count of <$200/mm^3$ is of itself AIDS-defining, in this system, patients in categories A3, B3, C1, C2, and C3 all have AIDS.

Table 38.2 1993 CDC revised classification system for HIV infected patients

Clinical categories

A Asymptomatic, acute HIV infection, or persistent generalized lymphadenopathy (PGL)

B Symptomatic disease; not A or C conditions

C AIDS indicator conditions (see Case 51)

CD4+ cell counts

1 $500/mm^3$ or greater

2 $200–499/mm^3$

3 Less than $200/mm^3$

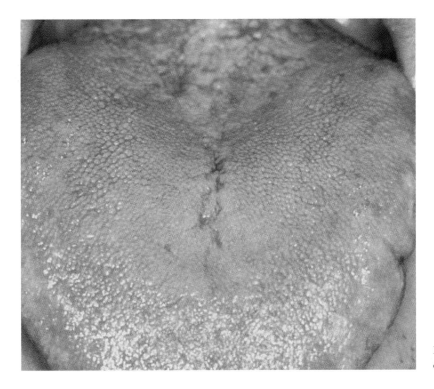

Fig. 38.1 Tongue showing oral hairy leucoplakia.

Q How should the progression of Jane's HIV infection be monitored?

A She should be assessed clinically at regular intervals to allow early diagnosis and management of any of the protean complications of HIV infection. More specifically, the state of her HIV infection should be monitored by serial measurement of: (1) peripheral blood viral load and (2) CD4 cell count.

Viral load measurement is performed using highly sensitive quantitative molecular assays. The level of viraemia in the patient's peripheral blood is clearly predictive of the time to development of AIDS. The absolute number of circulating CD4-positive lymphocytes provides additional information upon which to base clinical decision-making. Declining numbers of CD4 cells is an indicator of a poor prognosis. Guidelines on the use of anti-retroviral therapy (discussed in detail in Case 51) define thresholds for viral loads above which, and CD4 counts below which, treatment should be actively considered.

Q Should Jane be offered any anti-retroviral therapy at the time of her seroconversion illness?

A Possibly, but this is a difficult and as yet unresolved issue. In untreated patients, the viral load will settle down within 6–12 months after the acute infection to a level known as the 'set-point'. The level of this set-point is known to be predictive of the time to development of AIDS. There is an argument that aggressive anti-retroviral therapy at the time of initial infection may result in a lower set-point viral load and therefore a better long-term prognosis. However, this theoretical advantage of early therapy has to be set against considerations of adherence to long-term therapy, potential toxicity, and development of resistance (discussed in more detail in Case 51). Current UK recommendations are that patients wishing to embark on early therapy should be enrolled into clinical trials, with the hope that some of the imponderables regarding the value of this line of action can be properly evaluated.

Box 38.1 Oral hairy leucoplakia (OHL)

- Whitish lesions on oropharyngeal mucosal surfaces, usually on the side of the tongue
- May resemble oral candidiasis
- Caused by extensive replication of Epstein–Barr virus in epithelial cells
- May occur in any immunosuppressed patient, although rare in absence of HIV infection
- Lesions resolve with aciclovir therapy, but may recur once therapy is stopped

Jane asks about the possibility of passing her infection to her children, should she have any.

Q What information can you give her about the risk of vertical transmission?

A Although mother-to-baby transmission of HIV infection may occur, with appropriate management of the pregnancy and delivery, this is now largely a preventable disease. The management of HIV-infection in a pregnant woman is discussed in detail in Case 60.

The diagnosis and management of AIDS are discussed in detail in Case 51.

Summary: Human immunodeficiency virus (HIV) infection

Routes of infection
Vertical (mother-to-baby); sexual; blood and blood products

Diagnosis
Detection of anti-HIV—may take 3 months to appear after contact. Detection of HIV RNA—requires sensitive genome detection assays

Stages of infection
CDC classification based on clinical status and CD4 cell count; AIDS is defined by the presence of certain illnesses or a CD4 count < 200/mm^3

Case 39 Suprapubic pain and haematuria in Gavin, a 35-year-old sales executive

Gavin, a 35-year-old sales director, presents to his GP with suprapubic pain when passing urine, which contains blood. He has no past history of these symptoms nor of urethral discharge and has no relevant previous medical history. Gavin is on no medication and his wife, Hannah, and their four children are well.

Q What is this condition and what may cause it?

A Gavin has haematuria (frank blood *per urethram*) and, with the presence of pain, probably has haemorrhagic cystitis, which is usually characterized by obvious blood on micturition. The possible causes of this are:

- bladder carcinoma—diagnosed on cystoscopy and histology
- cyclophosphamide—a chemotherapeutic agent that results in severe ulceration and may lead to bladder contraction
- irradiation—following treatment for bladder carcinoma
- cystitis—relatively rare in uncomplicated cases but may occur as part of 'honeymoon cystitis' in females following sexual intercourse (see Case 34)
- Reiter's disease—abnormal host response to a number of infecting agents, such as chlamydia (see Case 36), *Salmonella*, *Shigella*, and *Yersinia* (see Case 69). Characterized by urethritis, arthritis, uveitis, and, occasionally, skin lesions. Hyperacute cystitis with haematuria is occasionally part of the presenting illness
- schistosomiasis—a helminth infection due to a trematode (fluke) seen in travellers to the developing world and seen endemically there also
- adenoviruses and polyomaviruses—occasionally (see Cases 8 and 40).

It transpires that Gavin had been to Egypt as part of an export sales drive for his company some weeks ago. During the visit he had taken a pleasure trip down the Nile and had bathed in the river. Culture of his urine is negative for bacterial pathogens.

Q What diagnosis is suggested from the history, and how might it be confirmed?

A Schistosomiasis due to *Schistosoma haematobium* is very possible in the light of recent travel to Egypt and the history of bathing. Peripheral blood eosinophilia may also point to a parasitic cause. A diagnosis may be confirmed by microscopic examination of concentrated or filtered urine for ova. Alternative approaches include bladder biopsy to demonstrate granulomata, examination of faeces for ova and parasites, or a rectal biopsy when gastrointestinal symptoms are prominent, and, finally, serology, which is only available through reference laboratories.

Microscopy shows over 100 pus cells/mm^3 and ova of *Schistosoma haematobium* (see Fig. 39.1) with the characteristic terminal spine. Gavin is

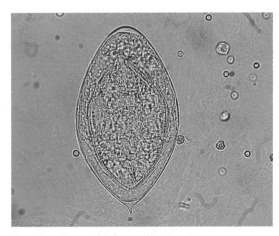

Fig. 39.1 Ovum of *S. haematobium* in urine.

prescribed one dose of praziquantal (an effect-ive antischistosomal agent), his symptoms resolve, and a follow-up urine sample is clear.

Q How is schistosomiasis acquired?

A The organisms, present in fresh water, gain access through the skin. There are a number of species responsible for a variety of clinical syn-dromes (see Box 39.1). Humans are the principal host, with the snail as the intermediate host. Eggs are excreted in the urine or faeces of humans where sanitation standards are poor, hatch in fresh water, and are then taken up by the snail, in which cer-cariae (fork-tails) develop. These are subsequently released into the fresh-water habitat from which people become infected via the skin.

Q What follow-up is required in Gavin's case?

A Usually, treatment is effective, symptoms resolve fairly quickly, and a follow-up sample of

---

Box 39.1 Species, geographical distribution, and clinical syndromes caused by schistosoma

- *S. haematobium* (Egypt, Middle East, Africa)
- *S. mansoni* (Middle East, Africa, Latin America, West Indies)
- *S. japonicum* (Far East)
- Also *S. intercalatum*, *S. mekongi*

- Purpuric papular skin rash—'swimmers itch' (*S. mansoni, S. haematobium*)
- Cystitis (*S. haematobium*)
- Katayama fever, a serum-sickness-like syndrome with fever, eosinophilia, lymphadenopathy, and splenomegaly
- Cor pulmonale, infiltration of lungs leading to obstruction of blood flow (*S. japonicum*)
- Liver fibrosis, liver failure due to vascular obstruction
- Chronic schistosomiasis, diarrhoea, dysentery, immune-mediated disease

---

urine should be clear of ova. The presence of anti-bodies, i.e. positive serology, which may also indi-cate a positive diagnosis, will persist for some time as will the presence of fibrosis on histology of blad-der biopsy. The eradication of ova accompanied by a resolution of symptoms is the best indicator of successful therapy

Q What complications may ensue from untreated or undiagnosed urinary schistosomiasis?

A These arise mainly in the indigenous popu-lation, where facilities for diagnosis and treat-ment may be inadequate. Complications include:

- secondary bacterial infection and renal stones
- bladder granulomata and papillomata
- ureteric blockage with hydronephrosis
- bladder carcinoma

Q How may schistosomiasis be prevented?

A Irrigation and water conservation schemes in developing countries make control increasingly difficult, as snails are disseminated. Measures to control the snail population will reduce the risk of infection. Other measures include:

- introduction of modern sewage disposal facilities
- measures to encourage people not to urinate in fresh water
- avoidance of bathing or walking barefoot in fresh water by visitors to endemic areas
- research on immune response, leading to the development of a vaccine

Résumé for undergraduate students

Schistosomiasis is only seen in temperate climates in the returned traveller who has been exposed in endemic areas. It is an important infection in many tropical countries but should be considered in the differential diagnosis of many patients with haematuria.

Summary: Schistosomiasis

Presentation

Haematuria or diarrhoea and dysentery in the returned traveller

Diagnosis

Clinical suspicion and examination of urine, faeces, or biopsy material for ova

Treatment

One dose of praziquantal. Surgery occasionally required for complications

Case 40 Mark, a 42-year-old solicitor, has a lump on his penis

Mark, a 42-year-old solicitor, comes to the genitourinary medicine (GUM) clinic complaining of a small, painless lump on his penis. He is concerned that he may have developed genital herpes. He is unmarried, having split from his long-term girlfriend a year ago. He has had four casual sexual partners since then. He has no urethral discharge and no dysuria, and there are no other symptoms related to the genitourinary tract. His past medical history is unremarkable, although he does suffer from occasional cold sores. He is on no regular medication. Examination is normal apart from the physical sign shown in Fig. 40.1. There is no inguinal adenopathy.

Q What is the diagnosis?

A The appearance is that of a wart. The absence of vesicles or ulcers clearly distinguishes this from genital HSV infection.

Q Name the infectious agent responsible.

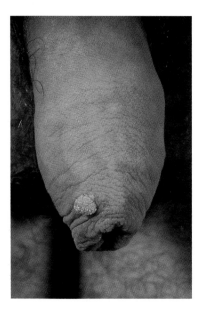

Fig. 40.1
Mark's penis.

A Human papillomavirus (HPV), sometimes referred to as wart virus.

Q How are papillomaviruses classified?

A Papillomaviruses contain a double-stranded DNA genome and belong to the papovavirus family. Papova is derived from 'papilloma–polyoma–vacuolar', which indicates that this family contains three distinct genera of viruses. The papillomaviruses are further classified into types, of which there are over 100 which infect humans. Unlike some other viruses (e.g. adenoviruses), this typing is not on the basis of antigenic differences, i.e. serotypes (which reside in the viral protein components), between strains, but is dependent on the degree of DNA sequence homology of the viral genome, i.e. genotypes.

Q At what anatomical sites may HPV infection occur?

A HPVs infect and replicate in squamous epithelium on both keratinized and mucosal surfaces. Infections are extremely common. Clinical presentation may be:

1. cutaneous
   - usually hands (verruca vulgaris) and feet (verruca plantaris, or plantar wart), but may occur elsewhere, e.g. face
   - most frequent in childhood and early adolescence
   - due to types 1–4

2. mucosal
   - single papillomas may occur in mouth, at any age; rarely recur after surgical excision
   - multiple papillomas associated with HPV types 6 and 11 are the most common benign epithelial tumours of the larynx, are more frequent in children than adults, and frequently recur after surgical excision

3. anogenital
   - an increasingly common sexually transmitted disease

- benign warts (condylomata acuminata) may occur on penis, vulva, urethra, cervix, perianal areas, due to types HPV 6 or 11
- malignant transformation in the cervix associated with HPV types 16 and 18 (and others)

Note. Manifestations of HPV infection are more common in immunosuppressed patients, e.g. renal transplant recipients have an increased incidence of skin warts and of squamous cell carcinoma arising from HPV infection.

Q How should you treat Mark?

A Warts may regress spontaneously, although this is unpredictable, and may take many months. Treatment of genital warts is, in general, unsatisfactory. Many lesions will recur, and this should be clearly explained to Mark before treatment is undertaken. The treatment options available for removal of small numbers of lesions are:

- podophyllin, or podophyllotoxin: must be applied carefully, as normal skin may be severely burned; should be washed off after 4 hours
- cryotherapy, e.g. with a slurry of cardice (solid CO_2) and acetone. May be painful!
- interferon therapy: injected either intramuscularly or intralesionally; still under evaluation
- surgery: persistent or extensive warts, or urethral warts or warts extending to the anal canal may be surgically excised

After appropriate discussion, Mark agrees to cryotherapy of his warts. He returns to the clinic 2 weeks later, and there are now no visible lesions. However, he has brought his current girlfriend with him, who is anxious that she may be at risk of cervical cancer.

Q What is the evidence linking cervical HPV infection with cancer of the cervix?

A There are a number of lines of evidence, suggesting that infection with certain HPV types (e.g. 16, 18) is a key step in the development of cervical malignancy.

- The epidemiology of carcinoma of the cervix strongly resembles that of a sexually transmitted disease
- Papillomaviruses are known to be oncogenic in animals
- A rare autosomal disease, epidermodysplasia verruciformis, is associated with multiple skin warts, and the development of squamous cell carcinoma, the malignant cells of which contain HPV (usually type 5)
- Over 90% of cervical carcinomas contain HPV DNA, most commonly of types 16 or 18. In most cases, this DNA is integrated into the host chromosomes
- At the molecular level, certain HPV-derived proteins can be shown to transform cells, i.e. induce uncontrolled cellular proliferation

Q How may HPV infection of the cervix be diagnosed?

A Evaluation of women with HPV lesions of the cervix is largely dependent on the detection of cytological abnormalities in cervical smears and on colposcopic examination and biopsy of suspicious lesions. Some authorities have suggested that screening women for the presence of HPV 16 DNA using genome amplification technology is more sensitive in detecting premalignant and malignant lesions of the cervix than is cytology. However, at present, this is a controversial subject, and women with genital warts and female partners of males with genital warts should be advised to have regular cervical smears.

Q The polyomaviruses were mentioned above as members of the papovavirus family. What diseases are caused by these viruses?

A Two polyomaviruses have been identified in humans—JC and BK viruses (named after the initials of the patients from whom they were first isolated). Most primary infections with these viruses occur in childhood, and are usually asymptomatic, although respiratory tract symptoms have been described. Both viruses are excreted in urine, and are rare causes of acute haemorrhagic cystitis (see

Case 39). Reactivation of JC virus infection in immunocompromised patients may result in progressive multifocal leucoencephalopathy (PML; see Case 51). In addition, simian virus 40 (SV40) is a pathogen of monkeys, but has been transmitted to humans, e.g. as a contaminant of polio vaccines prepared in monkey kidney tissue culture cells unknowingly contaminated with SV40. There are published data suggesting that SV40 infection may be a cause of human malignant diseases, e.g. some types of non-Hodgkin's lymphomas.

Summary: Genital papillomavirus infection

Presentation
Painless warts in genital area

Diagnosis
Clinical; HPV type can be determined by biopsy and genome analysis

Complications
HPV 16 and 18 are associated with cervical carcinoma

Treatment
None; topical podophyllin; cryotherapy; interferon; surgery

Self-assessment

1. Clinical manifestations of human papillomavirus infection include all but which one of the following?

(a) Laryngeal papillomatosis

(b) Cervical intraepithelial neoplasia

(c) Squamous cell carcinoma

(d) Plantar warts

(e) Condyloma lata

2. Which one of the following agents is not useful in the management of HPV infection?

(a) Podophyllotoxin

(b) Cryotherapy

(c) Aciclovir

(d) Alpha interferon

(e) Surgical excision

3. Characteristic clinical features of anogenital infection caused by herpes simplex viruses (HSV) include all but which one of the following?

(a) Higher recurrence rate with HSV-2 infection than with HSV-1

(b) Involvement of the cervix is more common in recurrent disease than primary disease

(c) Virus can be transmitted from an asymptomatic host

(d) Regional lymphadenopathy in primary attacks

(e) Mean time to healing of 14–21 days in primary attacks; 5–7 days in recurrent attacks

4. The differential diagnosis of genital ulceration includes all but which one of the following?

(a) Primary syphilis

(b) Chancroid

(c) Drug reaction

(d) Behcet's disease

(e) Trichomoniasis

5. In which one of the following diseases is a mucopurulent cervical discharge not a feature?

(a) Primary syphilis

(b) Gonorrhoea

(c) Pelvic inflammatory disease

(d) Primary genital herpes

(e) *Chlamydia trachomatis* infection

6. Which one of the following is not recognized as a complication of infection with *Neisseria gonorrhoeae*?

(a) Pharyngitis

(b) Urethritis

(c) Arthritis

(d) Myocarditis

(e) Conjunctivitis

7. Which of the following statements regarding acute HIV infection are true?

(a) The seroconverting illness is clinically similar to a glandular-fever-like illness

(b) Patients are always anti-HIV-positive at the time of presentation with an acute seroconverting illness

(c) Only around a quarter of HIV-infected patients give a history of an acute seroconversion illness

(d) The number of circulating CD4+ T cells is likely to be low at the time of an acute seroconverting illness

(e) HIV RNA is present in serum at the time of presentation with a seroconversion illness

8. Which *one* of the following is *not* a recognized route of transmission of HIV infection?

(a) Heterosexual intercourse

(b) Male homosexual intercourse

(c) Mother-to-baby

(d) Faecal–oral

(e) Transfusion of Factor VIII

9. Which antibiotic is the best choice in the community for the empirical or blind therapy of cystitis?

(a) Erythromycin

(b) Metronidazole

(c) Trimpethoprim

(d) Gentamicin

(e) Benzylpenicillin

10. Radiological investigations of the genito-urinary tract following urinary tract infection (UTI) are indicated in which circumstances?

(a) Infections caused by *Staphylococcus saprophyticus*

(b) Females in the 25–30 age group

(c) UTI accompanied by haematuria

(d) Presence of nocturia

(e) Acquired in another country

11. Which are the most commonly implicated bacteria in infection associated with continuous ambulatory peritoneal dialysis (CAPD)?

(a) Viridans streptococci

(b) *Staphylococcus aureus*

(c) Coagulase-negative staphylococcus species (CNS)

(d) *Staphylococcus saphrophyticus*

(e) Beta-haemolytic streptococci group A (*Strep. pyogenes*)

12. What does CAPD infection caused by *E. coli* suggest?

(a) Poor standards of hygiene by the patient

(b) A recent diarrhoeal illness

(c) Associated bacteraemia

(d) Bowel perforation

(e) Previous history of recurrent UTIs before CAPD

13. Reiter's disease following intestinal infection by *Campylobacter jejuni* is characterized by urethritis, arthritis, and which other factor?

(a) Endocarditis

(b) Hepatitis

(c) Uveitis

(d) Orchitis or oophoritis

(e) Pharyngitis/tonsillitis

14. Which of the following is a well recognized complication of schistosomiasis?

(a) Encephalitis

(b) Cor pulmonale

(c) Liver abscess

(d) Myocarditis

(e) Osteomyelitis

CHAPTER 5

Central nervous system

SECTION 5
Central nervous system

Case 41 Nigel, a 3-year-old boy with lethargy and a skin rash

Nigel, a 3-year-old boy, is referred to hospital with a 2-day history of lethargy, irritability, and poor feeding. On examination he is pyrexial and drowsy and has 2–3 purplish-red lesions on the trunk and extremities (Fig. 41.1) that, according to his parents, were not present when he was seen earlier by the family practitioner. There is no neck stiffness.

Q What is the most likely diagnosis? What investigations should be carried out to confirm it?

A Meningococcal septicaemia or bloodstream infection is the most likely diagnosis. Meningococcal disease may present with septicaemia, meningitis, or both. Septicaemia or bloodstream infection is the more serious manifestation of meningococcal disease as the mortality from meningitis is lower. Septic-

aemia is suggested by the presence of the skin lesions; the absence of neck stiffness does not exclude associated meningitis in Nigel. Blood cultures are essential, and two sets should be taken if at all possible. Cerebrospinal fluid (CSF) should also be obtained by lumbar puncture (LP) for biochemical and micro-

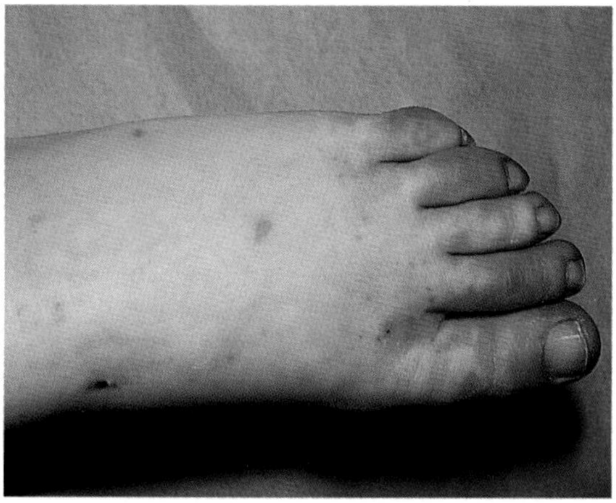

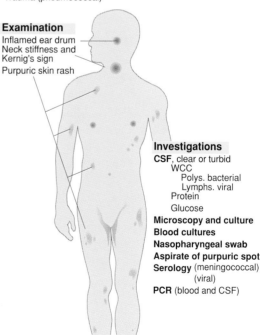

History
Duration of symptoms (>1 week suggests viral aetiology or TB)
Otitis media (*H.influenzae* possible)
Contact with a case recently (meningococcal)
Trauma (pneumococcal)

Examination
Inflamed ear drum
Neck stiffness and Kernig's sign
Purpuric skin rash

Investigations
CSF, clear or turbid
  WCC
    Polys. bacterial
    Lymphs. viral
  Protein
  Glucose
Microscopy and culture
Blood cultures
Nasopharyngeal swab
Aspirate of purpuric spot
Serology (meningococcal)
       (viral)
PCR (blood and CSF)

Fig. 41.1 Purplish-red lesions on foot.

Fig. 41.2 Diagnosis of meningitis.

Table 41.1 CSF features of bacterial, viral, and tuberculous meningitis

Aetiology	Protein	Glucose	Cytology
Bacterial	Very high, e.g. >6 g/l	< 60% blood level	Increased neutrophils, mainly
Viral	Elevated, e.g. 4 g/l	Normal	Increased lymphocytes
Tuberculosis	Elevated	< 60% blood level	Lymphocytes

biological analysis (Fig. 41.2) An LP is contraindicated if there is clinical evidence of raised intracranial pressure, such as rapid changes in pulse, blood pressure, and level of consciousness; papilloedema; or focal neurological signs. Microscopy of smears from the rash may provide a presumptive diagnosis if Gram-negative intracellular diplococci are seen . The biochemistry and cytology of the CSF may strongly indicate whether the infection is bacterial or viral in aetiology even if no organisms are seen on microscopy (Table 41.1).

Q What is the significance of age in predicting the likely aetiology of meningitis:

1. in this case?

2. in a 3-day-old neonate?

3. in a 25-year-old pregnant woman with a prodromal flu-like illness?

4. in a 75-year-old comatose man?

A Certain organisms are more likely to be involved at specific times in life, especially during the neonatal period. Bacterial meningitis is more common during childhood and early adulthood, and the most common cause is *Neisseria meningitidis* (the meningococcus). Capsulated *Haemophilus influenzae* type b or Hib (see Case 13) is now rare in those countries where vaccination against Hib is part of the routine childhood vaccination programme. *Streptococcus pneumoniae* (the pneumococcus) can cause meningitis throughout life (Table 41.2).

1. The age of the patient and the presence of a purpuric rash are very suggestive of meningococcal disease.

2. *Escherichia coli* and β-haemolytic streptococcus group B, which are part of the normal vaginal

Table 41.2 Aetiology of acute meningitis

Bacteria

- *N. meningitidis*
- *S. pneumoniae*
- *E. coli* (neonatal)
- Group B streptococcus (neonatal)
- *L. monocytogenes* (pregnant women, neonates; see Case 58)
- Staphylococci (often trauma- or surgery-associated)
- *Treponema pallidum*
- *Leptospira* species
- *Haemophilus influenzae* type b (unvaccinated children)

Viruses

- Enteroviruses (see Case 3)
- Mumps (see Case 65)

flora, are the most likely causes but are rare outside the neonatal period (>1 month old).

3. Viral meningitis is much more common than that due to bacteria. Likely viral causes include enteroviruses (coxsackieviruses, echoviruses, and polioviruses; see Case 3), mumps, and occasionally herpes simplex. *Listeria monocytogenes* must be considered as a possible cause during pregnancy or postpartum, and in the neonate (see Case 58). This opportunist pathogen may be acquired from the ingestion of certain foods, e.g. soft cheeses, pâté, or cook–chill foods that have been inadequately prepared. Consequently,

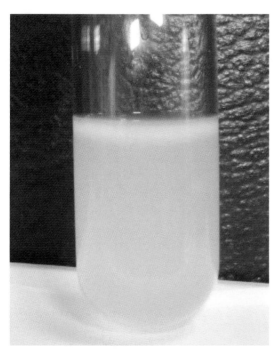

Fig. 41.3 Cloudy or turbid CSF is very suggestive of bacterial meningitis.

pregnant women should be advised to avoid these for the duration of pregnancy.

4. *S. pneumoniae* is relatively more common in the elderly, and this organism, together with the presence of coma, heralds a poor prognosis.

Nigel's CSF, obtained from lumbar puncture at presentation, is cloudy (Fig. 41.3) and contains 540 white cells/mm^3 (90% polymorphs) and 5 red blood cells/mm^3. CSF protein is 8 g/l and glucose 0.3 mmol/l (blood glucose, 5.7 mmol/l). The Gram stain reveals Gram-negative intracellular diplococci (Fig. 41.4). Nigel's blood cultures are also positive for Gram-negative diplococci within 24 hours of being taken.

Q Which of the above CSF values are abnormal? What type of meningitis is this and what is the likely pathogen?

A A cloudy or turbid CSF, together with raised white cells (normal, <5/mm^3) with neutrophils pre-

dominant, a raised protein (normal, 1.5–4.0 g/l), and a glucose concentration less than 60% of the blood level is highly suggestive of bacterial rather than viral meningitis. The organisms seen on the Gram film of both the CSF and blood are almost certainly *N. meningitidis*. Later, small grey colonies from both were growing on chocolate and blood agar; they were oxidase-positive and biochemically confirmed as *N. meningitidis*. This confirms the diagnosis of meningococcal septicaemia and meningitis.

Causes of meningitis that present with an 'aseptic' CSF pattern, i.e. raised white cells with lymphocytes predominant and slightly raised protein but normal glucose, include viruses (e.g. enteroviruses, mumps), *Treponema pallidum* (syphilis), leptospirosis, and tuberculosis (high CSF protein; glucose usually low; presentation not so acute, see Table 41.1). Occasionally, the predominant cells may be lymphocytes rather than polymorphs in the very early stages of meningitis caused by bacteria.

Q If the microscopy and culture of blood and CSF are negative for *N. meningitidis*, what other investigations might confirm the diagnosis?

A Analysis of CSF and blood by the polymerase chain reaction (PCR) is now routine in many countries with facilities for this (Fig. 41.5). It is especially useful in patients who have received antibiotics before or on arrival to hospital. In addition to confirming a diagnosis of meningococcal infection, molecular analysis can determine which meningococcal group is the likely cause. Isolation of meningococcus from the nasopharynx is suggestive of the aetiology but may only represent carriage. Finally, serology has less of a role in the diagnosis with the arrival of PCR but may be used retrospectively to confirm a diagnosis.

Q What is the antibiotic of choice here?

A Intravenous penicillin for 10–14 days is the treatment of choice for meningococcal septicaemia and meningitis. Penicillin is also indicated to treat pneumococcal meningitis, although resistance to penicillin is being increasingly reported and is a particular problem in Spain and South

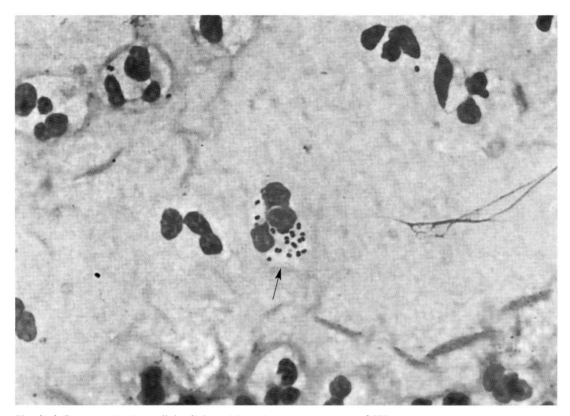

Fig. 41.4 Gram-negative intracellular diplococci (arrow) seen on microscopy of CSF are indicative of meningococcal meningitis.

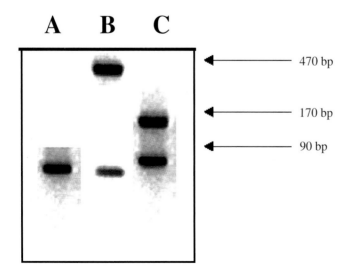

| A | B | C |

470 bp

170 bp

90 bp

Fig. 41.5 Multiplex PCR for the detection of meningococci. Lane A, Meningococci positive (serogroups X, Y, and W135); lane B, meningococci positive (serogroup B); lane C, meningococci positive (serogroup C). bp, Base pairs.

Africa. Blind therapy, where the aetiology is either unknown or *H. influenzae* (up to 20% β-lactamase positive) is possible, i.e. patient <5 years of age and unvaccinated, is a third-generation cephalosporin such as cefotaxime or, alternatively, chloramphenicol.

Q Was it preferable in this instance to delay starting treatment pending investigations?

A The rapid development of a purpuric rash indicates meningococcal septicaemia, which is a medical emergency as death may occur within minutes. Intravenous penicillin should be administered *before* a lumbar puncture is carried out or even before blood cultures can be taken, even if this means that an organism will not be grown from either specimen. This is one of the rare instances where treatment should precede microbiological investigations.

Q Is there any other therapeutic intervention that should be considered in the management of bacterial meningitis?

A There is recent evidence that corticosteroids administered early during the course of treatment have a beneficial effect on outcome resulting in reduced mortality. Therefore, dexamethasone should be started with or just before the first dose of antibiotics and continued for 4 days, especially if pneumococcal meningitis is suspected on clinical grounds or on the basis of initial microscopy results.

Nigel was started on high-dose intravenous penicillin and gradually improved over the next 48–72 hours. Pamela, his mother, expressed some concern as to the risk to his brother Lenny, aged 2, and sister Cynthia, aged 7.

Q What measures, if any, can be taken to minimize the risk to Nigel's close contacts?

A Chemoprophylaxis should be administered to all close contacts and vaccination may be indicated depending upon aetiology or type of organism (see Box 41.1).

Where the cause is due to Group A or C *N. meningitidis*, non-vaccinated close contacts should be vaccinated.

Box 41.1 Prevention of meningitis

Chemoprophylaxis

1. Meningococcal septicaemia or meningitis
   - Rifampicin: × 2 days
   - Ciprofloxacin: alternative
   - For all close contacts, i.e. family members, those sharing accommodation with the index case, 'kissing partners', and the index patient. This prevents acquisition by contacts and spread if already acquired. Treatment of the index case with penicillin does not always eradicate nasopharyngeal arriage. Not usually indicated for medical or nursing staff caring for the patient

2. *Haemophilus influenzae*
   - Rifampicin: × 4 days
   - For close contacts if there is an unvaccinated child under 5 in the household

Vaccination

A conjugated Group C *N. meningitidis* vaccine was recently introduced in many countries as part of the routine childhood vaccination programme and this has been followed by a fall in cases due to this group. However, most cases in temperate climates are due to *N. meningitidis* group B, for which there is as yet no effective vaccine. Close contacts or fellow class members of schoolchildren should be vaccinated if there are two or more cases due to group A (for which there is a vaccine, usually given to those travelling to areas of the world where group A is more common, e.g. Middle East) or group C (in unvaccinated individuals)

Vaccination should also be considered in any individual travelling to an endemic area, e.g parts of the Middle East

Conjugated polysaccharide *Haemophilus influenzae* type b (Hib) is now recommended for all infants from 2 months of age, and is indicated in close contacts of non-vaccinated children exposed to a case of meningitis or other form of invasive disease

Summary: Meningitis

Presentation

Headache, vomiting, fever, irritability, drowsiness (especially children), rash (indicates meningococcal septicaemia, which has a higher mortality than meningitis)

Diagnosis

CSF for microscopy, biochemical analysis, and culture, plus blood cultures, PCR, and serology

Management

- Intravenous penicillin (meningococcal + pneumococcal) or cefotaxime (aetiology unknown or if haemophilus likely) with dexamethasone, especially if pneumococcal infection likely

- Rifampicin to index case and contacts

- Prevention by vaccination (haemophilus and some strains of meningococcus)

Case 42 Mr Aldridge, a 45-year-old accountant with odd behaviour and a fever

Mr Aldridge, a 45-year-old accountant, is brought to the casualty department by his wife. Earlier in the day, he was found wandering in his local park, muttering unintelligibly to himself. His wife feels that, as the day has passed, he has become more and more detached from what is going on around him, although he has been able to answer direct questions. When you talk to Mr Aldridge, you find it difficult to elicit sensible answers, and in between his responses he appears very drowsy. His past medical history, taken from his wife, reveals no serious illnesses in the past, and he is on no regular medication. However, he has been complaining over the past few days of feeling generally unwell, and yesterday he returned home early from work with a headache and a fever, for which he took some paracetamol. On examination, he has a temperature of 37.9°C but, apart from his decreased level of consciousness, you find no other abnormal physical signs.

Q What is your differential diagnosis?

A The most striking features about Mr Aldridge are his recent behavioural changes and impaired level of consciousness. In the absence of any localizing signs, the most likely diagnosis is encephalitis, of which there is a multitude of possible causes. The prodromal illness and fever are suggestive of an infectious aetiology, of which viral encephalitis is the most common, but other diagnoses including tuberculous meningoencephalitis, cerebral abscesses, tumours, or strokes cannot be ruled out at this stage.

Q What viral causes of encephalitis are you aware of?

A Viral causes of encephalitis are listed in Table 42.1.

Q As can be seen from Table 42.1, the most common cause of sporadic viral encephalitis in the UK is herpes simplex virus (HSV). Does herpes simplex

encephalitis (HSE) represent a primary infection with HSV?

A Primary and secondary infections with herpesviruses are explained in Case 4. HSE may be a man-

Table 42.1 **Causes of viral encephalitis**
Herpes simplex virus types 1 and 2
The most common causes of sporadic viral encephalitis
Any age, including newborn (neonatal herpes; see Case 63)
Mumps virus (see Case 65)
Meningoencephalitis
Measles virus (see Case 6)
Post-infectious encephalitis
Subacute sclerosing panencephalitis
Varicella-zoster virus (see Case 7)
Post-infectious encephalitis (after chickenpox)
Zoster encephalitis as a complication of herpes zoster
Enteroviruses (see Case 3)
Direct viral invasion of brain substance
Influenza virus (see Case 17)
Post-infectious encephalitis
Rubella virus (see Case 59)
Panencephalitis as part of congenital rubella syndrome
Rabies virus (see Case 45)
Arthropod-borne viruses (geographically localized; the following examples do not exist in the UK), e.g. tick-borne encephalitis (Eastern Europe), Japanese encephalitis (South-east Asia, China), St Louis encephalitis (USA), and West Nile virus (see Box 42.1)
Nipah virus (see later)

ifestation of primary infection, but is much more commonly due to a secondary (re-activated) HSV infection.

Q As HSV is the most common infectious cause of encephalitis, would it be useful to know whether Mr Aldridge has any past or recent history of herpetic disease, i.e. recurrent cold sores, or genital herpes?

A No. A history of past or present external herpetic infection is of no discriminatory value in assessing the diagnosis of HSE. Patients with HSE give a past history of herpetic disease no more frequently than the general population. The presence or absence of a recurrent herpetic lesion at the time of presentation similarly gives no useful information about whether the virus has spread to the brain. Cold sores in particular can be misleading, as these may arise as a consequence of any intercurrent illness.

Q What is the pathogenesis of the damage to the brain in HSE?

A There are many important unanswered questions in relation to the pathogenesis of HSE, not the least being how does virus spread to the brain. However, it is clear that virus *is* present at the site of the affected tissue. The histological picture is one of acute haemorrhagic necrosis, which arises either as a direct result of virus-induced cell death, or possibly because of the host immune response to virus-infected cells.

Q How can you prove a diagnosis of HSE?

A Diagnosis is difficult, and there are a number of approaches.

1. *Neuroimaging.* Any part of the brain can be affected in HSE, but the most common site is the frontotemporal region—this underlies the bizarre behavioural changes that may be present in the history. The lesions in the brain are almost always focal—neurological imaging techniques such as computerized tomography (CT) or magnetic resonance imaging (MRI) scan (or even electroencephalography (EEG), if the former two are not available) should reveal this. The presence of a focal lesion seen by brain imag-

ing in a patient with an encephalitic illness should really be regarded as HSE unless proven otherwise.

2. *Lumbar puncture.* The cerebrospinal fluid (CSF) is rarely, if ever, normal in HSE, but the changes are not specific—red cells are often present, and any white cell pleocytosis is not necessarily severe. Intact virus particles are not often present in CSF and, therefore, viral culture is almost always negative. However, it is possible to demonstrate the presence of HSV DNA in a CSF sample using a genome amplification technique such as the polymerase chain reaction (PCR) assay. HSE was one of the first clinical situations in which the exquisite sensitivity of PCR was of major diagnostic benefit. PCR assays can also be fairly rapid—at least results can be generated in a single working day. Thus, this is the diagnostic method of choice *if* you have access to a laboratory with the capability of performing HSV PCR.

3. *Serology.* This relies on the demonstration of a rise in serum anti-HSV antibody titres, and of intrathecal synthesis of such antibodies. The major drawback to this approach is that it may take several days, if not weeks, for positive results to develop.

4. *Brain biopsy.* Virus can be detected at the affected site by immunofluorescence with appropriate monoclonal antibodies, by electron microscopy, or by isolation in tissue culture. However, most clinicians feel that this invasive procedure cannot be justified.

Q How, therefore, would you investigate Mr Aldridge?

A Investigations should include:

• a full blood count

• urea and electrolytes

• blood glucose

• a serum sample for viral serology. This can be paired with a later sample if need be, and various antibody titres assayed

- a throat swab in virus transport medium and a faecal sample for viral culture; these may provide the only clue to a diagnosis of enteroviral encephalitis
- cerebral imaging, as Mr Aldridge's pathology is most likely to be cerebral, e.g. CT or MRI scan
- lumbar puncture, provided raised intracranial pressure has been excluded

You admit Mr Aldridge to hospital, and order a CT scan, the results of which are shown in Fig. 42.1. A full blood count is normal, as are urea and electrolytes and blood sugar. A lumbar puncture is performed, yielding the following information.

- Slightly blood-stained fluid
- $700 \times 10^6/l$ red blood cells
- $43 \times 10^6/l$ white cells, 60% lymphocytes
- No organisms seen. Culture results to follow.
- CSF sugar, 3.6 mmol/l (blood sugar, 5.0 mmol/l)
- Protein. 5.0 g/l

Q How do you interpret these results?

A CSF is almost always abnormal in HSE, but the changes are not specific. The above lumbar puncture results are compatible with a diagnosis of HSE

(see above). The most common CSF abnormality in HSE is the presence of red cells, reflecting the haemorrhagic necrosis within the brain substance caused by the virus. The protein is on the high side, indicative of inflammation.

The CT scan shows focal areas of low attenuation in both temporal lobes containing flecks of haemorrhage and exerting a mass effect. The most common site of involvement of HSE is the temporal lobe and bilateral involvement is not unusual. Therefore, this also supports the diagnosis of HSE.

Q What is the treatment of herpes simplex encephalitis?

A Aciclovir, administered intravenously in high dose (see Appendix 3). This antiviral agent has potent anti-HSV activity, preventing viral replication.

On the basis of the CSF findings and the CT scan a provisional diagnosis of herpes simplex encephalitis is made, and Mr Aldridge is started on intravenous aciclovir, 10 mg/kg three times a day.

Q Should you have awaited laboratory confirmation of the diagnosis before initiating therapy?

A No. It is vital that specific antiviral therapy be started as soon as the diagnosis is suspected. Delay

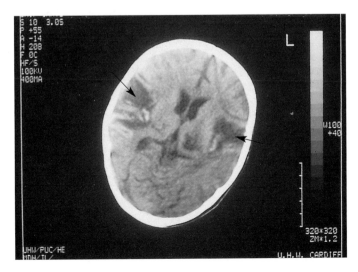

Fig. 42.1 Mr Aldridge's CT scan. Arrows point to areas of low attenuation in the frontotemporal regions.

in onset of therapy may have dire consequences in terms of residual morbidity on recovery.

Five days later you ring the laboratory to check on the progress of the various samples sent, and you are told that the serum sample taken on the day of admission contained no anti-HSV as determined by a complement fixation test (CFT), and the cultures inoculated with the CSF are not showing any cytopathic effect (CPE).

Q In the light of this new information, should the diagnosis be revised?

A No. The initial diagnosis of HSE was eminently correct. Mr Aldridge gave a classical history, the CSF findings were compatible with the diagnosis, and the CT scan revealed focal haemorrhagic lesions in the temporal lobes. In reality, most cases of HSE will in fact be much harder to diagnose than this one.

The absence of anti-HSV antibodies, determined by a relatively insensitive technique (CFT) in the acute serum sample, does not influence the diagnosis. Failure to isolate HSV from the CSF is the norm, not the exception in HSE. This result therefore also has no bearing on the diagnosis.

Mr Aldridge improves considerably following his admission to hospital, and the initiation of aciclovir therapy. By day 5, his temperature has settled, his speech has improved, and he shows no further episodes of bizarre behaviour.

Q Should you now consider stopping his aciclovir?

A No. There are reports of relapses of HSE following cessation of antiviral therapy, and there is also evidence from repeated lumbar punctures that HSE may be a more chronic disease than hitherto suspected. Hence it is advisable to continue therapy for a minimum 10-day course, even in the presence of the excellent response shown by Mr Aldridge.

Q The differential diagnosis of viral encephalitis shown in Table 42.1 mentions West Nile and Nipah viruses. Where might you find these, and why have they been in the news recently?

A These infections are referred to as 'emerging' infections, i.e. they have been described only recently, or they have appeared recently in a new geographical location. The salient features of West Nile virus infection are shown in Box 42.1. Nipah virus is named after the place where it was first discovered, as the cause of an epidemic of an encephalitic illness affecting humans (mainly pig farmers) and pigs in Malaysia in 1999. The natural host is most likely the fruit bat. The mode of transmission to humans is uncertain, but requires close contact with contaminated tissue from infected animals.

Box 42.1 West Nile virus

- Virology. A flavivirus, related to Japanese and St Louis encephalitis viruses
- Epidemiology. Viral reservoir is found in wild birds, which also act as the mode of geographical spread through migration
- Endemic in Africa, the Middle East, parts of Asia
- Introduced in 1999 into the USA, where it is now endemic
- Spread by the bite of an infected mosquito
- Clinical. Most infections, e.g. 80%, are asymptomatic.
- More severe disease presents with fever, rash, headache, and muscle weakness
- Most severe cases (< 1 in 100, and usually the elderly or immunosuppressed) develop encephalitis, which can be fatal
- Prevention. Requires mosquito control programmes. Experimental vaccines being developed

Summary: Herpes simplex encephalitis (HSE)

Presentation

Variable. May include fever, decreasing conscious level, focal neurological signs, speech and behavioural changes

Diagnosis

Clinical, with evidence of a focal lesion by any brain imaging technique. Rapid virological diagnosis by PCR assay of CSF for HSV DNA if available

Treatment

Immediate high-dose intravenous aciclovir for at least 10 days unless diagnosis is revised

Case 43 Jim, a 72-year-old man with progressive headache

Jim, a 72-year-old man, complains of a severe progressive headache over 1 month. There is no accompanying vomiting or photophobia, and he has otherwise been in good health until now. He does not smoke and drinks only occasionally. His close family have noticed that he is more lethargic of late, and he has also been observed having short-term memory lapses. On examination Jim has a temperature of 37.5°C and a pulse rate of 80/min. There is no neck stiffness, papilloedema, focal neurological signs, or abnormalities of any of the other organ systems. Following referral to hospital, he is admitted for further investigations.

Q What is the likely differential diagnosis?

A The recent onset of severe and progressive headache is ominous and suggestive of intracranial pathology. This includes:

- a cerebral neoplasm (primary or secondary)
- cerebrovascular accident; cerebral infarction
- meningitis; encephalitis
- chronic subdural haematoma
- subdural empyema
- brain abscess

Sinusitis, arthritis of the spine or jaw, and temporal arteritis might present with some of the features described above, but exclusion of intracranial pathology is essential first.

Q What initial investigations are indicated?

A A full blood count, serum urea and electrolytes, and erythrocyte sedimentation rate (ESR) or plasma viscosity, although non-specific, should exclude a connective tissue disorder (e.g. temporal arteritis) and may indicate systemic disease or point to an infective process. A lumbar puncture is required to exclude meningitis and is not contraindicated here (see Case 41 for contraindications). A heavily blood-stained cerebrospinal fluid

(CSF) that persists during the procedure, or xanthochromia, may indicate a recent intracranial haemorrhage. A computerized tomography (CT) or magnetic resonance imaging (MRI) scan, however, is likely to be the most useful investigation in confirming intracranial pathology, and many would prefer to carry this out in advance of a lumbar puncture in case of raised intracranial pressure not evident clinically. Other investigations, such as skull X-rays, arteriography, isotope brain scans, and electroencephalograms (EEG), have largely been superseded by the sensitivity of CT and MRI scans.

The initial results of investigations are: haemoglobin, 12.5 g/l; white cell count, 9.5×10^9/l (60% polymorph neutrophils); platelet count, 250/mm^3; and an ESR of 40 mm/h. Serum urea and electrolytes are normal. Lumbar puncture results in clear CSF under normal pressure with 3 red blood cells/mm^3, 85 white cells/mm^3 (50% polymorphs), a protein of 11 g/l (normal, 1.5–4 g/l) and a CSF glucose of 3.2 mmol/l (serum, 4.5 mmol/l). Gram and Ziehl–Neelsen stains are negative and there is no growth from bacterial, including mycobacterial, and viral cultures. The CT scan is shown in Fig. 43.1.

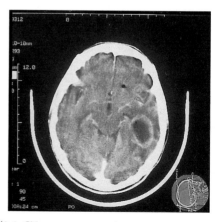

Fig. 43.1 CT scan at presentation.

Q Comment on the results of these investigations. What is the likely diagnosis?

A The ESR is unremarkable for a 72-year-old man and precludes the diagnosis of temporal arteritis. The CSF is abnormal (pleocytosis, elevated protein) but does not indicate specific pathology. In the absence of recent antibacterial agents, bacterial meningitis is unlikely and, despite the failure to isolate a virus from CSF culture, viral encephalitis is still possible, with herpes simplex the most likely (see Case 42). The CT scan suggests a mass in the temporal lobe that is circumscribed by ring enhancement and surrounded by cerebral oedema, all highly suggestive of a brain abscess. MRI is said to be more sensitive than CT, and may in addition detect satellite lesions, but it is not always available. Figure 43.2 highlights important predisposing risk factors in the pathogenesis of cerebral abscess.

Jim is taken to the operating theatre and undergoes a craniotomy: 3 ml of purulent fluid are removed from the right temporal lobe.

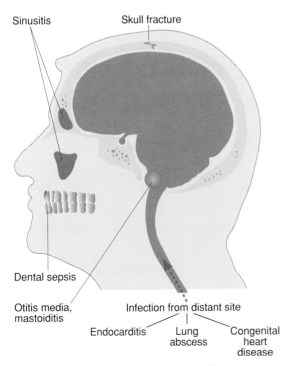

Fig. 43.2 Predisposing factors in cerebral abscess.

Labels: Sinusitis, Skull fracture, Dental sepsis, Otitis media, mastoiditis, Endocarditis, Infection from distant site, Lung abscess, Congenital heart disease

Gram's stain of this reveals numerous pus cells and Gram-positive cocci in chains (Fig. 43.3).

Q What is the likely microbiological aetiology?

A Gram-positive cocci in chains are very indicative of streptococci, and here one of the *Streptococcus anginosus* group, previously known as *Str. milleri*, is the most likely pathogen. These bacteria are part of the normal respiratory and gastrointestinal flora, grow best under microaerophilic conditions (sufficient CO_2), are characteristically associated with brain and liver abscesses, and on artificial media such as blood agar have a sweet caramel-like aroma. Other possibilities include anaerobic streptococci, viridans streptococci such as *S. mitis*, and *S. pneumoniae* (see Table 43.1).

Q What antimicrobial agents should be started pending the results of culture and sensitivity testing?

A In general, where an abscess can be drained antibiotics may not be required, provided all the infected material has been removed and the patient has no systemic evidence of infection. This does not strictly apply here, because of the inaccessibility of the infected site and the consequences of relapse requiring further surgery or drainage with considerable associated morbidity. The choice of agent is governed by the likely pathogen, the antimicrobial sensitivity pattern, and the ability of the agent to cross the blood–brain barrier and achieve adequate concentrations in brain tissue. Certain antimicrobial agents, such as the aminoglycosides, do not cross the blood–brain barrier in appreciable concentrations, even in the presence of inflammation or meningitis. Chloramphenicol and the third-generation cephalosporins reach relatively high concentrations in the CSF and brain, as does metronidazole, which will cover most anaerobes. Whilst awaiting the results of culture, a combination of high-dose intravenous cefotaxime and metronidazole would be a sensible choice. Cefotaxime is preferred to penicillin G, or ampicillin to cover Gram-negative bacilli, which may not be visible on the Gram's stain. A summary of antibiotics used in treating CNS infections and their characteristics is provided in Table 43.2.

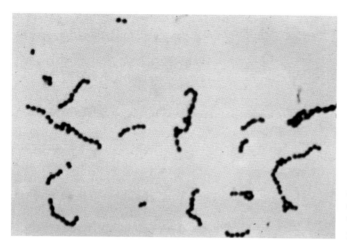

Fig. 43.3 Gram-positive cocci in chains, very suggestive of streptococci, seen on microscopy of pus.

Table 43.1 Aetiology of brain abscess according to anatomical location

Site	Predisposing factors	Organisms
Frontal	Sinusitis	Streptococci, *Bacteroides*,
	Dental sepsis	*Staphylococcus aureus*, *Haemophilus* spp.
Temporal	Otitis media	Streptococci, *Bacteroides* spp.,
	Mastoiditis	*Enterobacteriaceae*
Frontal, temporal, parietal, etc.	Trauma Penetrating wound	*S. aureus*, *Clostridia* spp.
Multiple	Infective endocarditis	*S. aureus*, viridans streptococci
	Congenital heart disease	*Fusobacteria*
	Lung abscess	*Nocardia*

Table 43.2 Antibiotics used to treat CNS infections, including brain abscesses

Antibiotic	Penetration into CNS	Comment
Cefotaxime	Good, especially if inflamed	Used for meningitis and brain abscess
Benzylpenicillin/flucloxacillin	Good, especially if inflamed	Used for meningitis and brain abscess
Metronidazole	Good	Anaerobic brain abscesses
Chloramphenicol	Very good	Replaced by cefotaxime due to toxicity
Gentamicin	Poor	Intrathecally for Gram-negative meningitis
Vancomycin	Poor	Intrathecal use for CSF shunt-associated infections

A pure growth of streptococci, one of the *S. anginosus* group, sensitive to penicillin and the cephalosporins, is isolated from the material aspirated during surgery. Jim makes a slow but gradual recovery and, on discharge from hospital 4 weeks later, is much less lethargic and fully orientated. The CT scan just before discharge shows considerable resolution of the initial abnormality but with residual ring enhancement, but at 6 months it is reported as normal.

Q How long should Jim remain on antibiotics?

A There are no hard data indicating how long treatment should be continued in this case. As the isolate is sensitive to penicillin, the cefotaxime should be replaced by high-dose intravenous penicillin, which will reduce the cost of treatment and is less likely to result in superinfections arising from a broad-spectrum cephalosporin. Intravenous treatment should be continued for 2–3 weeks and should be followed by oral amoxycillin for approximately another 4 weeks, i.e. 6 weeks in total. The duration of treatment and how long parenteral therapy should be continued depends a great deal, however, on the organism, its sensitivity pattern, operative findings—in particular how much of the infected material could be removed—and the initial response to antibiotics. Consequently, the treatment regimen needs to be tailored to individual circumstances in many patients. Because of the seriousness of the condition and the consequences of relapse, the duration of therapy may be longer than required, but there is a dearth of clinical trials in this area to guide us.

Q What is the prognosis from brain abscess?

A Since the arrival of antibacterial agents mortality has fallen from about 50% to approximately 10%. An adverse outcome is dictated by a number of factors (see Box 43.1). The incidence of seizures following diagnosis and treatment ranges from 30 to 70%, and there may be a role in many cases for prophylactic anticonvulsant therapy. Prognosis is also influenced by underlying disease and aetiology: fungal abscesses, e.g. *Candida albicans*, *Aspergillus* spp., often reflect severe immunosuppression and neutropenia, and antifungal agents do not achieve high concentrations in brain tissue.

Box 43.1 **Risk factors predicting an unfavourable outcome from brain abscess**

- Delayed diagnosis
- Posterior fossa location
- Multiple, deep or multiloculated lesions
- Rupture into the ventricles
- Coma (> 50% mortality)
- Fungal aetiology

Summary: **Brain abscess**

Presentation

Headache, drowsiness, change in personality that may come on over weeks or months

Diagnosis

Exclusion of other causes of intracranial pathology, e.g. tumour. Definitive diagnosis now is by CT or MRI scan

Management

Aspiration of pus by craniotomy or by burr hole, and intravenous antibiotics for 2–3 weeks followed by oral antibiotics for approximately another 2 weeks

Case 44 John, a 75-year-old man with muscle weakness

John, a 75-year-old man, is referred to the medical outpatients department with a 4-day history of muscle weakness and cramps, especially of the lower limbs, and difficulty in swallowing solids. He smokes 5–10 cigarettes a day and drinks occasionally at week-ends. He is on hydrochlorthiazide for mild hypertension and temazepam for difficulty in sleeping. On examination he is apyrexial, his blood pressure is 160/90 mmHg, and his pulse rate is 90/min. There is generalized abdominal rigidity but with normal bowel sounds and increased muscle tone, which is most marked in the adductor muscles of the upper limbs. Sensation is normal.

Following admission to hospital for investigation and management, his symptoms worsen over the next 2 days. There is increased clenching of the fists, extension of the lower limbs, and, later, difficulty in swallowing liquids. On the third day following admission John has a respiratory arrest, is resuscitated, and immediately transferred to the intensive therapy unit (ITU). There he is ventilated and a chest X-ray shows patchy consolidation of the superior segments of the right upper lobe, suggestive of aspiration pneumonia.

Q What is the most likely diagnosis?

A A combination of increased muscle tone and rigidity, difficulty swallowing, and respiratory muscle paralysis of fairly recent origin suggests tetanus, which is caused by a toxin, tetanospasmin, released by *Clostridium tetani*. The diagnosis of tetanus is usually made on clinical grounds, other possible causes having been excluded by lumbar puncture (normal cerebrospinal fluid (CSF)) and a negative computerized tomography (CT) scan. The classic features, including lockjaw and *risus sardonicus* (sardonic smile), however, may often be absent. A history of trauma with isolation of the bacterium

from the infected site may help in diagnosis, but in many cases this is absent. A history of immunization in a child or a booster dose of the vaccine within the last 5 years makes the diagnosis unlikely.

Q How is tetanus acquired?

A Tetanus is acquired in the developed world from wounds, especially if there is devitalized tissue, contaminated by soil containing clostridial spores, such as following a gardenering or road traffic accident. Neonatal tetanus may be acquired in other parts of the world where the umbilical cord gets contaminated during childbirth.

Q What other conditions might explain this combination of signs and symptoms?

A The above clinical picture describes abnormalities of the peripheral and bulbar motor systems. A number of possibilities arise:

- oculogyric crisis due to phenothiazines; temazepam is unlikely to cause this
- hypocalcaemic or alkalotic tetany; excluded by serum calcium and blood pH
- intracranial mass or haemorrhage; exclusively motor presentation makes this less likely
- strychnine poisoning; excluded by history or toxic screen
- meningitis; absence of fever and nuchal rigidity make this less likely

Q What other conditions resulting in neuroparalytic disease may be caused by *Clostridium* spp.?

A Botulism, an unusual form of food poisoning caused by toxins released by *C. botulinum*, also causes muscle weakness. There are important autonomic abnormalities, more prominent than in tetanus, such as reduced salivation, ileus, and urinary retention. The main features of botulism are shown in Box 44.1.

Q What are the principles of management for a patient with tetanus?

A Patients require immediate referral to hospital and usually admission to an ITU for ventilation. As this condition is toxin-mediated and it is difficult to counteract the effects of tetanospasmin once it is within the neuronal axons (see Fig. 44.1), the primary objective of management is to avoid the complications of paralysis until the toxin levels fall. Benzodiazepines such as diazepam reduce anxiety, sedate, and act as a central anticonvulsant. Anti-arrhythmic agents may be required to treat unstable cardiac rhythm, and antibiotics are indi-cated to treat complicating infections such as pneu-monia. Wound debridement and penicillin are indicated early on if there is a history of trauma, but often patients present some time after this when there is no evidence of a wound. Human tetanus immunoglobulin, administered intramus-cularly, will oppose the action of any tetanospasmin that has not entered the nervous system, but there is little evidence to support the injection of this antitoxin around the site of the initial wound or injury, as by the time of diagnosis there will be no toxin remaining locally. Finally, parenteral or enteral feeding and good nursing care to prevent decubitus ulcers, venous thrombosis, and pul-monary embolism are essential features of overall management.

Q What is the prognosis for this patient?

A Mortality is highest at the extremes of life. The majority of children with neonatal tetanus die, but this probably reflects more their poor social and nutritional background. Approximately 40% of those over 50 years of age die, and this is largely influenced by the presence of pre-existing disease such as ischaemic heart disease, and the quality of intensive care in preventing complications following prolonged ventilation. Muscle spasms usually persist for 10 days or so, but in the absence of the complica-tions referred to above recovery is usually complete.

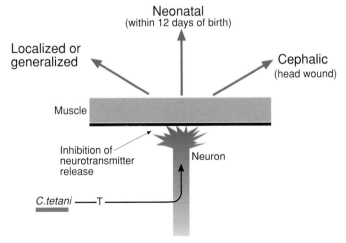

Fig. 44.1 Pathogenesis and classification of tetanus.

Table 44.1 **Guidelines for the use of toxoid and tetanus immunoglobulin**

Time of previous effective vaccination or booster	Tetanus vaccine required?		Tetanus immunoglobulin required?	
	Clean wounds	Other wounds	Clean wounds	Other wounds
<5 years ago	No	No	No	No
5–10 years ago	No	Yes	No	No
>10 years or unknown	Yes	Yes	No	Yes

John requires prolonged ventilation owing to aspiration pneumonia and adult respiratory distress syndrome (ARDS). He subsequently develops renal failure and requires dopamine to maintain blood pressure. Two weeks following admission John dies of multiple organ failure.

Q How is tetanus prevented?

A There is an effective vaccine available for use in the prevention of tetanus—this is not the case in botulism. This is usually administered in childhood as part of a triple vaccine with diphtheria toxoid and bordetella (acellular vaccine) at 2, 3, and 4 months, with boosters at 4–5 and 15 years of age. Adequate immunity is believed to persist for approximately 10 years. In the light of the age of the patient described above, it is probable that he was never vaccinated or had not received a booster in the last 10 years. Alternatively, antibody levels may have declined with advancing age. Wound debridement and the aspiration of pus are also important measures in prevention, and penicillin is indicated if the wound is likely to be infected with anaerobic bacteria. A patient presenting to the accident and emergency department may also require tetanus immunoglobulin at the time of wound debridement (see Table 44.1).

Summary: Tetanus

Diagnosis
Largely clinical from motor signs present in the limbs and bulbar muscle groups, other possible causes having been excluded. History of wound not always present and isolation of *C. tetani* rare

Management
Supportive, e.g. ventilation, artificial feeding, etc. Also intramuscular tetanus immunoglobulin and penicillin if bacterium likely to be still present; toxoid vaccine with boosters every 5–10 years is protective

Case 45 Andrew, a 20-year-old student with fever, nausea, and headache

Andrew, a 20-year-old student, presents with a 5-day history of fever, malaise, anorexia, nausea, and headache. He also reports difficulty in sleeping and, when he does sleep, he is disturbed by vivid nightmares. Over the same period, he has noticed a tingling sensation in a patch of skin on his left arm. He has no significant past medical history and is on no regular medication. On examination, he is febrile, but there is little else of note, apart from a ragged healed scar on his left arm, which Andrew confirms is the site of abnormal sensation.

Q What are your initial impressions of Andrew's presentation?

A Most of the symptoms and signs described here are very non-specific, and not suggestive of any particular pathology, but the history of abnormal sensation arising in a scar is of interest.

On further enquiry, it transpires that Andrew was bitten by a dog 3 months ago whilst backpacking in South America. Apart from thoroughly washing the area of the bite, he took no further action.

Q What diagnosis should you now consider?

A The obvious worry now is that Andrew may be suffering from rabies. Clinical rabies presents with a non-specific prodrome, lasting 2–7 days, which may include all of the symptoms mentioned, as well as vomiting, diarrhoea, sore throat, cough, and myalgia. Many patients also report behaviour disturbances, including hyperactivity, insomnia, hallucinations, anxiety, and aggression. Abnormal sensation in the site of a previous bite occurs in about 50%. The history of a bite is therefore critical, but a bite some 3–6 months previously may easily be forgotten by the patient, and the tell-tale scar may be missed by the physician.

You admit Andrew to hospital for observation, and conduct some diagnostic tests (see below) which confirm a diagnosis of rabies. Over the next 3 days he becomes increasingly restless and agitated, exhibiting purposeless movements of his limbs in response to tactile and auditory stimuli. He suffers intense spasms affecting the muscles involved in swallowing and accessory muscles of respiration, lasting for 10 seconds or so, and accompanied by frothing at the mouth. The frequency and severity of these spasms initially increase, but begin to decline after 2 days, when Andrew's conscious level declines into coma, and he dies 24 hours later.

Q Why is rabies sometimes referred to as 'hydrophobia'?

A Hydrophobia is manifested by uncontrollable violent jerking movements as fluid is brought to the mouth, leading to the onset of a spasm that may be accompanied by retching, vomiting, and generalized convulsions. It is evident in about 50% of cases of rabies. The fear of precipitating such spasms accounts for the hydrophobia. Spasms may also be precipitated by other stimuli, such as eating or a draught of air (aerophobia).

Q How may rabies be classified clinically?

A As follows:

- 'Furious' rabies, the more common form, as suffered by Andrew, is characterized by hyperexcitability, spasms, and hydrophobia
- 'Dumb' rabies presents with an ascending paralysis that may be clinically indistinguishable from the Guillain–Barré syndrome

However, these syndromes may overlap. Dumb rabies poses the greatest diagnostic problems. There may be a typical prodrome, with paralysis often involving the bitten limb first, before spreading rapidly and symmetrically.

Q What is the pathogenesis of rabies infection?

A This involves a number of stages:

1. *Entry of virus*. Intact skin is impermeable to the virus, but infection may occur across undamaged mucous membranes. Rabid animals have virus present in saliva, and so can spread infection by inoculating virus at the site of a bite or by licking abraded skin

2. *Viral replication*. Occurs initially in muscle cells at the site of the bite

3. *Ascent to the central nervous system (CNS)*. Following release from muscle cells, virus enters peripheral nerves via the neuromuscular junction and is translocated in their axoplasm to the spinal cord, and thence rapidly to the brain

4. *Spread within the CNS*. There is extensive viral replication within the brain, although curiously this results in very little gross structural damage

5. *Descent from the CNS*. Virus travels back down axoplasmic routes to sites throughout the body, including salivary glands, myocardium, lung, liver, skin, retina, and cornea. Involvement of the salivary gland mucosal epithelium results in virus being shed in salivary secretions from where it may be transmitted to others. Patients with infectious virus in their bodily secretions thus pose an infection risk to those involved in their care. Human-to-human transmission is, however, a rare occurrence

The incubation period prior to the development of disease is highly variable (up to a year, but on average 30–90 days). The shortest periods are seen in children, and in bites close to the central nervous system, i.e. head rather than foot wounds.

Q What factors influence the transmission of rabies from animal to man?

A Bites from rabid animals do not always cause disease. Factors that may influence this process include:

- the severity of the bite (may determine viral dose)

- the site of the bite—head and neck bites carry the greatest risk

- mortality is almost certainly higher for wounds inflicted through bare, rather than clothed, skin

Q What is the likely outcome of a patient suspected of rabies?

A Despite the best efforts of modern intensive care and experimental treatment with antiviral and immunomodulatory drugs, the prognosis of a patient presenting with rabies is bleak. The disease is almost invariably fatal within a short time period.

Q How can the diagnosis be confirmed?

A There are a number of possible approaches.

1. Ante-mortem
   - Demonstration of virus by specific immunofluorescence in corneal impressions (taken by gently abrading the cornea with a microscope slide) or skin biopsy (best taken from the neck or face)
   - Culture of virus from saliva or other bodily secretions. This requires access to a laboratory that has the necessary containment facilities to allow safe culture of rabies virus
   - Detection of antibodies to rabies virus in an individual who has not received vaccine

2. Post-mortem
   - Histological examination of brain tissue for the presence of Negri bodies, i.e. intracytoplasmic eosinophilic inclusions in nerve cells (see Fig. 45.1)
   - Immunofluorescent detection of rabies antigen in brain
   - Transmission of virus to laboratory animals
   - Electron microscopic detection of virus particles (which have a bullet-shaped morphology; see Fig. 45.2)

An additional approach to the demonstration of the presence of virus in bodily secretions or tissues is via genome amplification, e.g. reverse transcriptase polymerase chain reaction (RT/PCR).

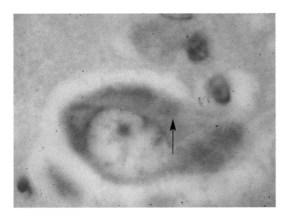

Fig. 45.1 Histological section showing Negri body (arrow).

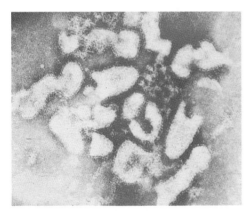

Fig. 45.2 Electron microscope picture of rabies virus.

Q Where, and in which animals, is rabies endemic?

A Rabies is enzootic in all continents except Australasia and Antarctica. There are other relatively disease-free areas (e.g. UK, Japan), mostly islands where stringent quarantine regulations are enforced.

All warm-blooded animals are susceptible to the virus, including bats and birds. Urban rabies is prevalent mostly in feral and domestic dogs. Sylvatic rabies involves a wide range of species (e.g. foxes, skunks, racoons), the predominant animal varying in different geographical areas.

Bat rabies has been of particular interest recently, as within the last 6 years there have been two reported instances of rabies in bats in the UK and, in 2002, a fatal case of bat rabies was reported in a bat handler in Scotland, the fourth case worldwide. The risk to humans is low, but anyone bitten or scratched by a bat, even in the UK, should seek advice about post-exposure prophylaxis (see below).

Q Could Andrew's fatal attack of rabies have been prevented?

A Yes. Both active (rabies vaccines) and passive (human rabies immunoglobulin) immunization against rabies are available, safe, and effective. Rabies vaccination has a long and chequered history. Vaccines derived from virus grown in nervous tissue are poorly immunogenic, and give rise to post-vaccination encephalitis in almost 1 in 1000 vaccinees. These are being replaced by safer vaccines grown in tissue culture (see below), but the latter are more expensive.

Q Who should be offered rabies vaccine?

A Pre-exposure (i.e. prophylactic) vaccine is indicated for certain occupational groups who, in the course of their work, regularly handle imported animals, e.g. at animal quarantine centres, zoos. Vaccine should also be offered to workers going abroad to enzootic areas, e.g. veterinary staff, zoologists.

Vaccine can also be administered as post-exposure prophylaxis (see below).

Q What is the correct management of a patient bitten by a possibly rabid animal?

A This includes:

1. Immediate thorough cleansing of the wound

2. Initiation of a course of post-exposure vaccination as soon as possible (see Table 45.1)

3. Individuals with high-risk exposures, e.g. deep or multiple bites, bites on the face, neck, or hands, should also be given a stat dose of human rabies immunoglobulin, one-half infiltrated around the wound itself, the remainder by intramuscular injection. This provides antibodies during the early critical period before development of active immunity

The above regimen, when properly administered, is highly successful in preventing rabies. The

Table 45.1 Post-exposure rabies vaccination

- Vaccine consists of virus grown in human diploid cells and inactivated by beta-propiolactone
- WHO recommendations are for a course of six intramuscular injections (deltoid muscle) on days 0, 3, 7, 14, 28, and 90 where day 0 is the day of the first dose, preferably also the day of the potential exposure
- Injection should *not* be into the gluteal region as vaccine failure may arise due to the poorer immunogenicity of vaccine injected into fat

immune response induced by this regimen acts to prevent entry of virus into nerve cells. The sooner it is initiated, the better, as once virus infection of nerve cells has taken place, the immune response has no effect.

Résumé for undergraduates

Rabies is a zoonotic disease caused by a virus, transmitted by bites and saliva from rabid animals, resulting in a fatal encephalomyelitis. It is preventable by appropriate use of active and passive vaccination.

Summary: Rabies

Presentation

Non-specific prodrome (malaise, headache, tingling at site of bite) followed by either 'furious' rabies (hyperexcitability, spasms, hydrophobia) or 'dumb' rabies (ascending paralysis)

Prognosis

Universally fatal once clinically evident

Prevention

Pre-exposure: vaccination. Post-exposure: vaccination following *any* possible exposure, plus passive immunization if risk of infection is high

Case 46 Mr Grundy, a 62-year-old histopathology biomedical scientist who has become forgetful and disorientated

Mr Grundy is brought to your surgery by his wife. He is 62 years old and works in the local hospital as a histopathology biomedical scientist. He had been well until 6 weeks ago, since when he has become increasingly anxious and forgetful, with difficulty in speaking and walking. On direct questioning, Mr Grundy appears somewhat confused and disorientated. He exhibits a number of multifocal myoclonic jerks on examination. He has evidence of both a receptive and expressive dysphasia.

You admit Mr Grundy to hospital for further investigation. Routine investigations, including urea and electrolytes, liver function tests, and blood gases, are normal. During the next 2 weeks, he becomes unsteady on his feet, with a number of falls, and his mental state deteriorates to one of dementia, with memory loss, impaired judgement, and a decline in virtually all aspects of mental function. There is no family history of dementing illnesses. Computerized tomography (CT) scan and cerebrospinal fluid (CSF) examination are normal. His electroencephalogram (EEG) reveals repetitive high-voltage polyphasic discharges.

A clinical diagnosis is made (see below). No treatment is offered, and Mr Grundy's condition continues to deteriorate. He dies 2 months after admission to hospital. Postmortem studies of his brain reveal the abnormalities shown in Fig. 46.1 (compare with Fig. 46.2).

Q What is the diagnosis?

A The striking features of Mr Grundy's illness are his relentlessly progressive dementia and ataxia. Routine investigations ruled out a metabolic cause of his presentation (e.g. liver, renal, or respiratory failure). There are a large number of dementing illnesses (e.g. Alzheimer's disease, Lewy body dementia), but the history of myoclonic jerks, plus the abnormal EEG, are suggestive of classical Creutzfeldt–Jakob disease (CJD). The majority of patients with CJD present with deficits in higher cortical function, which progress to a state of profound dementia. A minority may present with cerebellar or visual defects, which are usually followed rapidly by the onset of dementia. Over 85% of patients exhibit myoclonus, which persists in sleep, and may be elicited by sudden stimuli such as loud noises or bright lights.

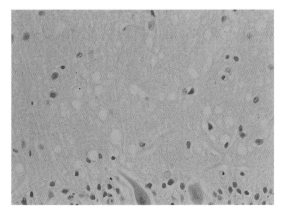

Fig. 46.1 Cerebral tissue from Mr Grundy.

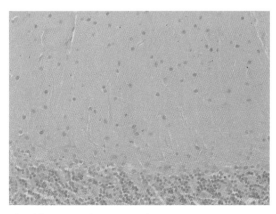

Fig. 46.2 Tissue from normal brain.

The brain histology of Mr Grundy confirms the diagnosis, by showing the spongiform change characteristic of this disease. Higher power studies would confirm that these changes are due to vacuolation within the nerve cells, rather than *between* them (as might occur in Alzheimer's disease, due to rapid loss of neurons from the brain).

Q Is CJD caused by an infectious agent?

A Yes ... and no (see below)! Inoculation of CJD brain into an experimental animal results in transmission of the disease—hence the classification of CJD as infectious—but the agent responsible is not one of the common groups of infectious pathogens, e.g. bacteria, viruses.

Q To what class of diseases does CJD belong?

A CJD is one of a group of diseases of humans and animals that share a number of distinctive features and are known by a variety of names:

- *transmissible dementias* (transmissible to experimental animals; dementia is the pre-eminent feature of the disease in humans)
- *spongiform encephalopathies* (neuronal vacuolation in brain produces spongy appearance)
- *prion diseases* (prions believed to be the causative agents; see below)
- *slow infections* (prolonged incubation period, infectious)

Q Name the known diseases of humans and animals that constitute this particular group.

A These diseases include:

Disease	Host species
Scrapie	Sheep, goats
Transmissible mink encephalopathy	Mink
Chronic wasting disease	Mule deer and elk
Bovine spongiform encephalopathy (a.k.a. 'mad-cow disease)	Cows
Kuru	Humans (cannibals)
Creutzfeldt–Jakob disease	Humans
Gerstmann–Straussler–Sheinker syndrome (very rare)	Humans

The salient features of these diseases are:

- pathology is largely confined to the CNS
- prolonged incubation period
- once disease presents, a progressive and fatal clinical course
- reactive astrocytosis and vacuolation of neurons on histology
- transmissible to experimental animals by intracerebral inoculation of diseased tissue

Q What is unusual about the causative agents of these diseases?

A The infectious agent is believed to consist entirely of protein! The term prion was coined to describe this novel agent, 'prion' being originally derived from the phrase 'proteinaceous infectious particle'. This radical hypothesis is based on the following lines of evidence.

- Infectivity of scrapie brain in experimental animals is resistant to a wide range of physical and chemical treatments that destroy nucleic acids, but is, however, affected by treatments that destroy or alter protein molecules
- Despite intensive efforts by many research groups, no one has succeeded in identifying any nucleic acid in the scrapie agent
- A protein of molecular weight 27–30 kDa (also referred to as prion protein, or PrP 27–30) whose concentration parallels the infectivity of experimental inocula has been identified in scrapie brain. This protein is resistant to proteolytic digestion, and is therefore also referred to as PrP^{res}. It is in fact a breakdown product of a larger protein of molecular weight 33–35 kDa (PrP 33–35).

The concept that injection of a protein molecule into a recipient animal can cause increased production of that protein, i.e. that the protein has the wherewithal to direct its own replication, challenges the very foundations of molecular biology. The gene encoding the prion protein is in fact a normal cellular gene, the product of which appears to exist in two versions, known as isoforms. The normal cellular isoform is referred to as PrP^C, whilst the abnormal (or scrapie) isoform is PrP^{Sc}. PrP^C is completely sensitive to protease digestion, whereas PrP^{Sc} is only broken down by proteases as far as PrP 27–30.

The current hypothesis as to how PrP 27–30, when injected into a normal cell, is able to induce its own production is that it causes the normal PrP^C to change into PrP^{Sc}. The latter eventually becomes digested by cellular proteases—but only as far as PrP 27–30—which therefore causes more production of PrP^{Sc} from PrP^C, and hence accumulation of more PrP 27–30, and so on. This is illustrated diagramatically in Fig. 46.3.

Thus, experimental inoculation of material containing the scrapie isoform will result in transmission of disease, as the abnormal isoform of PrP is generated in the recipient brain. A key question that is currently unanswered is what is the physical difference between PrP^C and PrP^{Sc}? In sporadic CJD, the gene encoding PrP is identical to that in non-affected patients, indicating that the difference does not simply reside in the amino acid sequence of the two forms of the protein. Presumably, the difference between the two isoforms occurs as a posttranslational event but, as yet, the nature of that event has not been identified.

The answer given above to the question 'Is CJD caused by an infectious agent?' was 'yes … and no!'. This is because in 10–15% of cases of CJD there is a family history, and the disease is hereditary. Analysis of the PrP gene in families thus afflicted shows that the prion gene does contain differences,

e.g. insertion of repeat sequences, or point mutations. The effect of these differences must be to increase considerably the likelihood of spontaneous conversion of PrP from the normal to the scrapie isoform.

Q How may accidental human-to-human transmission of CJD occur?

A CJD brain is infectious, and prions are unusually resistant to inactivation by conventional means (e.g. autoclaving at 121°C). Thus, any article contaminated by CJD tissue can inadvertently transmit the disease if it is subsequently inoculated into another patient. Such transmission has been described via:

- contaminated intracerebral EEG electrodes and other neurosurgical instruments
- corneal grafts (indicating that the abnormal prion must be present in the cornea)
- dura mater grafts
- human pituitary-derived growth hormone (given usually to children as replacement therapy) and follicle-stimulating hormone (FSH; given to women as treatment of infertility). Such human-derived hormones are no longer used

Iatrogenic transmission of CJD accounts for a tiny minority of CJD cases, but arouses considerable public interest—see Fig. 46.4.

Q Was Mr Grundy's occupation significant?

A Certain health-care professionals are more likely than the general population to be exposed to CJD-infected material, e.g. neurosurgeons, pathologists, and biomedical scientists. Cases of CJD have been described in such individuals, although at present there is no evidence that these occupational groups

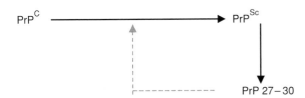

Fig. 46.3 Generation of PrP^{Sc}

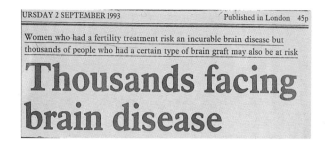

URSDAY 2 SEPTEMBER 1993   Published in London   45p

Women who had a fertility treatment risk an incurable brain disease but thousands of people who had a certain type of brain graft may also be at risk

Thousands facing brain disease

Fig. 46.4 Newspaper headline on follicle-stimulating hormone (FSH)-exposed women.

are overrepresented. However, it is clear that appropriate guidelines to reduce the risk of occupational exposure to these agents should be instigated.

Whether sporadic CJD arises through genuine transmission of the infectious agent, or through a chance event resulting in endogenous production of PrP^{Sc} is unclear. The latter seems a more likely explanation.

Q Are 'mad cows' safe to eat?

A Bovine spongiform encephalopathy (BSE), or 'mad cow disease', arose in the UK (first case described in 1986) due to the practice (now banned) of feeding ruminant offal to cows. Whether BSE is due to transmission of scrapie from sheep to cows, or whether there has always been an endogenous bovine agent, which has become amplified through the feeding cycle, is not clear. The epidemic in cattle does demonstrate that the infectious agent is transmissible through the oral route.

In 1996, a new variant of CJD was described in the UK, now known as vCJD. This was recognizable as a distinct entity because of several features, including the unusually young age of presentation (e.g. less than 40, while classical CJD is very rare in the under-60s, unless iatrogenically transmitted) and the very florid nature and signature distribution of plaques of abnormal prion protein present in the brain of sufferers. There is now an abundance of sophisticated laboratory evidence in favour of the hypothesis that vCJD has arisen through oral ingestion by humans of the agent responsible for the bovine epidemic of spongiform encephalopathy. How many cases of vCJD in humans will arise from consumption of infected bovine material

remains uncertain. Prion diseases, as mentioned above, have a long incubation period, and mathematical models of the outbreak of human disease give results varying from an optimistic few hundred to a pessimistic hundreds of thousands.

The BSE epidemic in cows has all but subsided to zero, following the ban on using ruminant offal to feed cows in the late 1980s. Several additional safeguards have also been put in place to minimize the risk of transmission of disease to humans, including the specified offal ban (whereby bovine offal is regarded as unfit for human consumption, as it may contain the abnormal prion protein) and steps taken to prevent nervous tissue contamination of meat destined for human consumption.

Q Are there any other possible routes of spread of this disease into and within the human population?

A Unfortunately, yes.

- There is a worry that the BSE agent may have crossed into sheep. Whilst there is good epidemiological evidence that scrapie in sheep is not directly transmissible to humans, this situation is different, as it involves a new agent that has already crossed at least one species barrier (bovine to human). Thus, it is conceivable that in the UK we have been exposed to infected ovine tissue, as well as bovine.

- We have no idea how many humans are in the incubation phase of vCJD. The pathogenic prion may be present in tissues other than the brain of such individuals—indeed, it has already been demonstrated in the tonsils and appendix of patients who underwent surgery at a time before their diagnosis of vCJD was made or even suspected. Given the remarkable resistance of prions to conventional forms of sterilization, it is possible that the disease will be spread inadvertently through, for instance, contaminated surgical instruments.

- The prion responsible for vCJD may be present in peripheral blood and therefore the infection may be spread via blood transfusion.

These are nightmare scenarios. It is to be hoped that they do not transpire. In the first edition of this book we wrote 'Several expert governmental committees have assessed the risk of transmission of BSE to humans via the oral route, and have concluded that such a risk is miniscule. Others disagree. Time will tell!' That particular nightmare has already eventuated.

Résumé for undergraduates

Prions are a new class of infectious agents that appear to be 'protein only'; they are associated with a number of diseases of animals and humans, including Creutzfeld–Jakob disease (CJD). The hallmark pathological feature of prion diseases is spongiform change within the brain. The recent epidemic of bovine spongiform encephalopathy (BSE; aka mad cow disease) in the UK has led to the transmission of the BSE prion to humans, manifesting as a variant form of CJD, known as vCJD.

Summary: Creutzfeldt–Jakob disease

Presentation
Progressive dementia, ataxia, myoclonus

Diagnosis
Spongiform pathology and presence of PrP 27–30 within brain seen at post-mortem

Causative agent
Prion, may consist entirely of protein. Product of normal gene, with posttranslational modification. May catalyse its own formation

Iatrogenic infection
May arise from contaminated neurosurgical instruments, human pituitary-derived hormones, dura mater grafts

Variant CJD
A new disease, due to transmission of the bovine agent to humans through consumption of contaminated food

Self-assessment

1. Which one of the following statements regarding herpes simplex encephalitis is true?

(a) The presence of active orolabial herpes is a useful diagnostic indicator of the cause of the encephalitis

(b) The parietal lobes are most often affected

(c) Culture of CSF is positive in less than 5% of cases

(d) Brain biopsy is always needed to confirm the diagnosis

(e) Neuroimaging does not usually reveal focal lesions

2. Which of the following are recognized causes of viral encephalitis?

(a) West Nile virus

(b) Measles virus

(c) Rabies virus

(d) Coxsackie B viruses

(e) Mumps virus

3. Which one of the following statements regarding rabies is not true?

(a) Post-exposure prophylaxis of a high-risk exposure includes both passive and active immunization

(b) Rabies vaccine should not be administered into the gluteal muscle

(c) Rabies vaccine used in the UK contains live attenuated virus

(d) Rabies virus is endogenous in the UK bat population

(e) Rabies encephalomyelitis is characterized by the formation of Negri bodies in infected cells

4. Which one of the following statements regarding rabies is not true?

(a) Can be transmitted to humans via bat-bites

(b) May have a prolonged incubation period, e.g. up to a year

(c) Is almost invariably fatal once symptoms develop

(d) Is transmitted to the brain via the bloodstream

(e) Can be diagnosed by immunofluorescent staining of corneal impression smears

5. Iatrogenic CJD has been associated with which of the following?

(a) Contaminated EEG electrodes

(b) Corneal transplantation

(c) Dura mater grafts

(d) Human growth hormone

(e) Human follicle-stimulating hormone

6. Which of the following statements regarding spongiform encephalopathies is not true?

(a) The causative agent of CJD has been shown to contain a limited amount of DNA

(b) Routine autoclave procedures are not sufficient to eliminate infectivity of CJD

(c) The scrapie isoform of PrP cannot be completely digested by proteinase K

(d) Variant CJD arises as a result of infection with the BSE agent

(e) The average age of patients with vCJD is about 20 years younger than that of those with classical CJD

7. Which one of the following diseases of the central nervous system is thought to have a viral aetiology?

(a) Alzheimer's disease

(b) Progressive multifocal leuco-encephalopathy (PMLE)

(c) Creutzfeldt–Jakob disease

(d) Kuru

(e) Parkinson's disease

8. In which one of the following samples may a Gram film reveal the presence of Gram-negative intracellular diplococci with 'pus' cells, indicating a well recognized infection?

(a) urine

(b) intraabdominal pus

(c) cerebrospinal fluid (CSF)

(d) sputum

(e) postoperative wound swab

9. A CSF specimen with raised white cells, predominantly lymphocytes, is characteristic of which pathogen causing infection of the CNS?

(a) *Neisseria meningitidis*

(b) *Haemophilus influenzae* type b

(c) *Listeria monocytogenes*

(d) *Streptococcus pneumoniae*

(e) *Leptospira* spp.

10. Which of the following bacteria is the most likely cause of brain abscess secondary to infective endocarditis?

(a) *Staphylococcus aureus*

(b) *Staphylococcus epidermidis*

(c) *Escherichia coli*

(d) *Streptococcus milleri/anginosus* group

(e) *Bacteroides fragilis*

11. Which antibiotic penetrates well into brain tissue and therefore renders it useful in the treatment of brain abscesses?

(a) Gentamicin

(b) Ciprofloxacin

(c) Cefotaxime

(d) Trimethoprim

(e) Erythromycin

12. Which species of clostridia is associated with food poisoning?

(a) *C. difficile*

(b) *C. botulinum*

(c) *C. tetani*

(d) *C. sporogenes*

(e) *C. septicum*

13. Which of the following patients require tetanus immunoglobulin as part of traumatic wound management?

(a) 3-year-old with a clean wound

(b) 4-year-old girl with a dirty wound

(c) 7-year-old boy with a clean wound

(d) 45-year-old man with a dirty wound

(e) 35-year-old female with a clean wound

6

CHAPTER 6

Systemic infections

SECTION 6
Systemic infections

Case 47 Mary, a 35-year-old engineer with nausea, weakness, and rigors

Late on Friday evening Mary, a 35-year-old engineer, is taken to the accident and emergency department of her local hospital following consultation with her GP by phone. That afternoon she had become feverish, nauseous, and generally weak. Later, she had experienced two episodes of rigors. Four years previously she had a breast lump, which was benign, removed and during her two pregnancies had had recurrent urinary tract infections. A week before this presentation she complained of dysuria and frequency, and was prescribed oral ampicillin for presumed cystitis.

Q What is the most likely diagnosis and which physical sign may confirm this?

A Pyelonephritis is the most likely diagnosis, often characterized by renal angle tenderness with fever.

On examination Mary looks flushed and has a temperature of 40°C and a tachycardia of 120/min. General physical examination, including that of the breasts and axillary lymph nodes, is normal apart from acute tenderness in the costovertebral or renal angle. There is protein and blood in a urine sample.

Q What investigations are indicated to confirm the diagnosis?

A A midstream sample of urine (MSU) should be examined microscopically for white and red cells, and cultured. Blood for culture should also be taken (Box 47.1). A white cell count may reveal a polymorph leucocytosis, which would be consistent with a bacterial infection.

Q How many blood culture sets should be taken?

A Two sets of blood cultures (i.e. four bottles, two per set), preferably at different times, should be taken. A negative result if one set only is taken may be false due to intermittent bacteraemia. Furthermore, the isolation of a skin bacterium, e.g. *Staphylococcus epidermidis*, may represent a false-positive result if only one set is taken, owing to contamination. In general, the greater the volume of blood cultured, the higher the diagnostic yield. It is rarely necessary, however, to take more than two sets, except with a fever of undetermined origin (see Case 53) or infective endocarditis (see Case 49).

Box 47.1 Steps in the taking of blood for culture

- Hands should be washed and gloves worn
- Inspect skin for suitable peripheral vein and disinfect (e.g. chlorhexidine in alcohol)
- Remove caps from top of blood culture bottles (usually two per set) and disinfect bung with alcohol
- Withdraw 10 ml of blood (for one set) and inject blood equally into both bottles
- Take blood culture bottles to the laboratory immediately or place in incubator (Fig. 47.1)

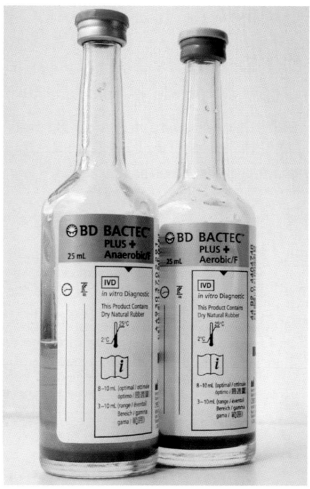

Fig. 47.1 A set of blood culture bottles, i.e. two (aerobic and anaerobic).

Q Is the yield of positive cultures from children, especially small infants, less than that from adults?

A No. It is clearly undesirable to take large volumes of blood from small children but this is compensated for by a higher number of organisms per ml of blood compared with adults. In bacteraemic adults, 1 colony-forming unit (cfu) per ml is the norm, but in infants 10–100 times more organisms may be present.

On admission, blood cultures and an MSU are taken and Mary is prescribed a first-generation cephalosporin, cephradine, which is administered orally. A lactose-positive oxidase-negative coliform is isolated from the MSU, in which there are numerous pus cells seen, and Gram-negative bacilli are seen in blood cultures. Mary's antibiotic therapy is changed as she remains symptomatic.

Q What is the likely identity of the organism in the urine and blood?

A The most common cause of urinary tract infection (see Case 34) is *Escherichia coli*, a lactose-positive coliform (see Box 47.2). The positive MSU and blood cultures confirm that Mary has pyelonephritis (upper urinary tract infection with bacteraemia).

Q What is the difference between 'bacteraemia' and 'septicaemia'?

A The terminology is a little confusing here! Strictly speaking, 'bacteraemia' refers to the presence of bacteria in the bloodstream and does not imply anything about the clinical state of the patient. Furthermore, transient clinically insignificant bacteraemia is a relatively common everyday occurrence, e.g. following defecation or while brushing teeth. The transient nature of these episodes, the low virulence of the bacteria involved, and the presence of an intact immune system ensure that there are usually no clinical consequences.

In contrast, 'septicaemia' implies that the presence of bacteria in the blood is accompanied by clinical consequences, such as high fever, rigors, low blood pressure. With septicaemia there are greater numbers of dividing bacteria in the blood, which are more likely to be pathogenic. In recent years the terms 'bacteraemia' and 'septicaemia' have been replaced by the term 'bloodstream infection', especially in North America. Whichever term is used, *E. coli* is the most common cause (see Table 47.1) and may be community- or hospital-acquired.

Q What is the most frequent primary source of bloodstream infection (BSI) ?

A The urinary tract is implicated as the source in about 30% , and this is especially true when *E. coli*,

> ### Box 47.2 *Escherichia coli*
>
> - A motile Gram-negative bacillus that grows well on non-selective media
> - Virulence may be related to the presence of certain K antigens, especially in urinary tract infection (UTI)
> - Predominates amongst the aerobic flora of the intestine, especially the colon
> - May also be found in the lower urinary and genital tracts, and occasionally in the upper respiratory tract
> - Causes UTI (see Case 34), septicaemia, neonatal meningitis (see Case 41), intraabdominal infection (see Case 26), and diarrhoea (see Case 25)

Klebsiella spp., *P. aeruginosa*, or other Gram-negative bacteria are involved. Other sources include:

- respiratory tract 15%, *Str. pneumoniae*, *S. aureus*
- gastrointestinal tract 10%, *E. coli*, *Salmonella*, etc.
- biliary tract 10%, *E. coli*
- intravascular lines 5%, coagulase-negative staphylococci (e.g. *S. epidermidis*), *S. aureus*

In a proportion of cases, however, no source can be detected clinically, microbiologically, or following extensive radiological investigations.

Table 47.1 **Aetiology of clinically significant bacteraemia (bloodstream infection)**

Organism	Hospital (HA) or community (CA) acquired	Incidence (% of total cases)
Escherichia coli	HA = CA	29
Staphylococcus aureus	HA > CA, 2:1	19
Streptococcus pneumoniae	CA > HA, 10:1	13
Klebsiella spp.	HA > CA, 3:1	7
Pseudomonas aeruginosa	HA > CA, 10:1	5
'Viridans' streptococci	CA > HA, 3:1	4
Coagulase-negative staphylococci	HA > CA, 20:1	4
Miscellaneous	Varies with the organism	19

Q Is BSI always present in septic shock?

A With a greater understanding in recent years of the pathogenesis of septic shock (see Fig. 47.2) it is apparent that this is a spectrum of conditions that may or may not be accompanied by the presence of bacteria in the bloodstream. A patient may have overwhelming sepsis with negative blood cultures because of recent antibiotics, intermittent bacteraemia, or endotoxaemia without BSI. Other terms used to describe patients with serious sepsis, especially if requiring intensive care (see Case 26), include:

- pyaemia: chills and fever due to an abscess
- sepsis syndrome: clinical evidence of infection, with tachypnoea, tachycardia, hyper- or hypothermia, and evidence of inadequate organ perfusion (e.g. hypoxaemia, oliguria)
- septic shock: sepsis syndrome with hypotension (systolic blood pressure <90 mmHg) in the absence of other causes
- fungaemia and other factors may also precipitate septic shock

Q Comment on the choice of antibiotic and route of administration in the treatment of Mary's condition.

A BSI is a potential medical emergency because of complications such as shock and multiple organ failure. Consequently, parenteral antibiotics active against the likely pathogens are indicated and, if the source or organism is not known, a broad-spectrum agent should be used. Initial treatment with oral antibiotics is therefore not appropriate, and cephradine is not optimal here because of the possibility that the bacterium may be resistant.

Q What alternatives are there?

A Mary should be changed to an intravenous second- or third-generation cephalosporin (such as cefuroxime, cefotaxime), co-amoxyclav, an aminoglycoside (e.g. gentamicin), or a fluoroquinolone (e.g. ciprofloxacin), all of which are appropriate in pyelonephritis as approximately 40–50% of coliforms will be resistant to ampicillin and the earlier cephalosporins such as cephradine. Supportive measures are also important , especially where complications have ensued (see Table 47.1).

Mary is treated with intravenous co-amoxyclav as the *E. coli* isolated from blood and urine is resistant to ampicillin, cephradine, and trimethoprim. After 72 hours she is apyrexial, her other symptoms have largely resolved, and she is changed to oral co-amoxyclav, which is continued to give a total duration of antibiotic treatment of 10 days. Before discharge from

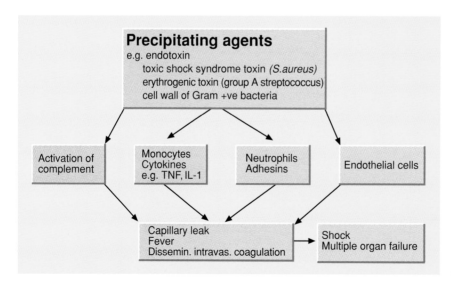

Fig. 47.2 Pathogenesis of septic shock.

Table 47.1 Management of clinically significant bacteraemia

Supportive therapy

- Fluids, e.g. intravenous colloids, saline, etc.
- Inotropes, e.g. dobutamine with monitoring
- Organ support, e.g. ventilation, haemofiltration

Removal of infected focus

- Surgery to drain abscess
- Removal of infected intravascular catheter
- Wound debridement

Antibiotics

- Must be intravenous at least initially and in high dose
- *Broad spectrum*: if aetiology unknown and focus cannot be removed, e.g. cefotaxime + metronidazole for intraabdominal sepsis
- *Narrow spectrum*: when organism known, e.g. flucloxacillin for *S. aureus*

Immunotherapy

- ? Corticosteroids: no current evidence of benefit
- ? Monoclonal antibodies, e.g. antiendotoxin (HA-1A), which is not effective; cytokine antagonists being evaluated

Q What is the mortality from clinically significant bacteraemia or BSI?

A Around 30% of patients die directly or indirectly from BSI. Underlying diseases, e.g. malignancy, or accompanying life-threatening conditions, e.g. multiple severe trauma, also contribute to an unfavourable outcome. Factors associated with a high mortality include:

- extremes of age, i.e. very young (premature neonate) or the elderly (>75 years)
- white cell count, i.e. <4 or >30 × 10^9/l
- polymicrobial infection, e.g. *E. coli* and *S. aureus* from pneumonia with BSI
- shock at initial presentation
- significant or severe underlying disease, e.g. diabetic ketoacidosis
- inappropriate or inadequate initial antibiotics

Summary: Bloodstream infection

Presentation
Fever, rigors, shock with or without symptoms related to original focus of infection, e.g. cough, sputum, chest pain with pneumonic BSI

Diagnosis
Usually confirmed by isolating organisms from blood cultures

Management
Reverse shock with intravenous (IV) fluids, IV high-dose antibiotics (broad-spectrum if aetiology unknown or pending). No role for corticosteroids

hospital arrangements are made for investigation of her genitourinary tract (see Case 34), to detect renal tract abnormalities that might explain her recurrent urinary tract infections.

Case 48 Bill, a 65-year-old man with vomiting, abdominal pain, and fever

Bill, a 65-year-old man, presented to hospital with vomiting, right-sided abdominal pain, and fever. At laparotomy a mass was detected in the ascending colon, with perforation of the bowel and generalized peritonitis. The tumour was resected and a right hemicolectomy performed. Histological examination revealed a poorly differentiated adenocarcinoma. His postoperative course was characterized by fever, a leucocytosis (white cell count $24 \times 10^9/l$) and a wound infection caused by *Staphylococcus aureus* and *Bacteroides fragilis*. Despite a 10-day course of intravenous cefotaxime, flucloxacillin, and metronidazole, he remains pyrexial with a temperature of 39–40°C and is generally unwell 2 weeks after surgery. He is unable to tolerate oral feeds, is being fed parenterally via a central line, and he also has a urinary catheter.

Q What are the possible causes of the persistent fever and leucocytosis?

A Infection is the most likely cause. Possible sites of infection include the wound, abdomen (persistent peritonitis or an intraabdominal abscess requiring drainage), intravascular line, bloodstream (i.e. bacteraemia), urinary tract (especially as he is catheterized), and chest. Other possible causes include the effects of the tumour, deep venous thrombosis or pulmonary embolism, and a drug-related fever.

Q What steps should be taken to identify the source and aetiology of the probable infection?

A Despite the antibiotics, a full septic screen should be taken, which includes two to three sets of blood cultures, a wound swab or pus (preferable to a swab if present), urine, sputum if productive cough, and removal of intravascular lines for culture if line infection is possible. These specimens should be taken just before antibiotics are given, when serum and tissue antibiotic levels are at their lowest, to maximize the chances of isolating a pathogen. A chest X-ray may help to exclude lower respiratory tract infection, and an ultrasound examination or an isotope or computerized tomography (CT) scan may help diagnose an intra-abdominal collection.

The initial results of Bill's investigations are as follows: blood cultures are sterile after 48 hours; a scanty growth of an enterococcus is isolated from the wound swab; a catheter urine specimen is sterile; *Candida albicans* is isolated from a pharyngeal swab; and respiratory commensals only are grown from a mucoid specimen of sputum. The chest X-ray reveals right basal atelectasis but no gross evidence of infection, and both an ultrasound and CT examination of the abdomen are negative for an intraabdominal collection. Topical nystatin is prescribed for the oral candidiasis and the antibacterial agents are discontinued.

Q Was it a good decision to stop the antibiotics?

A Yes. If the patient is clinically stable, it is reasonable to discontinue antibiotics now after 10 days, reassess the clinical situation, and reculture. Prolonged courses of antibiotics result in the selection of resistant bacteria and superinfections. Enterococci, as isolated here, rarely cause wound infection but are selected for by the use of cephalosporins to which they are resistant.

Q Is the oral candidiasis likely to be the cause of his persistent pyrexia?

A Oral or vaginal candidiasis is quite common in patients who have been on antibiotics owing to selective pressures on the normal flora, but rarely result in systemic signs or symptoms. Colonization or superficial infection is not a reliable predictor of systemic candida infection, except perhaps with *C. tropicalis* in immunocompromised patients during an outbreak.

Three days later it is noticed that the site of the central line is inflamed and pus is present. A sample of this is sent to the microbiology laboratory for culture and repeat blood cultures are taken. The following day the laboratory calls to say that yeasts are present in one of the blood culture bottles (Fig. 48.1).

Q Is the presence of yeasts in only one set of blood cultures likely to represent contamination?

A The isolation of *Candida* from blood cultures should always be regarded as significant until proven otherwise. Although yeasts may colonize the skin, especially in a patient who has been on broad-spectrum antibacterial agents, they should not be considered as contaminants in the blood, as is often the case with coagulase-negative staphylococci (e.g. *Staphylococcus epidermidis*), micrococci, and diphtheroids. Furthermore, Bill has a number of risk factors for systemic candida infection or candidaemia (see Table 48.1).

Table 48.1 Risk factors for systemic candida infection

- Immunocompromised state, e.g. neutropenia, malignancy, corticosteroids
- Presence of a foreign body, e.g. intravascular catheter (see Fig. 48.2), urinary catheter
- Major surgery, e.g. bowel resection, ruptured aortic aneurysm
- Broad-spectrum antibacterial agents, e.g. cephalosporins such as cefotaxime, quinolones such as ciprofloxacin
- Extensive burns
- Parenteral nutrition

Q What should be done next to confirm this diagnosis?

A Further blood cultures should be taken and, where possible (i.e. if an intraarterial or triple-

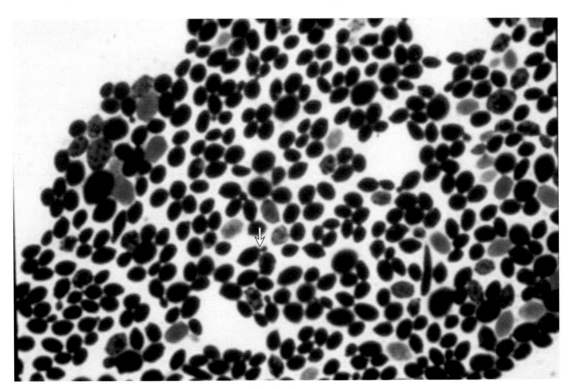

Fig. 48.1 Budding (arrow) yeasts (Gram-positive) in blood cultures.

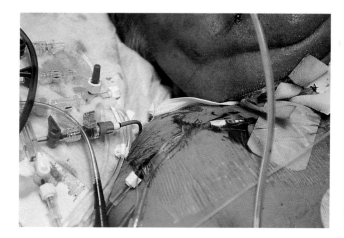

Fig. 48.2 Central line, a possible source of candidaemia.

lumen intravenous catheter is present), these sets should be taken through the catheter if this is suspected as the source. Isolation of *Candida* from pus taken around the catheter site and from the tip of the central line, when removed, will also confirm this as the likely source. Removal of the infected line tip is necessary for effective eradication.

Q How is systemic candida infection usually diagnosed?

A Clinical suspicion in patients with one or more risk factors is the first requirement for early diagnosis. Laboratory confirmation may be achieved by:

- blood cultures: only about 50% of blood cultures are positive in candidaemia. Specialized techniques such as lysis centrifugation (releases yeasts from inside white cells) are recommended by some as these increase the yield, but these are not always available

- tissue biopsy: skin lesions may occasionally accompany candidaemia and yeasts may be isolated from these or visualized on histology. Similarly, internal organs such as the liver and kidneys may be biopsied if these are involved

- antibody detection: some patients may develop serum precipitins to *C. albicans*, but this is dependent on a normal immune response, which may be absent in immunocompromised patients. The presence of antibodies is suggestive but not diagnostic

- antigen detection: during candidaemia a variety of metabolites (e.g. d-arabinitol) or antigens (e.g. enolase, mannan) may be detected in the serum of systemically infected patients, but the presence of these is usually transient and may be missed when the sample is taken.

- polymerase chain reaction (PCR): an ultra-sensitive technique for the detection of genomic material, which is increasingly being used in the diagnosis of many other infectious conditions and offers considerable promise for the future

The last three approaches, i.e. antibody detection, antigen detection, and PCR, are not routinely available except in reference laboratories or research centres.

Q What options are there for the treatment of systemic candida infection?

A Intravenous amphotericin B with or without flucytosine is still considered the treatment of choice for systemic candida infection. Renal failure due to amphotericin B, acquired candida resistance to flucytosine, liver toxicity or bone marrow failure with flucytosine, and the many side-effects of amphotericin B, such as rigors, thrombocytopenia, hypokalaemia, hypomagnesaemia, and rising creatinine, are significant problems.

Liposomal or colloidal amphotericin B are more effective because higher doses can be administered with a lower incidence of side-effects. These compounds are, however, more expensive. The triazole drugs, fluconazole and itraconazole have a role to play in the treatment of oesophagitis and some systemic candida infections, but should not be regarded as agents of choice, especially in the severely immunocompromised host. Furthermore, some *Candida species*, e.g. *C. krusei*, are resistant to fluconazole. These agents are, however, increasingly used in the treatment of less severe fungal infections such as superficial (i.e. oral, vaginal, and skin) candidiasis. Newer agents such as voriconazole and caspofurgin remain to be fully evaluated.

Q What other systemic candida infections do you know of?

A *Candida* spp. can infect almost any organ in the body but endocarditis, meningitis, and infection of the liver and spleen are especially difficult to treat. Some features of these and other infections are outlined in Box 48.1.

The central line is removed and *C. albicans* is isolated from the tip and pus at the site. Repeat blood cultures are also positive. Bill is started on intravenous fluconazole but remains pyrexial. Later that week he starts to vomit, his abdomen becomes distended, his urine output declines, and his serum urea and creatinine increase. He undergoes a laparotomy, which reveals that the bowel anastomosis has broken down, with resultant peritonitis. In the intensive therapy unit, he rapidly goes downhill with respiratory failure due to the adult respiratory distress syndrome (ARDS), renal failure, and jaundice. He dies shortly afterwards, 3 weeks after admission. At postmortem, micrometastases from his bowel tumour are detected in his liver and a vegetation, from which *C. albicans* is isolated, is seen on his tricuspid valve.

Box 48.1 **Other deep-seated candida infections (may be accompanied by candidaemia)**

Infection	Clinical features	Comments
Peritonitis	Cloudy dialysate with CAPD (see Case 35)	Removal of catheter required
	Usually following bowel surgery	Antifungal agents not essential if adequate drainage
Urinary infection	Often asymptomatic if lower renal tract involved in catheterized patient	Removal of catheter usually followed by clearance
	Renal abscess may be a feature of disseminated candidiasis	Poor prognosis if immunocompromised
Hepatosplenic candidiasis	Fever of undetermined origin in leukaemic/neutropenic patient with elevated liver function tests	Diagnosis made by liver scan or biopsy. Prolonged antifungal chemotherapy required
Endocarditis	Occasional cause of endocarditis. Acute presentation with fever and emboli in at-risk patient, e.g. intravenous drug abuser	Multiple blood cultures may be sterile and echocardiogram often negative (see Case 49)
Arthritis, osteomyelitis, meningitis, ophthalmitis	Localized signs and symptoms	Often associated with trauma and diagnosed on tissue culture. Prognosis variable

Q Is it surprising that Bill died despite the fluconazole?

A The prognosis from candidaemia is disappointing when the underlying state of the patient is poor. The development of multiple organ failure heralds an especially poor prognosis and makes treatment more difficult. It is unlikely that conventional or liposomal amphotericin B, although perhaps preferable, would have altered the outcome here.

Q Which patients should be considered for prophylactic antifungal chemotherapy?

A This is a difficult question. The increasing number of patients at risk of systemic candida and systemic fungal infections (see Box 48.2) has stimulated interest in targeting certain patients for chemoprophylaxis, e.g. those with neutropenia. Oral fluconazole is often prescribed as part of a selective gut decontamination regimen for the duration of the risk period, i.e. just before the onset

---

Box 48.2 Other systemic fungal infections

Disease	Pathogen	Location	Features
Aspergillosis	A. *fumigatus*, A. *flavus* (moulds; Fig. 48.3)	Worldwide	Pneumonia, disseminated disease, aspergilloma, allergic lung disease
Cryptococcosis	C. *neoformans* (true yeast)	Worldwide	Meningitis, occasionally respiratory or disseminated
Histoplasmosis	H. *capsulatum* (dimorphic fungus)	River valleys of eastern USA	Pneumonia disseminated in AIDS
Coccidioidomycosis	C. *immitis* (dimorphic fungus)	USA and Mexico	Respiratory, skin, or subcutaneous involvement

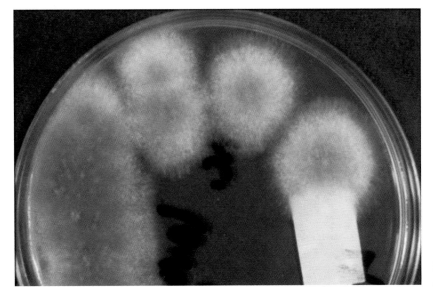

Fig. 48.3 Culture plate of *Aspergillus fumigatus*.

of neutropenia and until the white cell count begins to increase. Itraconazole has been used prophylactically for neutropenic patients at risk of invasive aspergillosis, e.g. during building construction work, when there will be dissemination of fungal spores.

Summary: Systemic candida infection

Presentation
Fever with or without localizing signs in an at-risk patient, e.g. neutropenia, broad-spectrum antibiotics, leukaemia

Diagnosis
Blood cultures (positive in only 50%); isolation from deep site, e.g. liver biopsy; serum positive for antibodies, antigens, or metabolites (where available)

Management
Correction of underlying risk factors (if possible); intravenous amphotericin B or fluconazole

Case 49 Eric, a pyrexial 76-year-old surveyor with a heart murmur

Eric, a 76-year-old retired surveyor, is seen in the medical outpatients clinic for evaluation of persistent fever, malaise, anorexia, and weight loss. He has been fit and healthy throughout his life, During the past 3–4 months, however, he and his wife Doris have noticed that he has 'slowed up', and that he has been hot and sweaty on occasions. He has no respiratory symptoms and there has been no change in bowel habit. On examination he has a tachycardia of 100/min and a temperature of 37.5°C, but his blood pressure and respiratory rate are normal. He has extensive gum disease and dental hygiene is poor. There is a soft diastolic murmur at the sternal border but examination of the lungs, abdomen, and rectum is normal. There is no lymphadenopathy.

Q Is this man sufficiently ill to warrant admission to hospital?

A Yes. Although Eric is not critically ill he requires observation and investigation, which is best done in hospital.

Q What diagnosis should be considered first?

A Infective endocarditis. The combination of fever, systemic symptoms such as weight loss or fatigue/lassitude, and a changing or recently diagnosed murmur should immediately alert one to this diagnosis. A minority of patients have a history of a recent precipitating procedure, such as dental extraction, and there may be no record of damaged heart valves such as that following rheumatic valve disease (see Fig. 49.1).

Q How may a diagnosis of infective endocarditis be confirmed?

A Three sets of blood cultures should be taken, at least 30 minutes apart and preferably from differ-

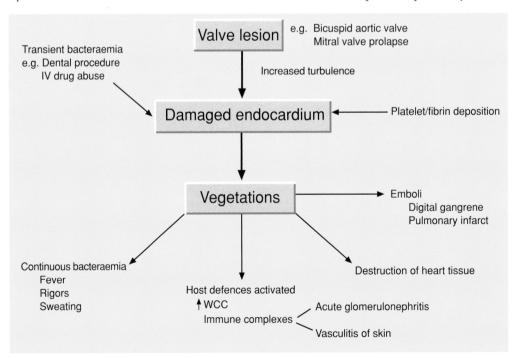

Fig. 49.1 Pathogenesis of infective endocarditis.

ent sites. It is usual in endocarditis for all three to be positive, as a continuous bacteraemia is typical of this condition (see also Case 47). Sometimes it may be necessary to take more than three sets, e.g. if the patient has recently been on antibiotics or if a fastidious organism is suspected as the cause. It is important to delay antimicrobial therapy if possible until a microbiological diagnosis has been made, to ensure that the most appropriate treatment is started. Vegetations seen on an echocardiogram are very suggestive of infective endocarditis, but a negative result does not exclude the diagnosis because in early disease they may not be visible or they may be difficult to see in right-sided disease. Increasingly, transoesophageal as opposed to transthroacic, echocardiography is used as it is more reliable. Other contributory investigations include a full blood count (raised white cell count due to bacterial infection, anaemia due to chronic disease), erythrocyte sedimentation rate (ESR), C-reactive protein (CRP; considered to be more specific than an ESR for bacterial infection), urinalysis (haematuria indicative of glomerulonephritis; see Fig. 49.1), and an immunology profile that might include C_3 and C_4 levels (both low), C_3 degradation products (elevated), and assays for the presence of immune complexes.

Q What are the Duke criteria?

A The Duke criteria, which originated from Duke University in North Carolina, USA, try to standardize the diagnosis of infective endocarditis based on the results of the clinical features and investigations described above. Two major criteria (i.e. typical organism from blood cultures, positive echocardiogram), one major and three minor criteria (e.g. predisposition to endocarditis, fever, etc.), or five minor criteria are required to make a diagnosis of definite endocarditis.

Q What is subacute bacterial endocarditis (SBE) and is it different from infective endocarditis?

A In the pre-antibiotic era, SBE was characterized by a prolonged illness of 3–6 months with many of the classic clinical manifestations, such as Osler's nodes, Roth spots. This illness was due to low-grade pathogens such as 'viridans' streptococci. This was in contrast to acute bacterial endocarditis caused by more virulent bacteria such as *Staphylococcus aureus* or *Streptococcus pyogenes* (β-haemolytic streptococci group A), where the course of the illness was uniformly fatal within a matter of days to weeks. This clinical distinction is less relevant now, and the term 'infective endocarditis' is used to encompass both of the previously used terms.

Q What groups of organisms are most commonly implicated in the aetiology of infective endocarditis?

Table 49.1 Organisms implicated in the aetiology of infective endocarditis

Organisms	Incidence (%)
Streptococci	65
'Viridans'	50
Enterococci	10
Others	5
Staphylococci	20
S. aureus	14
Coagulase-negative	6
Others, e.g. Gram-negative bacilli, fungi	5
No organism identified	10

A Streptococci, especially 'viridans' streptococci (see Case 5), and *Staphylococcus aureus* are the most common causes (see Table 49.1).

Eric is admitted to a bed in the cardiology division for observation and evaluation. He is persistently pyrexial over the next 48 hours and, although his white cell count is normal, he is mildly anaemic (haemoglobin (Hb), 9.7 g/dl). *Streptococcus mitis* is isolated from three sets of blood cultures (six bottles). The echocardiogram reveals an aortic valve with regurgitation, and a vegetation with an abscess (see Fig. 49.2). Urinalysis and a complement profile are normal.

Q What is *S. mitis* and where may it have come from?

A *S. mitis*, usually an α-haemolytic 'viridans' streptococcus, is a normal inhabitant of the oral cavity and the upper respiratory tract. It accounts for 15–20%

of infective endocarditis and may gain access to the bloodstream during dental procedures, such as tooth extraction or even during scaling. Eric's extensive gum disease is likely to be significant as a possible source. In the majority of patients, however, no predisposing event is identifiable.

Q What is the role of the microbiology department in the management of endocarditis?

A This includes:

- isolation and identification of the organism to indicate the possible source (e.g. 'viridans' streptococci from the oral cavity, *S. bovis* from a bowel tumour) and what measures may be necessary to prevent recurrence (e.g. dental hygiene)

- sensitivity testing, including minimum inhibitory concentrations (MIC) as well as routine tests to assess how sensitive the bacterium is, especially to penicillin. Dosages of anti-

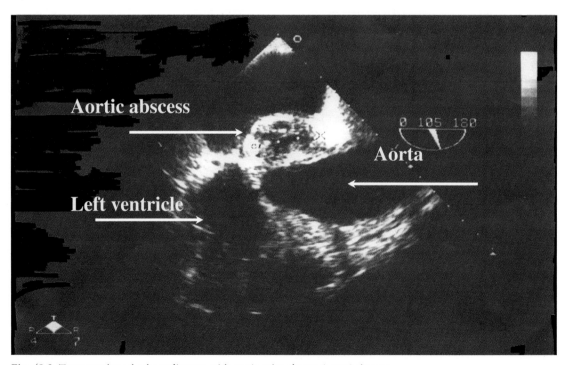

Fig. 49.2 Transoesophageal echocardiogram with aortic valve abscess (arrow) that may follow vegetation.

biotics will be influenced by what serum concentrations are required to kill and not just inhibit the bacteria

- antibiotic assays. Because of the low therapeutic index of aminoglycosides and vancomycin, key agents used in treatment, it is essential to monitor serum levels regularly to ensure adequate but non-toxic levels (see Case 26)

- CRP (often assayed in immunology or biochemistry departments) may be used to monitor response to treatment.

The isolate of *S. mitis* has an MIC to penicillin of 0.03 mg/l, i.e. very sensitive. Eric is started on high-dose intravenous (IV) penicillin and gentamicin. Eric's temperature gradually falls over the next 10 days, and his general condition improves.

Q Why is gentamicin used when the isolate is very sensitive to penicillin?

A The aminoglycosides, including gentamicin, have poor activity against streptococci on their own but act synergistically when combined with a β-lactam antibiotic such as penicillin. This probably relates to different modes of action: penicillin disrupts the cell wall, facilitating the entry of gentamicin into the cell and its action on protein synthesis. Synergistic antibiotic activity is important in eradicating bacteria from the vegetations.

Q What is the normal duration of therapy for infective endocarditis?

A Where a 'viridans' streptococcus is very sensitive to penicillin, 2 weeks of IV therapy may be adequate if uncomplicated. With a less sensitive isolate, e.g. an enterococcus, 4 or even 6 weeks of IV treatment is recommended. Four weeks of parenteral treatment with flucloxacillin and an aminoglycoside (for 1 week) is recommended for staphylococcal endocarditis. Vancomycin or teicoplanin are indicated if there is allergy to penicillin or if resistant bacteria (e.g. methicillin-resistant *S. aureus*) are responsible. These are, however, only general guidelines and therapy should be individu-alized to the patient's circumstances, the causative organism, the response to treatment, and underlying cardiac abnormality.

Q What is the mortality from infective endocarditis?

A Since the start of the antibiotic era mortality has declined significantly to around 30%, largely due to earlier diagnosis, more aggressive treatment, and surgery. The outlook is better for native valve as opposed to prosthetic valve endocarditis (see Box 49.1) and the prognosis is also influenced by the aetiology (staphylococcal and Gram-negative endocarditis have a higher mortality), the age of the patient, presentation (significant cardiac decompensation and embolic phenomena herald a poorer outcome), and response to treatment. Other recent changes in the epidemiology of infective endocarditis include:

- endocarditis in intravenous drug abusers (right-sided relatively more common) due to *S. aureus*, yeasts, or *Pseudomonas aeruginosa* is increasingly common

- clinical presentation characterized by fewer of the classic stigmata, such as splinter haemorrhages, Osler's nodes, due to earlier diagnosis and treatment

- now more a disease of the elderly rather than the young or middle-aged, due to increasing life expectancy and the declining incidence of rheumatic fever

---

Box 49.1 Prosthetic value endocarditis (incidence 2%)

Early (within the first 3 months of surgery)
- Organisms acquired during surgery and hence preventable
- Staphylococci predominate; 70% mortality

Late (occurs 3 months or later after surgery)
Aetiology similar to that of native valve endocarditis; 10% mortality

- 'viridans' streptococci account for proportionally fewer cases and enterococcal and staphylococcal infection increasing in incidence.

Newer microbes, often difficult or impossible to isolate on routine laboratory media and hence diagnosed using molecular techniques, such as *Bartonella henselae* (seen in immunocompromised patients), and *Tropheryma whipplei* as part of Whipple's disease, are being described. These should be considered especially in patients with 'culture-negative endocarditis' (Box 49.2).

Two weeks after the start of antibiotics, however, Eric's temperature spikes to 38.5°C, but his general condition, including cardiac status, remains unchanged.

Q What are the possible reasons for the recurrence of Eric's pyrexia?

A Possible explanations:

- extensive infection of the valve ring and adjacent structures, requiring surgery and immediate valve replacement
- metastatic infection involving bones, kidneys; more likely with *S. aureus* endocarditis than with streptococcal infection

---

Box 49.2 'Culture-negative endocarditis'

Refers to cases of infective endocarditis where no organism is isolated or an atypical cause is identified

Causes

- Recent antibiotics, especially if taken for > 3 days
- Fastidious organisms, e.g. haemophilus–actinobacillus–cardiobacterium–eikenella–kinge
lla (HACEK) group, *Brucella* spp. (see Case 53), *Legionella* spp. (see Case 19), *Bartonella* spp., *Tropheryma whipplei*
- Fungi, e.g. *Candida* spp. in drug abusers, *Aspergillus* following valve surgery
- *Coxiella burnetii* (Q fever) and *Chlamydia psittaci*, both diagnosed serologically

---

- systemic or pulmonary emboli, the latter more common in right-sided infection, as with IV drug abusers
- drug hypersensitivity or allergy
- a second infection, e.g. intravascular line
- antibiotic resistance: relatively rare when patients are on combined treatment

Most patients respond fairly quickly to IV antibiotics if the organism isolated is sensitive to conventional antibiotics. In culture-negative endocarditis it is always possible that treatment is not appropriate or that a rare cause is responsible (see Box 49.2). Failure to respond to treatment or recurring pyrexia require a careful and multidisciplinary approach involving cardiologist, microbiologist, infectious diseases physician, and cardiac surgeon (urgent valve replacement may be required).

Eric is assessed for local or systemic spread of infection, clinically and by echocardiogram. Repeat blood cultures are negative. The site of the peripheral line through which he is receiving the IV antibiotics is a little inflamed. Consequently, the line is removed and a central one inserted for the duration of IV antibiotic therapy. *S. epidermidis*, resistant to penicillin, gentamicin, and flucloxacillin but sensitive to vancomycin, is isolated from the removed peripheral vascular catheter tip and the fever resolves without a change in his antibiotics. During his hospital stay, he is seen by a dentist for assessment of his gum disease and referred on for further management of this. After parenteral penicillin and gentamicin his treatment is changed to oral amoxycillin, and 3 days later Eric is discharged from hospital to be followed up in the clinic.

Q What advice should Eric be given regarding future visits to the dentist?

A He should receive prophylactic antibiotics when undergoing dental extractions, scaling, or periodontal surgery. Patients with prosthetic valves, patients with a previous attack of endocarditis, and patients due to have a general anaesthetic who have damaged heart valves are all at increased risk. These patients should receive parenteral amoxycillin at induction and orally 6 hours later, plus gentamicin 120 mg at induction. Other at-risk patients, i.e. those with rheumatic or congenital heart disease and mitral valve prolapse, should receive high-dose oral amoxycillin, i.e. 3 g 1 hour before the procedure. Clindamycin is preferred for patients allergic to penicillin.

Summary: **Infective endocarditis**

Presentation
Fever in a patient with a new or changing murmur, pyrexia of unknown aetiology, embolic phenomena

Diagnosis
Clinical features and repeated positive blood cultures with or without a positive echocardiogram

Management
Intravenous followed by oral antibiotics for 4 or more weeks, with close liaison among all involved in management

Case 50 Margaret returns from Africa with a fever and headache

Margaret arrives in the accident and emergency department at 3 o'clock in the morning, with a high fever, headache, and backache. She first felt ill on the previous day, with nausea, vomiting, and anorexia, and what she describes as bouts of shivering and feeling cold. She is 25 years old, a qualified nurse, and has been working at a mission hospital in Zimbabwe for the previous 6 months, returning to England 4 weeks ago. Prior to her departure from England, she received vaccinations against hepatitis A and typhoid, and she had been taking mefloquine prophylaxis against malaria, although she admits to having missed occasional doses. She was previously fit and well and on no regular medication. On examination, her temperature is 39.6°C and she has a tachycardia of 120/min, but there are no other physical signs.

Q What is your differential diagnosis and initial management?

A Malaria must be the first consideration in a patient developing fever within a year of visiting an endemic area, despite the history of prophylaxis. Other possibilities include bacterial meningitis (Case 41), influenza (Case 17), typhoid (Case 27).

Q Should you admit Margaret to hospital?

A Yes. A diagnosis of malaria constitutes a medical emergency. There are a number of life-threatening complications of malaria, the risks of which increase with delay in instituting appropriate therapy. Thus, besides admitting Margaret to hospital, you should order a range of blood tests, and call out the on-call microbiologist or haematologist to perform the relevant diagnostic tests, despite the unsocial hour.

Q What is the cause of malaria?

A Infection with one or more of the four plasmodia that infect humans:

- *P. falciparum* (malignant tertian malaria; throughout the tropics, especially Africa, South-east Asia, South America)
- *P. vivax* (common cause of benign tertian malaria; Indian subcontinent, Africa, South-east Asia)
- *P. ovale* (uncommon cause of benign tertian malaria; Africa)
- *P. malariae* (quartan malaria; throughout tropical world)

Q How is the diagnosis of malaria made in the laboratory?

A By examination of unfixed thick films stained by Field's stain, and thin blood films stained at pH 7.2 by Giemsa or Leishman stains. The thick films are for the rapid detection of parasites especially if these are few in number, whilst the thin films allow identification of the species of plasmodium. The films must be examined by an experienced observer using oil immersion ($\times$ 1000) magnification. Even if initial films are negative, malaria remains a possible diagnosis, and repeat films should be taken. In addition, most laboratories can also perform enzyme immunoassay-based tests for detection of plasmodial antigens, which are sensitive and reasonably specific.

Parasites are seen on a thick film from Margaret. The appearance of a thin film is shown in Fig. 50.1.

Q What does this show?

A Multiple red cells infected with ring forms (see below) of a plasmodium parasite. The high frequency of red cell parasitaemia, and the absence of mature forms of the parasite (on thin film) make this most likely to be *P. falciparum*.

Q Are you surprised that Margaret has malaria, even though she was taking prophylaxis?

A No. Mefloquine prophylaxis is estimated at best to be around 90% effective. In addition, Margaret missed some of her doses, which will reduce the

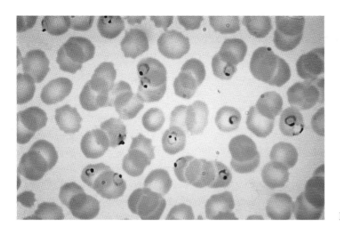

Fig. 50.1 Thin film of Margaret's blood.

protective efficacy. Finally, there is the possibility of infection with mefloquine-resistant organisms, although, to date, such resistance has only very rarely been described.

Q What is the treatment of malaria?

A This consists of:

1. Specific antimalarial chemotherapy must be given as soon as a diagnosis of malaria is suspected.

   • Severe or complicated disease due to *P. falciparum* should be assumed to be chloroquine-resistant and treated with oral (or intravenous, if imparied consciousness) quinine sulphate plus oral pyrimethamine-sulfadoxine (Fansidar®) or doxycycline, with subsequent oral maintenance therapy. Chloroquine is the drug of choice for *P. vivax*, *P. ovale, and P. malariae* infections. Intravenous administration is indicated for severe cases, especially with heavy parasitaemias, but care is necessary because of potential cardiotoxicity. *P. vivax* and *P. ovale* infections must also be treated with primaquine, to eliminate the reservoir of organisms in the liver (see below) and thereby prevent late relapses. Care should be taken with the latter drug to exclude G6PDH (glucose-6-phosphate dehydrogenase) deficiency; otherwise the dosage must be adjusted accordingly.

   • Drugs for uncomplicated infection, given orally, include quinine (given with pyromethamine–sulphadoxine or doxycycline), mefloquine, Malarone® (atovaquone plus proguanil), or Riamet® (artemether with lumefantrine). All these drugs may exhibit cardiotoxicity; mefloquine may cause neuropsychiatric side-effects. Tetracycline, clindamycin, and pyrimethamine–sulfadoxine have some activity, but are unreliable when used alone. Patients should not be treated with the same drugs they were taking as prophylaxis, as the organisms may be resistant to those agents.

2. Supportive therapy for the various life-threatening complications (see below)

You initiate therapy with intravenous (IV) quinine sulphate. Later that night, you receive the following results:

Hb 7.3 g/dl (mean corpuscular volume (MCV), normal); 10% reticulocytes

white cell count, 4.5×10^9/l

platelets, 57×10^9/l

urea, 25.2 mmol/l (normal range 2.5–7.0 mmol/l)

electrolytes, normal

glucose, 2.6 mmol/l (normal range 3.3–5.4 mmol/l)

Margaret is now sweating profusely, and her fever is declining. She manages to pass a small urine sample, which is very dark in colour. However, she has become drowsy and difficult to communicate with.

Q What complications of malaria may now be developing?

A These are:

- Anaemia—due mainly to acute haemolysis and cytokine-induced suppression of bone marrow function

- Acute renal failure—usually oliguric; dark urine arises from free haemoglobin and malarial pigment filtered from blood into urine

- Cerebral malaria—seizures, impairment of consciousness, coma

- Hypoglycaemia—due to depletion of liver glycogen from decreased oral intake prior to seeking medical attention; glucose consumption by the large number of malarial parasites; hypoglycaemic effects of inflammatory cytokines; stimulation of insulin release by quinine. Glucose levels should be checked hourly during IV infusions of this drug

Rare complications include pulmonary oedema, disseminated intravascular coagulation, severe impairment of liver function, shock with systolic blood pressure <70 mm Hg, splenic enlargement (chronic *P. falciparum*, *P. vivax*)

Q What is the pathogenesis of the multiorgan failure seen in severe *P. falciparum* malaria?

A The pathogenesis of many of the complications of malaria is not fully understood. The most important factors are:

- cytoadherence of parasitized red cells to endothelial cells in the small vessels of brain, kidneys, and other affected organs, leading to occlusion and impairment of organ function. The ability to sequester infected red cells in the microcirculation is unique to *P. falciparum*, which explains both why this species causes malignant disease and the absence of mature forms of *P. falciparum* in peripheral blood smears

- induction of cytokine release from macrophages. Tumour necrosis factor (TNF)-alpha levels are increased in severe *P. falciparum* malaria. Cytokines have a wide range of inflammatory effects

- at the tissue level, the roles of nitric oxide and free radicals in causing oxidative damage are the subjects of current research

Q What is the route of infection of malaria?

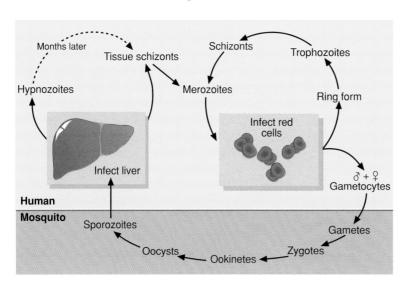

Fig. 50.2 Life cycle of malaria parasite.

A Malaria is spread by bites of female anopheline mosquitos. Plasmodia have a complicated life cycle, involving replication within both the mosquito vector and the human host (see Fig. 50.2).

1. *Sporozoites* acquired from the mosquito infect hepatocytes, where they mature to form *tissue schizonts* or become dormant *hypnozoites* (*P. vivax*, *P. ovale*)

2. *Tissue schizonts* produce several thousand *merozoites*, which are released into the bloodstream and infect red cells

3. Each *merozoite* matures through an asexual cycle of 48–72 hours involving a *ring form*, *trophozoite*, and *schizont*, ultimately producing 8–24 new *merozoites*, which are released as the red cells lyse, thus initiating another cycle of red cell infection

4. Some parasites within red cells differentiate into male and female *gametocytes* (sexual forms)

5. These sexual forms are taken up during a blood meal by the mosquito, where the sexual cycle involves formation of *gametes*, *zygotes*, *ookinetes*, *oocysts*, and ultimately *sporozoites*, which migrate to the salivary gland, ready to be injected into the next human host

The hypnozoites (see (1) above) may remain dormant for several months before eventually maturing to tissue schizonts, and initiating a clinical relapse. This exo-erythrocytic liver cycle is not part of the life cycle of *P. falciparum*. Thus, late relapses do not occur with this plasmodium, and there is no need for a course of primaquine to eliminate liver organisms. The same is possibly true of *P. malariae*.

Q What do the terms 'tertian' and 'quartan' mean?

A These terms refer to the periodicity of malarial fevers and their meaning is related to the red cell cycle. The malarial paroxysm of fever typically includes a 'cold or chilling stage', then a 'hot stage' coincident with red cell lysis and release of merozoites and lasting several hours, and, finally, a 'sweating' phase with resolution of fever and

marked fatigue. These classical patterns of fever take some cycles to develop, and patients may therefore present before the pattern is evident. In addition, since erythrocytic parasites of *P. falciparum* do not become synchronized, typical tertian fevers are unusual in falciparum malaria and their absence should not mislead the diagnosis.

Q How may malaria be prevented?

A Elimination of the mosquito vector would prevent transmission of disease. Swamp drainage and use of insecticides has resulted in a degree of success in some areas.

For travellers to endemic areas, the four principles of prevention are:

1. be aware of the risk of malaria

2. take appropriate antimalarial prophylaxis

3. avoid being bitten by mosquitos, e.g. by using bed-netting (impregnated with insecticide if possible), insect repellents, covering skin at dusk

4. seek urgent medical advice in the event of a fever or 'flu-like illness' within a year of travel, remembering to relate the travel history

Q When should chemoprophylaxis begin?

A Shortly *before* travel (in case of unacceptable side-effects, and to ensure adequate levels on arrival in an endemic area). It should be continued religiously throughout the period of travel, and for at least 4 weeks after return. The exact choice of drugs is a complex issue, with the emergence of drug-resistant plasmodia and the toxicity of some of the recommended agents. Expert advice should be sought. Guidelines are issued and updated at intervals by national or other bodies. Typical regimens include

- chloroquine (weekly) alone
- chloroquine (weekly) plus proguanil (daily)
- *mefloquine (weekly)
- *doxycycline (daily)
- *atovaquone plus proguanil (Malarone, daily)

(Regimens marked with an asterisk are appropriate for areas with known chloroquine-resistant plasmodia.) Chloroquine should not be taken long term (>5 years) because of the risk of retinopathy. Mefloquine should not be taken for more than 1 year.

Note that, as in the case of Margaret, prophylaxis may not be 100% effective, compliance may be less than optimal, and resistant strains may emerge; hence the need for other precautions to try and avoid infection.

Margaret had a stormy course in intensive care. Her parasitaemia disappeared after 4 days of therapy, and the antimalarial treatment was therefore terminated after 7 days. She eventually made a full recovery.

Summary: **Malaria**

Presentation
Cyclical fever, headache, nausea, diarrhoea, and vomiting, in patient with appropriate travel history

Diagnosis
Urgent; by examination of thick and thin blood films

Complications
Cerebral malaria; renal failure; anaemia; metabolic upset (hypoglycaemia, lactic acidosis)

Management
A medical emergency; initiate therapy, dependent upon likelihood of encountering resistant organisms

Case 51 Thomas, a 35-year-old teacher who is anti-HIV-positive

Thomas, a 35-year-old schoolteacher, is homo-sexual and first tested positive for anti-HIV 5 years ago. You see him at roughly 6-monthly intervals, and thus far there have been no additional medical problems. His CD4 count 6 months ago was 700/μl, and viral load 150 copies/ml. He now complains of a painful vesicular rash on the right side of his abdomen. On examination, you note the typical appearance of herpes zoster affecting the T10 dorsal root.

Q Does the presence of herpes zoster now mean that Thomas has AIDS?

A No. The different stages of HIV infection, as defined by the Centers for Disease Control (CDC) in the USA, were discussed in Case 38 (see Table 38.1). Herpes zoster, recurrent muco-cutaneous herpes simplex, oral candidiasis (see Fig. 51.1), and oral hairy leucoplakia (see Case 38) are all considerably more common in HIV-infected individuals than in age- and sex-matched controls. These manifestations reflect an underlying immuno-deficiency, and may herald the imminent onset of AIDS, but they are not of themselves AIDS-defining illnesses. For epidemiological and com-parative purposes, the complications of HIV

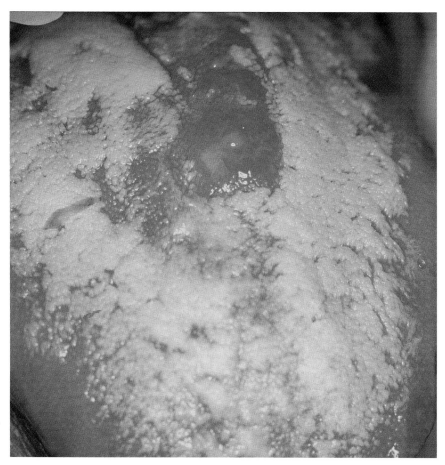

Fig. 51.1 Oral candidiasis.

infection are broadly categorized into infectious, malignant, and neurological. Common clinical manifestations in HIV-infected patients are listed in Table 51.1, which also shows which ones are AIDS-defining conditions. The relative frequency of these will vary in different patient groups. The spectrum of opportunistic infections particularly will reflect the pattern of infectious organisms extant in a given geographical location.

Some of the features of the opportunistic infections listed in Table 51.1 are provided in Table 51.2. The key features of Kaposi's sarcoma are shown in Box 51.1, and a typical skin lesion is seen in Fig. 51.5.

You treat Thomas's zoster rash with high-dose oral aciclovir (see Case 7) and, after 2 weeks, the rash resolves. His CD4 count is down to 250/μl, and his viral load is 12 000 copies/ml.

Q How should you manage Thomas now?

A The decline in CD4 count, the rise in viral load, and the symptomatic (but not AIDS-defining)

Table 51.1 Common clinical manifestations of AIDS. Those that are AIDS-defining are shown in bold

Opportunistic infections

Pulmonary

Pneumonia	*Pneumocystis carinii* (see Table 51.2)
	Cytomegalovirus (CMV; see Table 51.2)
	Cryptococcus neoformans
Tuberculosis	*Mycobacterium tuberculosis* (see Case 52)

Gastrointestinal

Oral and **oesophageal thrush**	*Candida albicans*
Oral hairy leucoplakia	Epstein–Barr virus
Oral ulcers, **oesophagitis**	Herpes simplex virus (HSV), **CMV** (see Table 51.2)
Diarrhoea	*Salmonella* species
	Shigella
	Giardia lamblia
	***Cryptosporidium* (chronic, > 1 month, see Table 51.2)**
	M. *avium* complex (see Table 51.2)
Colitis	**CMV (see Table 51.2)**

Central nervous system

Multiple brain abscesses	*Toxoplasma gondii* (see Table 51.2)
Meningitis	*Cryptococcus neoformans* (see Table 51.2)
Retinitis, encephalitis	**CMV (see Table 51.2)**
Progressive multifocal leucoencephalopathy (PML)	JC polyomavirus (see Table 51.2)

Table 51.1 *cont'd*	
Skin and mucous membranes	
Prolonged (>1 month), recurrent ulceration	Herpes simplex virus
Herpes zoster	Varicella zoster virus
Multiple skin lesions	*Cryptococcus neoformans*
Reticuloendothelial system	
Lymphadenopathy	*Toxoplasma gondii*
	M. *avium* complex
	Epstein–Barr virus (EBV)
Malignant disease	
Kaposi's sarcoma	
Non-Hodgkin's lymphoma, cerebral or peripheral	
EBV-associated lymphomas, e.g. polyclonal lymphoproliferation, Burkitt's lymphoma	
Carcinoma of the uterine cervix	
Hodgkin's lymphoma	
Squamous carcinoma	
Testicular cancers	
Basal cell cancer	
Melanoma	
Neurological disease	
Aseptic meningitis	may be HIV-related
HIV encephalopathy	**HIV**
Intracranial mass lesions	**Cerebral toxoplasmosis** (see Table 51.2)
	Primary CNS lymphoma
	Metastatic lymphoma
	Kaposi's sarcoma
	PML (see Table 51.2)
	CMV or HSV encephalitis
	Cerebral tuberculosis
Other	
Wasting syndrome of HIV infection	

intercurrent illness all suggest that Thomas is progressing towards AIDS. He should be recommended to start antiretroviral therapy.

Q What classes of antiretroviral drugs are available for treatment of HIV-infected patients?

Table 51.2 Features of seven common opportunist infections in AIDS

Cerebral toxoplasmosis

- Most common cause of intracranial mass lesions

- CT scan features include multiple ring-enhancing lesions. MRI scan is more sensitive

- Initiation of therapy (pyrimethamine with folinic acid, plus sulfadiazine) usually empirical

- Serology is of little diagnostic value

Cryptococcal meningitis

- Caused by *Cryptococcus neoformans*, a fungus

- Seen in CSF by India ink staining

- More reliable diagnosis by isolation of the organism or cryptococcal antigen detection

- Measurement of antigen titre useful in monitoring response to treatment and the emergence of relapsing disease

- Initial therapy with amphotericin B and flucytosine

Cryptosporidiosis

- Protozoan

- Cause of chronic (>1 month) diarrhoea

- Diagnosis by microscopy of faeces

- No proven form of therapy available

Cytomegalovirus

- Multisystem disease including one or more of the following: retinitis (the most common manifestation; see Fig. 51.2); leucopenia; hepatitis; pneumonitis; oesophagitis (see Fig. 51.3), colitis; painful peripheral neuropathy; encephalitis

- Disease may respond to ganciclovir (toxic to bone marrow), foscarnet (nephrotoxic), or

cidofovir (nephrotoxic). Long-term therapy is necessary to prevent reactivation

***Mycobacterium avium* complex disease**

- Causes fevers, night sweats, abdominal pain and diarrhoea, fatigue, and weight loss

- Hepatosplenomegaly, and diffuse lymph-adenopathy

- Continuous bacteraemia; therefore diagnosis by isolation from blood culture

***Pneumocystis carinii* pneumonia (PCP)**

- A fungus infection acquired early in life; only causes disease when host is immunosuppressed

- Reactivation results in intra-alveolar pneumonitis, life-threatening

- Clinical features include cough, fever, low oxygen saturation, and a chest X-ray with diffuse interstitial shadowing (see Fig. 51.4)

- Diagnosis by demonstration of *P. carinii* cysts in clinical material, e.g. by immunofluorescence or genome detection in induced sputum or bronchoalveolar lavage fluid

- Treatment is with high-dose co-trimoxazole or: pentamidine; clindamycin plus primaquine; dapsone plus trimethoprim

Progressive multifocal leucoencephalopathy (PML)

- Due to reactivation of polyomavirus infection (JC virus)

- Primary infection acquired in childhood

- CNS infection causes multiple white matter lesions

- May respond to cytosine arabinoside therapy

A Currently, there are four groups of drugs for the treatment of HIV-infected patients: the nucleoside analogue reverse transcriptase inhibitors (NRTI), of which six are licensed, e.g. zidovudine, lamivudine; the non-nucleoside analogue reverse transcriptase inhibitors (NNRTI; two licensed), e.g. efavirenz; and the protease inhibitors (PI; six licensed) e.g. nelfinavir, ritonavir. The latest addition to the anti-retroviral armoury, enfuvirtide, represents the fourth class of drugs, fusion inhibitors, i.e. drugs that inhibit the very early steps in the viral life cycle of binding to cellular receptors and entry into the host cell.

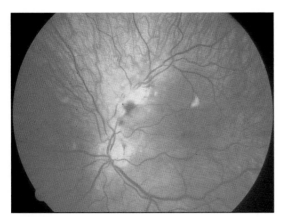

Fig. 51.2 CMV retinitis.

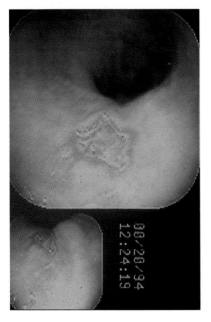

Fig. 51.3 CMV oesophagitis.

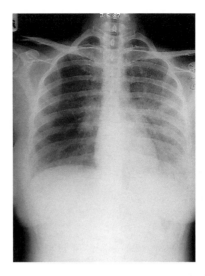

Fig. 51.4 Chest X-ray showing *Pneumocystis carinii* pneumonia.

Q How does resistance arise?

A Through the spontaneous generation of viral mutants, or variants, followed by natural selection of those variants. The molecular basis for antiretroviral resistance development is the subject of much study. All of the common mutations that give rise to reduced sensitivity to one or other of the currently used drugs have been characterized. Some of these mutations confer cross-resistance to other members of the same class of drugs; others are unique to specific agents. Yet others, whilst increasing resistance to one

Q Which drug should be used for initial therapy in a patient such as Thomas?

A This is a trick question, as one of the most important principles underlying antiretroviral therapy is that under no circumstances should therapy be with a single agent.

Q Why not?

A Because of the inevitable development of antiviral resistance.

Box 51.1 Kaposi's sarcoma

- The most common neoplasm affecting HIV-infected individuals
- Human herpesvirus type 8 invariably found in tumour tissue of all types of Kaposi's sarcoma
- Histology shows proliferation of abnormal vascular structures
- Skin is most common site—painless, non-pruritic firm nodular tumours; usually violaceous in colour
- Can involve any site—hard and soft palate, (see Fig. 51.5) gums of the mouth are other common sites
- Pulmonary involvement may be fatal

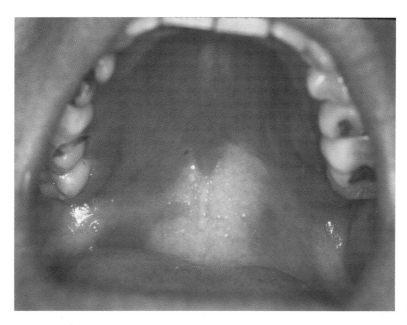

Fig. 51.5 Kaposi's sarcoma.

agent, may fortuitously increase the sensitivity of the virus to a different agent—the best example of this is the mutation at position 184 within the reverse transcriptase, which induces lamivudine resistance, but increases sensitivity to zidovudine.

Q How can the development of resistance be avoided?

A By treating patients with a multidrug regimen. This should reduce the chances of a single viral variant emerging that is simultaneously resistant to all of the drugs in the cocktail. Ideally, one would wish to use drugs that each act at a different site within the viral life cycle. However, at present this is possible only to a limited extent, as there are only three viral targets within the available armamentarium—the reverse transcriptase, the viral protease and the fusion/entry process.

Q What is HAART?

A This stands for <u>h</u>ighly <u>a</u>ctive <u>a</u>nti<u>r</u>etroviral <u>t</u>herapy. It was coined originally when the PI class of drugs was developed, and multidrug regimens were developed that led to greater than 3-log drops in viral load.

Q What are the important principles of selection of an antiretroviral therapy regimen?

A Patients should be treated with at least two, and preferably three, drugs whose resistance mutations do not confer cross-resistance to each other. Logical combinations would include drugs whose resistance mutations increase sensitivity to the other drugs.

Triple therapy regimens currently suggested include: three NRTI; two NRTI plus an NNRTI; two NRTI plus a PI; and possibly an NRTI plus an NNRTI plus a PI. Clearly, there will be a large number of possible drug combinations.

Additional factors to consider when choosing particular drugs are the side-effects profiles of each drug (these should not be additive) and the dosage patterns (i.e. the convenience of taking the regimen).

Q What is the therapeutic aim of initiating a patient on HAART?

A To reduce the viral load by as much as possible for as long as possible. The aim should be to render the peripheral blood viral load undetectable. Using modern ultrasensitive assays, this equates to a viral load less than around 40 copies/ml. With such low levels of viral replication, it is hoped that it will take a considerable time before resistant viral variants emerge.

Q What are the potential drawbacks to the use of antiretroviral drugs?

A All of the drugs in current use have side-effects. These may be minor in most patients, e.g. nausea, vomiting, diarrhoea, headache, and may regress once the patient has taken a few doses. However some patients may not be able to tolerate particular agents. More serious, possibly life-threatening, side-effects include pancreatitis, peripheral neuropathy, hepatic impairment, and hypersensitivy reactions. A worrisome development has been the appearance of a lipodystrophy syndrome (redistribution of body fat, hyperlipidaemia, glucose intolerance), seen most often, but not exclusively, in association with the PIs.

Q What other measures may be taken in the management of an HIV-infected patient?

A Despite the dramatic effects of HAART, antiretroviral therapy is not capable of curing a patient's HIV infection. Thus, there will always be the possibility of damage to the immune system, leaving the patient at risk of the various opportunistic infections and other diseases associated with AIDS. Once viral load begins to return or CD4 counts drop, the emphasis in patient management should be on prevention of these complications by appropriate prophylactic therapy. This may result in HIV-positive patients being on multiple antimicrobial agents, e.g. co-trimoxazole (for prevention of pneumocystis infection), aciclovir (for prevention of herpes simplex virus and varicella zoster virus reactivations), and fluconazole (for prevention of cryptococcal disease), in addition to specific anti-HIV drugs. The chances of drug interactions can only increase with such polypharmacy, and possible interactions between the antiretrovirals discussed above with the many other medications that HIV-infected patients may be taking add a further level of complexity to the management of such patients.

Q When should an HIV-infected patient be started on antiretroviral therapy?

A This is a difficult issue. The desire for early treatment should be balanced against the development of toxicity and also, the sooner drugs are started, the sooner resistant variants will appear. Factors to take into consideration include the viral load (if above

10 000 copies/ml, consider therapy) the CD4 count (consider therapy when this drops to <350/μl), and the clinical status of the patient. The initiation of therapy requires a considerable commitment from the patient. Compliance is essential, as failure to take optimal dosages will increase the risk of emergence of resistance, and, at least initially, the patient may feel worse on therapy than off it, due to the side-effects. It may take some time and juggling of drugs to find a successful regimen for an individual patient.

Q How would you monitor a patient on HAART?

A The key parameter to measure is the viral load. If viral load does not drop by more than a log after 4 weeks of HAART, one should suspect that that patient's virus is resistant to some or all of the components of his/her regimen, and alternatives should be tried. Serial measurement of the viral load will allow detection of reappearance of virus.

Q Why might viral load increase in a patient on HAART?

A The first answer would be because of the emergence of resistant viral variants. However, before launching into sophisticated resistance testing, one should first consider a more mundane possibility— that the patient has not been compliant with the regimen. Investigation of resistance is possible, e.g. by sequencing the virus to determine which mutations have occurred, but this is expensive and currently only carried out in selected reference laboratories. The options for a patient whose drug regimen appears to be failing include changing any or all of the components of his/her combination therapy.

Q What other effects may HAART have?

A In addition to suppression of viral replication and indeed presumably as a direct consequence of it, the immune systems of patients on HAART may demonstrate considerable recovery of both CD4 cell numbers and function—known as immune reconstitution. This may be so pronounced as to obviate the need for previously instituted prophylactic regimens, e.g. those against *Pneumocystis carinii* pneumonia or cytomegalovirus (CMV) retinitis.

Q What other steps in the viral life cycle might be suitable targets for the development of novel anti-HIV drugs?

A As mentioned above, the newest class of anti-HIV drugs is that of 'fusion inhibitors'. Small molecules have been developed to inhibit HIV binding to CD4 positive cells and one of those, enfuvirtide (also known as T-20), has been licensed. The other main target of interest is the viral integrase enzyme, which mediates incorporation of the HIV proviral DNA into the host cell chromosome.

Summary: Management of HIV infection

Natural history
Decline in CD4 count and immune function, leading to development of AIDS-defining illnesses

Routine monitoring
Viral load, CD4 count, clinical status

Antiretroviral therapy

- Use multidrug regimen
- Monitor efficacy by serial viral load measurement
- Side-effects—may be life-threatening
- Drug-resistant variants may eventually emerge
- If so, change one or all drugs of regimen
- Consider appropriate use of prophylactic therapy for opportunistic infections

Case 52 Karim, a 65-year-old cachectic man with fever

Karim, a 65-year-old man, is admitted to hospital because of a 2–3-month history of increasing lassitude, weight loss, anorexia, and intermittent pyrexia. Eight years ago Karim made an uncomplicated recovery from an inferior myocardial infarction, and non-insulin dependent diabetes mellitus was diagnosed 3 years before this presentation. His father died of tuberculosis at the age of 45 and one of his two brothers also has diabetes mellitus. On examination he is a pleasant, if slightly confused, cachectic man. His temperature is 38.5°C but his blood pressure, respiratory rate, and heart rate are all normal. The rest of his physical examination is unremarkable. There is no neck stiffness.

Q What initial investigations should be carried out?

A Full blood count (FBC), erythrocyte sedimentation rate (ESR), urea and electrolytes, electrocardiogram (ECG), blood sugar, and chest X-ray are initially indicated. Culture of urine, blood, and sputum (if available) should also be carried out. A lumbar puncture and/or computerized tomography (CT) scan may be considered because of Karim's confusion, to rule out intracranial pathology such as a cerebral abscess (see Case 43) or encephalitis (see Case 42).

The urea and electrolytes are normal and the FBC reveals a mild normochromic normocytic anaemia. Evidence of the previous myocardial infarct is present on the ECG and the random blood sugar is elevated, at 10 mmol/l. The chest X-ray (see Fig. 52.1) is abnormal.

Q What abnormality is seen on the chest X-ray?

A A pattern of fine opacities is present throughout both lung fields.

Q What is the differential diagnosis?

A The differential diagnosis includes

- lymphangitis carcinomatosis
- occupational lung disease

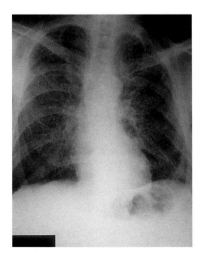

Fig. 52.1
Karim's chest
X-ray at
presentation.

Table 52.1 **Miliary tuberculosis**
Extensive haematogenous spread involving multiple organs that is most commonly seen in the very young or the elderly
Risk groups   Immigrants from the developing world, the socially deprived, alcoholics, intravenous drug users, patients with liver disease or cirrhosis, neoplasia, HIV disease, diabetes mellitus, and pregnancy
Features   • Fever, malaise, and weight loss occurring over 10–15 weeks   • Previous history of tuberculosis present in only 5%   • Meninges involved in 20% of cases   • Hyponatraemia if adrenals infected; raised alkaline phosphatase if liver involved

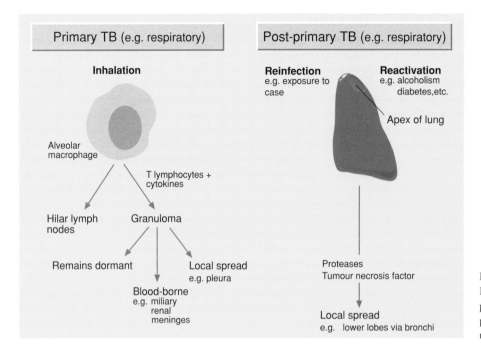

Fig. 52.2
Pathogenesis of
primary and
post-primary
tuberculosis.

- idiopathic pulmonary fibrosis
- sarcoidosis
- miliary tuberculosis

The appearance of the X-ray, the recent history of deteriorating health, and a positive family history of tuberculosis indicate that miliary disease (see Table 52.1 and Fig. 52.2) must be excluded.

Q How may the diagnosis be confirmed?

A Investigations to confirm the diagnosis should include:

- tuberculin skin test (see Box 52.1)
- microscopy (Ziehl–Neelsen (ZN), Fig. 52.3, or auramine stains) and culture of sputum (Fig. 52.4) or pulmonary lavage obtained at bronchoscopy, urine (24-hour collection), bone marrow, and liver biopsy material
- histological examination for caseating granulomata (see Fig. 52.5) of lung, lymph nodes, liver, etc.
- polymerase chain reaction (PCR)—increasingly used to confirm microscopy-positive specimens as *M. tuberculosis* as opposed to other species or

---

Box 52.1 Tuberculin skin tests (Heaf, Tine, or Mantoux)

- Purified protein derivative (starting at 1 and then moving to 10 and 100 IU if necessary) administered intracutaneously by a needle or 'gun' and read at 48–72 hours
- Positive result, which is graded, indicated by significant erythema, swelling, and induration around the puncture site (type IV hypersensitivity reaction)

Result and interpretation

Positive result

- Infection (current or previous)
- Previous vaccination (see below)
- Asymptomatic exposure to *Mycobacterium tuberculosis* or other mycobacteria in the past

Negative result

- Not infected, no previous exposure
- Very early infection
- Infection but negative response due to immunosuppression (e.g. HIV disease, steroids)
- Overwhelming infection suppressing the type IV immune response

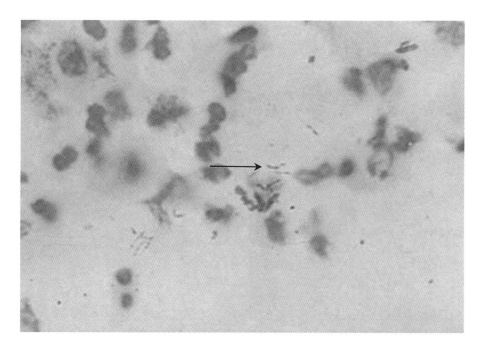

Fig. 52.3 Positive
microscopy
showing bacilli
(arrow) on ZN
stain of sputum
specimen.

(a)

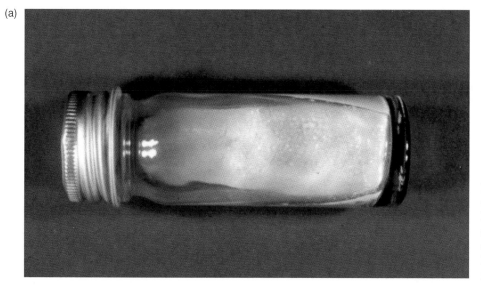

Fig. 52.4
(a) Traditional
Löwenstein–Jensen
solid media and
(b) automated
liquid system
increasingly used.

(a)

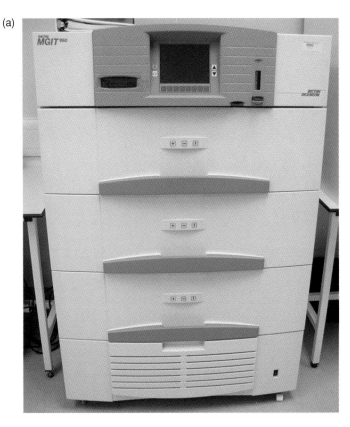

Fig. 52.4 (b) *Contd.*

in microscopy-negative specimens from normally sterile sites, e.g. cerebrospinal fluid (CSF), bone, where delayed diagnosis and treatment may be especially serious

A Heaf test carried out on Karim is strongly positive. Acid-fast bacilli are not seen on microscopy of either lung aspirates or biopsies obtained during bronchoscopy, but granulomata are seen in histological sections of lung and liver biopsies. *M. tuberculosis* (see Box 52.2) is isolated from lung and liver biopsies after 2–3 weeks' incubation on Löwenstein–Jensen medium.

Q What are the main principles of the treatment of tuberculosis?

A Unlike most other bacterial infections, this involves the use of more than one agent for a period

---

Box 52.2 Mycobacteria

- Non-motile, slowly growing curved rods (take 2–8 weeks to isolate on artificial media); obligate aerobes

- Possess a thick complex lipid-rich cell wall; will only take up carbol fuchsin following heating and difficult subsequently to decolorize with mineral acids or alcohol (acid-fast). *Not* therefore visualized with Gram stain

- Mycobacteria are pathogens of humans (e.g. *M. tuberculosis*) and animals (e.g. *M. bovis*) but are also found in the environment such as in water (e.g. *M. marinum*)

---

of months. Uncomplicated pulmonary tuberculosis is treated with four agents (e.g. rifampicin, isoniazid, pyrazinamide, and ethambutol) for an initial

(a)

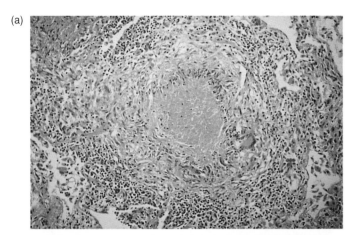

(b)

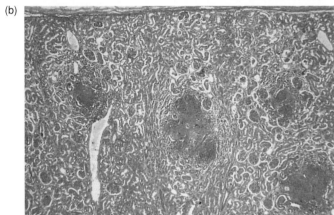

Fig. 52.5 (a) Caseating granuloma in lung with giant and epithelioid cells; (b) multiple granulomata in kidney.

2-month period to be followed by 4 months of dual therapy (e.g. rifampicin and isoniazid). Treatment is continued for longer if the disease is extrapulmonary, the isolate is resistant to one or more of the agents used, or there is non-compliance. Because of the widespread nature of infection in this patient, treatment should probably be continued for 9–12 months, and this should also minimize the incidence of drug-resistant tuberculosis. Table 52.2 includes some characteristic features of the common drugs used in the treatment of tuberculosis.

Q How common is drug-resistant tuberculosis?

A Multidrug-resistant tuberculosis (MDRTB), i.e. an isolate resistant to at least isoniazid and rifampicin, is still relatively uncommon in the UK and Western Europe, i.e. about 5% of isolates.

However, it may be seen in patients who do not comply with treatment, patients with HIV disease, or patients who acquired tuberculosis abroad where the incidence may be higher. There is much interest at present in the use of PCR to detect MDRTB rapidly to improve patient management and prevent spread.

Q What is the risk of Karim having transmitted tuberculosis to contacts?

A Karim's tuberculosis is not 'open', i.e. he does not have a productive cough that is Ziehl–Neelsen-positive or an open lesion in which acid-fast bacilli are seen. He is not therefore considered to be at as great a risk of transmitting tuberculosis as a patient with a productive cough with positive microscopy. However, even microscopy-negative patients with respiratory tuberculosis may be considered for

Table 52.2 Features of commonly used anti-tuberculosis drugs

Drug	Activity	Pharmacokinetics	Toxicity
Isoniazid	Highly bactericidal	Elimination depends on acetylator status	Hepatitis Neurotoxicity prevented by vitamin B6
Rifampicin	Intracellular activity	Good penetration to most organs	Induces hepatic enzymes
Ethambutol	Bacteriostatic	Concentrated in macrophages	Optic neuritis
Pyrazinamide	Intracellular activity	Good CSF penetration	Uncommon
Ethionamide	Bacteriostatic	Enteric coating improves absorption	Gastric irritation
Para-aminosalicylic acid (PAS)	Bacteriostatic	Metabolized in liver	Gastrointestinal tract effects

isolation, preferably in a negative pressure ventilated room, if they have MDRTB or it is suspected, if they are particularly ill, or if they have a productive cough.

Q Who are most at risk from 'open' tuberculosis?

A Family members, other household members with whom the patient lives, and friends and work colleagues who are in regular and frequent contact. Young contacts, i.e. those less than 35 years of age, can be screened with a Heaf test only, but if positive should have a chest X-ray. Those older than 35 may be screened with a chest X-ray at initial contact and possibly subsequently. Such contact tracing, which is usually carried out by public health authorities, emphasizes the importance of notifying diagnosed or suspected tuberculosis.

Q Is nosocomial spread common?

A Not usually. Although nosocomial spread may occur if the diagnosis of 'open' tuberculosis is unsuspected and therefore delayed, most contacts are at relatively low risk, but their doctors should be informed. Patients with suspected tuberculosis should be isolated in a side room or infectious disease unit until the result of microscopy is negative. Staff in hospitals in many parts of the world receive bacille Calmette–Guérin (BCG) vaccination (see Box 52.3) and are therefore relatively protected.

Where this is not routine, occupational acquisition is a recognized hazard and the use of masks or respirators is recommended, especially if aerosol dispersion is likely (e.g. suctioning of airways).

Q Is chemoprophylaxis indicated for any of Karim's contacts?

A No. This is reserved for some contacts of 'open' cases, including the patient's children and at-risk individuals, e.g. HIV-positive individuals, neonates, and other contacts who have not been vaccinated with BCG but who, following exposure, have become tuberculin skin test-positive and may therefore be incubating the infection.

Q What is the standard chemoprophylaxis regimen?

Box 52.3 BCG (Bacille–Calmette–Guérin) vaccine

- Live attenuated vaccine derived from *M. bovis*
- 75% protective in the UK but less elsewhere, e.g. India, because of exposure to other mycobacteria or malnutrition
- Excellent protection against disseminated (miliary) or meningeal tuberculosis
- Affords some protection against leprosy (see Case 12)

A This varies depending on the indication, i.e. contacts of newly diagnosed cases, tuberculin skin conversion thought to be due to exposure and not vaccination, infants of mothers with tuberculosis, and patients with HIV. However, most regimens involve 3–6 months of isoniazid alone or isoniazid and rifampicin in combination.

Q Which other organs or systems may *M. tuberculosis* infect?

A Tuberculosis can affect almost any system in the body, as may be deduced from its pathogenesis (see Fig. 52.2). Extrapulmonary tuberculosis, including miliary disease, is more common in immigrants than the indigenous population of most Western countries, and is a recognized cause of fever of unknown origin (FUO; see Case 53). The more common organs infected with tuberculosis include:

- lymph nodes: not an uncommon initial presentation of tuberculosis especially in children; previously often referred to as scrofula. Cervical glands are most commonly involved, and are usually painless

- genitourinary: recognized cause of 'sterile pyuria' and infertility or other gynaecological problems in females

- bones and joints: may present with septic arthritis or spinal abscess and tuberculosis should be excluded by Ziehl–Neelsen stain and culture of all bone and joint specimens

- brain: tuberculous meningitis should be suspected in any case of meningitis characterized by a high CSF lymphocyte count and a low CSF glucose (see Case 41). Delayed diagnosis contributes to the poor outcome.

Q What is meant by the term 'atypical mycobacteria', and what diseases do these organisms cause?

A In the past these were also referred to as 'environmental mycobacteria', as they are found in water, soil, etc., and it was assumed that they were harmless or of low pathogenicity. In recent years, however, they have been increasingly described as pathogens in the compromised host and cause a range of illnesses in a variety of patient groups. Consequently, they have also been referred to as 'opportunist mycobacteria'.

These bacteria may cause:

- lymphadenitis: most commonly seen during childhood and may be caused by *M. avium* complex or *M. scrofulaceum*; not unlike that due to *M. tuberculosis*

- skin lesions and ulcers: abscesses (*M. chelonei*) or 'fishtank granuloma' (*M. marinum*)

- pulmonary infection: similar presentation to that of tuberculosis but usually seen in previously damaged lungs, such as in patients with chronic obstructive or industrial lung disease (*M. kansasii*)

- disseminated infection: seen in severely immunocompromised states, such as the terminal stages of AIDS (*M. avium* complex; see Case 51)

Unlike *M. tuberculosis*, patient-to-patient transmission is extremely uncommon with these mycobacteria and attempts should be made to isolate the organism from repeat specimens because of the chance of specimen contamination, causing a false-positive result. Management often involves surgery. Antimicrobial chemotherapy is less predictable because many strains are resistant to a number of antimycobacterial agents *in vitro*, but these may be effective *in vivo*.

Summary: Tuberculosis

Presentation
Cough, respiratory tract infection (pulmonary), systemic signs and symptoms, e.g. fever, weight loss if miliary or extrapulmonary

Diagnosis
Microscopy and culture of specimens, histology, PCR (in certain circumstances), radiology, and skin testing (Heaf, Mantoux, etc.)

Management
Combination chemotherapy for 6 months or longer; chemoprophylaxis for at-risk groups

Case 53 Gordon, a 35-year-old Scottish vet with fever

Gordon is a 35-year-old Scottish vet who has been in hospital for 7 days for investigation of fever, malaise, and weight loss. Apart from fracturing his arm during a game of rugby 4 years earlier, he has never been ill or required admission to hospital. He is on no medication, has no relevant family history, and does not smoke. On initial examination his vital signs are normal. There are no skin rashes, enlarged lymph nodes, heart murmurs, or hepato-splenomegaly.

Q Does Gordon have an FUO (fever of unknown origin)?

A No. Strictly speaking, FUO (previously known as a PUO, referring to pyrexia) as originally described is an illness characterized by a fever of 38.5°C or higher on several occasions of more than 3 weeks' duration, despite appropriate investigations in hospital or as an outpatient. Gordon has only been an inpatient for 7 days and we are not told how high the fever is or long he has had it. The term is often loosely used to describe patients under investigation for shorter periods with a fever for which there is no obvious cause.

Q What other information might it be useful to know about Gordon?

A Specific questions Gordon should be asked are:

• What vaccinations has he received, e.g. BCG (bacille Calmette–Guérin) for tuberculosis (see Case 52)?

• What does his work as a vet involve: is he in direct contact with sick animals rendering him vulnerable to acquiring a zoonosis (see Box 53.1)?

• Has he been abroad recently, i.e. in the last year? If so, when, where, and for how long? Did he take malaria prophylaxis (see Case 50) if appropriate, or receive additional immunizations, e.g. typhoid (see Case 27)?

• Has anybody with whom he lives or has close contact, e.g. work colleagues, had a similar illness recently?

• What are his pastimes or hobbies, e.g. does he keep budgies or parrots (see Case 19) or walk through 'tick-infested forests' (see Case 11)?

• What is his life style? Does he have risk factors such as intravenous (IV) drug abuse which predispose him to acquiring HIV (see Case 38)?

Gordon has daily contact with farm animals, including cattle and sheep, but none of his veterinary colleagues have been ill recently. He has had a booster tetanus dose in the last year. He has not been abroad since a trip to Majorca 3 years earlier, and apart from rugby his only other hobby is collecting antique teapots! He

---

Box 53.1 Some features of zoonoses

Definition

Infections acquired by man through contact with animals (usually vertebrate) or animal products

How acquired

• Directly, e.g. farmer, vet in contact with cows or sheep

• Inhalation, e.g. infected droppings or excreta

• Saliva, e.g. bite or lick from a dog

• Faeces, e.g. chicken faeces contaminating eggs

• Urine, e.g. urine from animal contaminating recreational waters

• Blood/tissues, e.g. animal house attendants involved in research

Common examples

Tuberculosis (see Case 52), salmonellosis (see Case 23), brucellosis, leptospirosis, listeriosis (see Case 58), Q fever (see Case 19), rabies (see Case 45), Lassa fever (see Case 68), toxoplasmosis (see Case 64), leishmaniasis (see Case 55)

has never injected intravenous drugs and has been living with his current girlfriend for the last 2 years. He denies any homosexual encounters or other heterosexual relationships, apart from on one occasion 8 years previously when he was very drunk during a rugby tour! As far as he is aware his girlfriend has not had sexual intercourse with anybody else for the last 2 years and has no risk factors for HIV disease.

Q What aspects of the physical examination are especially important here?

A In addition to his vital signs, i.e. pulse, blood pressure, respiratory rate, and temperature (should be monitored initially every 4–6 hours), a comprehensive phyical examination should be carried out looking for evidence of anaemia, jaundice, weight loss, lymphadenopathy, and hepatosplenomegaly. Localizing signs in the respiratory tract and abdomen should also be sought. Particular attention should be paid to the presence of skin rashes and a new or changing heart murmur, indicative of endocarditis (see Case 49).

On repeat examination Gordon appears pale, but his vital signs are normal apart from an elevated temperature of 39°C. Fundoscopy is normal and there is no evidence of peripheral vein injection sites, indicative of IV drug abuse. There are no skin rashes, enlarged lymph nodes, heart murmurs, or hepatosplenomegaly. Rectal examination and examination of the external genitalia are normal. Repeat physical examinations over the next few days are unremarkable. He continues to remain pyrexial 3 weeks after admission for investigation, and by now has lost 3 kg.

Q What is the relevance of fundoscopy here?

A Fundoscopy is part of the normal physical examination and may reveal abnormalities such as exudates consistent with candidaemia (as may occur in IV drug abusers (see Case 48)), infective endocarditis, and cytomegalovirus infection (HIV disease).

Q What initial investigations should be undertaken in a patient with FUO?

A These may be classified as general and microbiological. General investigations include a full blood count (including blood film for atypical mononuclear cells or pathogens such as malaria, trypanosomes), erythrocyte sedimentation rate (ESR), C-reactive protein (CRP), urea and electrolytes, liver function tests, chest X-ray, electrocardiogram (ECG), and echocardiogram. These tests will both reflect the general state of Gordon's health and may point to specific areas requiring further investigation, e.g. abnormal liver function tests indicating the need for liver biopsy. Initial microbiological tests will include the following:

- blood cultures. At least two sets from different sites and taken at least half an hour apart. If endocarditis (see Case 49) is suspected, three sets should be taken, or more if the patient has recently been on antibiotics. If the patient remains pyrexial, repeat cultures should be taken

- urine microscopy and culture. Red blood cells and casts may be indicative of endocarditis, pyuria reflect a renal abscess, and a 24-hour collection should be made for Ziehl–Neelsen staining and tuberculosis culture

- serology. There is a multitude of tests that one might carry out to investigate infective causes of a FUO. 10–20 ml serum should be taken and 5–7 ml stored for later to serve as a baseline serum if initial screening tests are negative. Initial tests should include: monospot for infectious mononucleosis; complement fixation tests for *Mycoplasma pneumoniae*, *Chlamydia* spp., *Coxiella burnetii* (Q. fever), influenza, and adenoviruses; and serology for *Legionella pneumophila*. Serology for Lyme disease, brucellosis, leptospirosis, toxoplasmosis, and syphilis should also be undertaken early on.

- skin tests. A Heaf or Mantoux test for tuberculosis is important. Skin tests to detect anergy (present in sarcoidosis and HIV disease) may also be relevant, as may be skin tests to

Table 53.1 Some of the more common causes of FUO in temperate climates

Infective (incidence, 30%)	Neoplasia (incidence, 25%)	'Autoimmune' (incidence, 15%)
Occult abscess, e.g. liver	Hodgkin's disease	Systemic lupus
Endocarditis	Abdominal lymphoma	Polyarteritis nodosa
Tuberculosis	Renal-cell carcinoma	Polymyalgia rheumatica
Epstein–Barr virus	Atrial myxoma	Sarcoidosis
Toxoplasmosis		

diagnose hydatid disease (see Case 30) and histoplasmosis (see Case 48), if recently abroad in certain parts of North America or elsewhere.

Q What proportion of FUOs is due to infection?

A Approximately 30%, but this will vary according to the population or ethnic group, geographical location, i.e. temperate or tropical climate, and the age of the patient (see Table 53.1). In children under 6 years of age, viral respiratory infection is the most common cause, but after this connective tissue diseases such as juvenile rheumatoid arthritis are more common. After 14 years of age the aetiology reflects that of adults. In 30% of adults no aetiology is identified, and the remainder may be categorized into infective, neoplastic, and connective tissue or 'autoimmune'.

In the HIV-infected or neutropenic patient, opportunist pathogens such as *Pneumocystis carinii* (see Case 51) and systemic or fungal infections (see Case 48) are more likely. If the patient has been hospitalized for some time, nosocomial infections such as wound, catheter-associated urine, and intravascular line (see Case 35) infections are relatively more important. After extensive investigation and especially in some patients with a psychiatric disorder, a factitious temperature must be considered, e.g. self-injection with pyrogens, and the patient closely observed.

The results of Gordon's initial investigations are not very helpful. His ESR is elevated at 50 mm/h and his CRP is also high, at 25 mg/l (normal,

<10 mg/l) but full blood count, examination of repeat blood films, urea and electrolytes, liver function tests, ECG, echocardiography, ultrasound, and computerized tomography (CT) scan of the abdomen are normal. Magnetic resonance imaging and white cell labelled scans are also negative. Urinalysis and culture of three samples of urine are negative, as are blood cultures. He also undergoes a bone marrow biopsy, which reveals normal architecture and cells, and on routine culture is sterile. The Ziehl–Neelsen staining of the marrow biopsy is negative. His chest X-ray shows some 'tenting' of the right diaphragmatic pleura, but without a previous chest X-ray it is not clear whether this is long-standing or not. CT scans of his thorax are no more helpful and bronchoscopy is unremarkable. Bronchial aspirates are sterile and Ziehl–Neelsen stains are negative (tuberculosis culture negative so far). His Heaf test is moderately reactive, with 10 IU (see Case 52), but he has a scar (Fig. 53.1) indicating a previous BCG vaccination on his left upper arm.

Q What options should now be considered?

A There is often no obvious diagnosis following intitial and repeated investigations of FUO. The negative ultrasound and CT scans, with a normal white cell count, probably exclude an occult abscess, but a white cell-labelled scan is more sensitive. The normal biochemistry, e.g. liver function tests, is consistent with the absence of a malig-

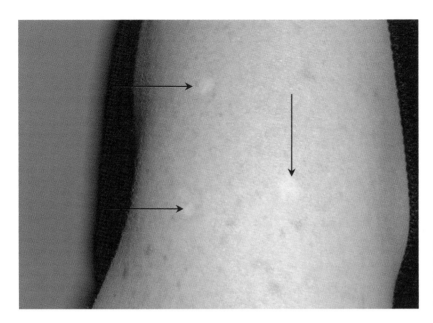

Fig. 53.1 Scar (arrows) on arm indicating previous BCG vaccination also worth checking for in a patient with a FUO.

nancy but non-Hodgkin's lymphoma may present like this if abdominal lymph nodes are involved without marked lymphadenopathy. The minor abnormalities on the chest X-ray and the positive Heaf test indicate that tuberculosis must be considered possible. The negative Ziehl– Neelsen stains and the negative culture results to date do not rule this out. Finally, we are not told the results of any investigations to exclude a connective tissue disorder or serology results.

Rheumatoid factor and antibodies to DNA, histones, non-histone antigens and nuclear antigens are negative, all of which probably excludes a connective tissue or 'autoimmune' disorder. A monospot is negative, as are antibodies to Epstein–Barr virus. Antibodies to the following from paired samples of sera are also negative: *Mycoplasma pneumoniae*, *Chlamydia* spp., *Legionella pneumophila*, *Coxiella burnetii* (Q fever), *Borrelia burgdorferi* (Lyme disease), adenovirus, influenza virus, *Toxoplasma gondii*, *Toxocara canis*, syphilis, and *Leptospira* spp. Following discussion with the patient he agrees to have an HIV antibody test, which is also negative. Three days later his case is dis-

cussed at the hospital's medical conference, where the physican looking after Gordon seeks advice from her colleagues about how to proceed from here. The negative rheumatoid factor and other immune parameters, it is agreed, point against a connective tissue disease. There is also a consensus that, because he is not acutely ill, has not lost a great deal more weight, and the various scans are negative, a malignancy is down the list of likely diagnoses.

There is much discussion about the abnormal chest X-ray and the positive Heaf test. These findings, combined with the elevated ESR and CRP, suggest to many present that an infective process, most likely bacterial, is present and the idea of a therapeutic trial with antituberculosis chemotherapy is favoured by some. Finally, just before the conference concludes, a recently retired general physician who is a regular attender at these conferences requests the results of one test outstanding, especially relevant here.

Q What test is he referring to?

A Serology for brucellosis (see Table 53.2). In a farmer, vet, or abattoir worker one must consider

Table 53.2 Brucellosis

- Caused by small fastidious Gram-negative bacilli, i.e. *Brucella abortus* (from cattle), *B. mellitensis* (from goats and sheep), and *B. suis* (from pigs). Acquired by contact with animal tissues, blood, e.g. abortions, or consumption of unpasteurized milk

- Acute illness; incubation period of 2–3 weeks with fever, headaches, sweating attacks, and arthralgia. May be recurrent or chronic, presenting with depression

- Diagnosis by serology (more than one technique required, e.g. complement fixation, agglutination) or culture (blood, liver biopsy), which is difficult and hazardous to laboratory staff

- Treatment is with tetracyclines for 3 months

Box 53.2 Q fever (query fever)

- Rickettsial disease caused by *Coxiella burnetii*, which is acquired by inhalation of aerosols or contact with animals

- Presents with FUO (often with splenomegaly), atypical pneumonia (see Case 19), or infective endocarditis (see Case 49)

- Diagnosis by demonstrating a rise in complement fixing antibodies to phase 1 (chronic disease or endocarditis) or phase 2 (Q fever or pneumonia) antigens

- A tetracycline is the treatment of choice

Box 53.3 Leptospirosis

- Caused by spirochaetes (*Leptospira icterhaemorrhagiae*, *L. canicola*, *L. hardjo*) from contact with rodent urine, livestock, or contaminated water such as during farming or water sports, e.g. canoeing (Fig. 53.2)

- Presents with fever and sometimes jaundice, proteinuria, and renal failure (Weil's disease)

- Diagnosis usually by demonstration of a rise in antibodies, but bacteria may be cultured with some difficulty from urine and blood

- Benzylpenicillin is the treatment of choice

this together with tuberculosis (see Case 52), Q fever (see Box 53.2), and leptospirosis (see Box 53.3).

The results of Gordon's brucella serology indicate a rise in antibodies to *Brucella abortus*: serum on admission had antibodies at a dilution of 1 in 16 (barely raised), but 2 weeks later this had risen to 1 in 256, indicative of acute brucellosis. He is started on oral tetracycline and a week later his temperature is almost normal. He is discharged home and arrangements are made for him to be seen in the outpatients in 3 weeks' time.

Q How long should Gordon receive antibiotics for, and what is the likely prognosis?

A Three months' treatment is usually adequate. In the past, combined treatment with a tetracycline and streptomycin has been advocated but it is doubtful whether this is more efficacious than tetracycline alone. Co-trimoxazole is an alternative for those patients who should not receive tetracycline antibiotics, e.g. growing children. The majority of patients with acute brucellosis respond but a minority develop recurrences or chronic brucellosis. Chronic brucellosis is difficult to diagnose clinically and serologically (elevated antibodies from acute infection may be lifelong), and the differential diagnosis includes many of the other causes of the chronic fatigue syndrome.

Résumé for undegraduate students

A fever (pyrexia) of unknown origin (FUO) that truly fulfils the criteria for this condition is not that common but presents a major diagnostic challenge. Its management requires a broad knowledge of medicine and an understanding of the less common causes of infection. Endocarditis, tuberculosis, and an occult abscess are the most common infective causes but less common casues must be considered depending on the history and the findings, if any, on physical examination.

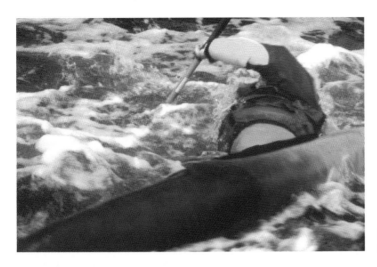

Fig. 53.2 Canoeing in fresh water, a risk for leptospirosis.

Summary: **Fever of unknown origin**

Presentation

Persistent temperature of 38.5°C for 3 weeks or more with no obvious cause after initial investigations. Physical examination is often completely normal

Diagnosis

Comprehensive history including that of occupation, family, travel, and pastimes with repeated physical examinations. The number and type of investigations are almost infinite but should be directed to the most likely cause, i.e. whether infective, neoplastic, or connective tissue disease

Treatment

Will depend upon the cause: antimicrobial chemotherapy if infective (a therapeutic trial, e.g. tuberculosis or endocarditis, may be necessary); chemotherapy for neoplastic disease; or immunosuppressive therapy, e.g. corticosteroids, for connective tissue or 'autoimmune' diseases

Case 54 **Complications of a road traffic accident in Brian, a retired 63-year-old barrister**

Brian is a 63-year-old retired barrister who was involved in a serious road traffic accident 3 months ago. He was in a head-on collision and sustained injuries to his chest (four fractured ribs), head (subdural haematoma with cerebrospinal fluid (CSF) leak), abdomen (lacerated liver, and lacerated spleen requiring removal), and lower limbs (compound fracture of his right femur). He spent 5 weeks in the intensive care unit (ICU) and was ventilated because of adult respiratory distress syndrome (ARDS) and bronchopneumonia. This was followed by 3 weeks in the orthopaedic ward for management of his fractured femur and a wound infection due to *Escherichia coli*, treated with oral co-amoxyclav. Tragically, Brian's wife died in the accident and he himself has had difficulty coping since.

At the orthopaedic clinic following discharge from hospital, Brian is apyrexial but there is some discharge at the leg wound site, where an intramedullary nail was inserted, and he complains of a dull ache there in the last couple of days. A wound swab is sent to the microbiology laboratory and a provisional report indicates that *Staphylococcus aureus* has been isolated, with sensitivities to follow. Brian has not been on antimicrobial agents for almost 4 weeks.

Q Is it surprising that Brian is on no antibiotics whatsoever?

A Yes. Brain had his spleen removed, and therefore he is at increased risk of fulminating infection with *Streptococcus pneumoniae* and other capsulated bacteria for the remainder of his life. Consequently, he should receive pneumococcal (see Case 18) and *Haemophilus influenzae* type B vaccines (see Case 13) and the meningococcal group C vaccine (see Case 41) also. Should he travel to a meningococcal-endemic area, e.g. the Middle East, a meningococcal vaccine that will protect him against non-group B strains preva-

lent there is especially important. Malaria prophylaxis is also essential when travelling to endemic areas. It is also widely recommended that he receive lifelong oral penicillin to protect against pneumococcal bacteraemia. His GP should be informed of his increased susceptibility to infection and, finally, he should always carry a card in case of emergency, indicating that his spleen has been removed.

Q What is the significance of the *S. aureus*?

A Staphylococci, especially coagulase-negative staphylococci such as *S. epidermidis*, are part of the normal flora of the skin. *S. aureus* readily colonizes or infects damaged skin or wounds (see Case 5), and isolation may represent a wound infection, but the significance of this bacterium here, especially from a swab, is difficult to interpret. A sample of the discharge fluid or wound debridement tissue is likely to be more representative of what is happening in the deeper tissues.

Brian is admitted to hospital. An X-ray of his right femur indicates increased sclerosis of the bone and periosteum beneath the site of the wound (Fig. 54.1 shows similar changes in a child) with accompanying soft tissue swelling. The *S. aureus* isolated from the swab is resistant to penicillin, flucloxacillin, erythromycin, and gentamicin. Brian is taken to the operating theratre, where the wound and underlying tissue are explored. A specimen of bone taken during debridement is sent to the microbiology laboratory and *S. aureus* with similar sensitivities is isolated.

Q What is the likely diagnosis?

A Brian almost certainly has osteomyelitis, as indicated by the radiological features and the isolation of a pathogen from tissue taken at operation. Other investigations that may contribute to this diagnosis include a peripheral white cell count,

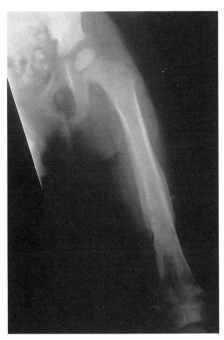

Fig. 54.1 X-ray of femoral osteomyelitis showing extensive sclerosis in a child.

Table 54.1 **Pathogenesis of osteomyelitis and septic arthritis**
Primary
• *Haematogenous*, usually acute disease, largely of childhood, with abrupt onset and systemic illness
• *S. aureus* (long bones), *H. influenzae* type B (< 5 years and not vaccinated), β-haemolytic streptococci
Secondary
• *Contiguous focus*, e.g. pressure sore, trauma, local signs
• *Vascular problems*, elderly patients involving feet, local signs, cellulitis
• Often polymicrobial, with *S. aureus*, coliforms, *Ps. aeruginosa*, anaerobes, etc.

erythrocyte sedimentation rate (ESR) or C-reactive protein (CRP), and magnetic resonance imaging (MRI) or computerized tomography (CT) scans.

Q How may osteomyelitis be classified?

A Bone and joints are remarkably vascular, especially during childhood and early adolescence, when infection is often blood-borne. Osteomyelitis and septic arthritis may be considered as acute or chronic, but a more useful classification is based upon pathogenesis (see Table 54.1). Patients with sickle cell disease are at greater risk of Gram-negative osteomyelitis due to infarction and deficient phagocytosis. Tuberculosis (see Case 52) usually arises from dissemination via the bloodstream, even if infection does not manifest for some years after the initial exposure. Bones commonly infected in tuberculosis are the spine, hips, and knees, reflecting the volume of blood flow there.

Q Are antibiotics required in non-acute, non-haematogenous osteomyelitis where infected tissue is removed during surgery?

A Yes. Although it is essential that as much infected tissue as possible be removed during surgical debridement (this also provides specimens for microbiological diagnosis), antibiotics are also necessary to eradicate any bacteria remaining. Few if any well-conducted clinical trials on the choice of antibiotics, routes of administration, or total duration of treatment have been carried out in osteomyelitis/septic arthritis, but the following recommendations can be made:

• acute osteomyelitis: 3–4 weeks antibiotics in total, with the first 2 weeks by the intravenous (IV) route

• chronic osteomyelitis: longer course required, 3–4 weeks IV followed by 1–2 months oral antibiotics

Q Is there anything unusual about the *S. aureus* recovered from Brian?

A The isolate is resistant to many of the commonly used antibiotics used to treat staphylococcal infection, including flucloxacillin, erythromycin, and gentamicin. In fact, it is an MRSA (methicillin-resistant *S. aureus*). Methicillin rather than flucloxacillin was originally used in the laboratory to assess susceptibility to the antistaphylococcal penicillins and resistance implies the unsuitability of all β-lactam agents in treatment. As some of these strains are resistant to almost all anti-staphylococcal antibiotics and are epidemic in distribution, other synonyms have been used, e.g. multiresistant *S. aureus* or epidemic MRSA (EMRSA); see Table 54.2. For many patients, iso-lation of MRSA from the skin or a superficial site represents asymptomatic colonization rather than infection requiring systemic antibiotic treatment.

Q Is it likely that Brian acquired the MRSA while at home?

A No. Methicillin-resistant *S. aureus* is pre-dominantly a hospital pathogen but may be seen in the community either in patients previously admitted to hospital or patients in long-stay insti-tutions. Brian probably acquired MRSA during his

previous admission to the ICU or orthopaedic ward, but it was not detected until now. MRSA is found worldwide and is especially prevalent in the larger tertiary referral hospitals, where vulnerable patients congregate from a wide variety of hospitals or geographical areas.

Q What options are available for the treatment of Brian's osteomyelitis?

A The glycopeptides, i.e. vancomycin and teico-planin, and fusidic acid, rifampicin, and co-trimax-ozole are useful here. These are usually effective as treatment when the patient's underlying state does not herald a poor prognosis, but none of these agents is very effective in eradicating skin carriage.

Brian is started on IV vancomycin, adminis-tered via a long line, and oral fusidic acid, to which the isolate is sensitive. Assays of serum taken after 2 days indicate subtherapeutic levels of vancomycin and the dose is therefore increased. Swabs of his nose, axilla, and peri-neum, i.e. screening swabs to detect MRSA, were positive. One week later he returns to theatre for further removal of infected bone tissue, from which MRSA is again isolated.

Q Are all staphylococci and *S. aureus* in particular susceptible to glycopeptides?

A No. Some species of coagulase-negative staphy-lococci, e.g. *S. haemolyticus*, are often resistant and, in recent years, strains of MRSA with reduced sus-ceptibility to vancomycin, sometimes referred to as heteroresistant (become resistant after exposure to vancomycin) have been described in the USA, the UK, and elsewhere. In some cases this may be purely a laboratory finding, without clinical relevance, whereas in other cases there is an impli-cation for treatment, i.e. no clinical or micro-biological response to vancomycin. The mechanism of resistance to vancomycin here appears to be thickeneing of the cell wall with increased accumu-lation of excess peptidoglycan. In 2002, isolates with high-level resistance to vancomycin, mediat-ed by *vanA*, probably transferred from vancomycin-resistant enterococci (VRE), were described in the

---

Table 54.2 Features of methicillin resistant *S. aureus*

MRSA

Implies resistance to methicillin, flucloxacillin, and other β-lactam agents. Some strains also resistant to aminoglycosides (e.g. gentamicin), macrolides (e.g. erythromycin), and quinolones (e.g. ciprofloxacin)

Resistance

Gene responsible (*mecA*) is chromosomal and results in the production of a penicillin-binding protein with low affinity for β-lactams and hence these antibiotics have little or no activity against MRSA.

Epidemiology

- Hospital-acquired; especially prevalent in ITUs and trauma units
- Common carriage sites include nose, axilla, perineum, and broken skin
- Spread is by contact, e.g. hands, and both patients and staff may be asymptomatic carriers
- Different EMRSA strains denoted by number, e.g. EMRSA 16, and characterized by similar genotype and often geographical distribution

USA. Isolates similar to this are likely to be seen in other countries in due course.

Q What measures, if any, need to be taken to prevent the spread of MRSA?

A Brian is heavily colonized, as indicated by the positive screening specimens for MRSA, and requires isolation, preferably in a single room with the door closed to prevent transmission to other patients if re-admitted to hospital. This is particularly important on an orthopaedic ward, where there may be other vulnerable patients with open wounds or with orthopaedic screws and nails.

Whenever he goes to theatre, personnel there need to be informed. Effective and thorough hand-washing (Fig. 54.2), however, remains the single most effective measure in preventing spread.

Q Is it necessary for staff to wear face masks when entering Brian's room?

A No. Protective clothing such as disposable plastic aprons and gloves (Fig. 54.3) will reduce the likelihood of transmission via hands or clothing. As this bacterium does not pose a threat to the health of staff or visitors and as it is furthermore highly unlikely to be acquired by inhalation, masks are unnecessary.

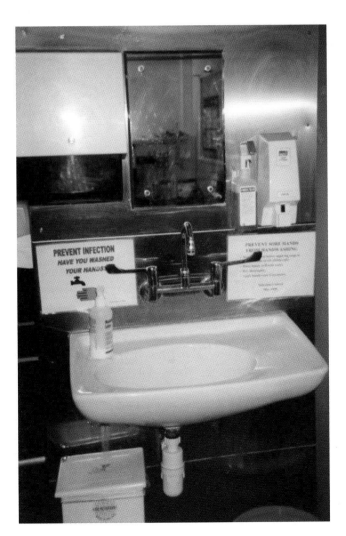

Fig. 54.2 Wash hand basin with elbow-operated taps and hand disinfectant dispenser and foot-operated bin.

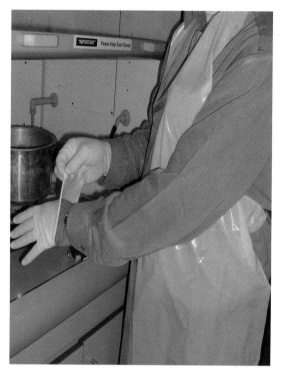

Fig. 54.3 Disposable aprons and gloves.

Q Does the isolation of MRSA from a repeat specimen indicate antibiotic failure?

A Probably no, although it is advisable that the sensitivity tests be repeated on the latest isolate, to exclude a vancomycin-heteroresistant strain. The presence of necrotic tissue with microabscesses may indicate poor antibiotic penetration to the infected site—hence the necessity of removing dead bone. It is possible, but less likely, that persistent or extensive skin carriage may lead to repeat inoculation of the operative site with MRSA.

Q What measures should be taken to eradicate skin carriage?

A Mupirocin, a topical antistaphylococcal antibiotic, may be applied to the nose, and chlorhexidine baths are also effective in reducing or eliminating skin carriage. Alternative topical agents include povidone–iodine and triclosan.

Brian receives a total of 2 months antibiotic treatment with vancomycin and fusidic acid. Clinical evaluation, laboratory indices (e.g. CRP and ESR), and X-rays of his femur indicate resolution of his osteomyelitis. A 5-day course of mupirocin applied to the nose, together with daily chlorhexidine baths, eradicates MRSA from carriage sites and later screening samples are negative. He is subsequently discharged, to be followed up at the orthopaedic outpatients.

Q Do the negative screening samples indicate that Brian no longer poses a risk of spreading MRSA?

A Unfortunately no. Our current understanding of MRSA suggests that we cannot be sure that patients, once colonized or infected but subsequently clear following treatment, will remain free of MRSA indefinitely. Patients such as Brian remain a potential risk and should be isolated and screened when subsequently admitted to hospital. It is therefore important that Brian's case notes indicate clearly that he is an MRSA carrier, and that other hospitals are informed before transfer or referral.

Q Should other patients or staff in contact with Brian be screened for MRSA?

A Large-scale screening is disruptive and expensive and often induces a state of near panic, especially among staff. Decisions on screening should be made by those responsible for infection control (microbiologists or infection control doctors and nurses) and will be influenced by the strain of MRSA, clinical area, extent of carriage and likely dissemination, and the type of ward or unit involved. Because the consequences of spread on an ICU or oncology ward are more serious, screening of patients or staff in these areas is more likely to be necessary than, for example, on a care of the elderly ward. Nonetheless, all patients known to be previously MRSA-positive in the past, or suspected of having been so, should preferably be screened on admission and isolated in a single cubicle while awaiting the results.

Q Does MRSA pose a risk to Brian's relatives or friends?

A No. Even if the MRSA were inadvertently transmitted to a healthy individual, colonization rather than infection requiring treatment would be the only likely consequence. Therefore MRSA-positive patients should be encouraged to socialize with friends and family in the normal way.

Summary: Osteomyelitis due to MRSA

Presentation
Local bone pain with possible discharge or sinus. Systemic symptoms and signs unusual

Diagnosis
Clinical, radiological, and microbiological evaluation. Tissue or deep aspirates rather than superficial swabs for culture essential. MRSA indicated by sensitivity pattern and more common in certain national or international areas

Management
Debridement with prolonged antibiotics, initially administered intravenously. MRSA requires patient isolation and infection control measures, especially hand-washing

Case 55 Fever, sweating, and weight loss in George, recently returned from East Africa

George is a 64-year-old retired businessman who returned to England 2 months ago from East Africa, where he had been working for the past 5 years. He is referred by his GP to the medical outpatients clinic because he has been unwell for the past month. He complains of intermittent fever, sweating attacks, weight loss of 3 kg, and increasing lassitude. His past medical history includes occasional episodes of malaria, for which he was treated in Africa, and a myocardial infarction 10 years previously. He is on no medication. On examination he has a temperature of 38°C, appears pale, and his liver and spleen are palpable. He is admitted to hospital for observation and investigation. His elevated temperature is characterized by a twice-daily elevation to 38–39°C and his initial investigations reveal an elevated erythrocyte sedimentation rate (ESR), a haemoglobin of 9.5g/dl, and a white cell count of 2.7×10^9/l.

Q What is the differential diagnosis?

A The combination of weight loss, increasing lassitude, an enlarged liver and spleen, and anaemia suggests possible malignancy, such as a lymphoma. Infection, especially one imported from abroad, must also be borne in mind. The possible infective causes include:

- malaria: a possibility no matter how long the interval between presentation and past exposure (infection with *Plasmodium vivax* and *P. ovale* may be recurrent) or history of chemoprophylaxis. In particular, malaria due to *P. falciparum* should be excluded because of its potential seriousness. Repeated blood films for examination of parasites (see Case 50) may confirm the diagnosis

- typhoid or paratyphoid fever: the normal incubation period is up to 3 weeks, and hence the

interval between departure from Africa and the onset of illness make this diagnosis less likely. Culture of blood and faeces are the diagnostic tests of choice (see Case 27)

- typhus: this and many other arthropod-borne illnesses (see Box 55.1), especially those caused by rickettsia, are often accompanied by a skin rash with fever, headache, and myalgia. Confirmation of the diagnosis is by serology

- schistosomiasis (bilharzia): hepatosplenomegaly may be seen with infection due to *Schistosoma mansoni*, a blood fluke (see Case 39), but this is often accompanied by abdominal pain or rectal bleeding. Biopsy of infected tissues, e.g. the rectum, or examination of urine for cysts may confirm the diagnosis

- miliary tuberculosis: disseminated tuberculosis is possible here. One should check for the scar of BCG vaccination (usually protects against disseminated disease), do a Heaf test, carry out a chest X-ray, and culture sputum, urine, and bone marrow for *Mycobacterium tuberculosis* (see Case 52)

- amoebic liver abscess: the absence of a history of diarrhoea does not exclude this infection, but a tender liver without splenomegaly is more common. Diagnosis may be confirmed by ultrasound examination and elevated antibodies to *Entamoeba histolytica* (see Case 30)

- Chagas' disease: also known as American trypanosomiasis (caused by *Trypanosoma cruzi*) and transmitted by a bite from the tsetse fly (see Box 55.1), but unlikely in George who has been to Africa not the Americas. Lymphadenopathy is more prominent and cardiac involvement may result in death

- kala azar: visceral leishmaniasis (caused by *Leishmania donovani*) is accompanied by hepatosplenomegaly and anaemia and has an

Box 55.1 Some arthropod-borne infections and their epidemiology (excluding leishmania)

Disease and organism	Vector	Reservoirs	Geographical distribution	Comments
Malaria, *Plasmodium, falciparum, vivax, ovale,* and *malariae*	Female mosquito	Humans	Most tropical and subtropical areas	Falciparum malaria is life-threatening (see Case 50) Resistance to prophylaxis increasing
Yellow fever, flavivirus	Mosquito	Humans, monkeys	Africa, South America	Effective live vaccine available
Dengue, flaviviruses	Mosquito	Humans	Africa, Southeast Asia	Like yellow fever, a cause of viral haemorrhagic fever (see Case 68)
West Nile encephalitis, flavivirus	Mosquito	Wild birds	Africa, Middle East, parts of Asia, USA	Recently introduced into USA (see Case 42)
Filariasis, *Wucheria bancrofti, Brugia malayi*	Mosquito	Humans	Asia, South America	'Respiratory tract infection', lymphoedema, fever
Typhus, *Rickettsia prowazecki*	Louse	Humans	Africa	Increases during war
Lyme disease, *Borrelia burgdorferi*	Ticks	Humans, deer	USA, Europe	Skin rash with multisystem disorder (see Case 11)
Epidemic encephalitis, alpha flaviviruses	Mosquito, ticks	Humans, sheep, rodents, cattle	North and South America	Different types defined geographically and by vector
Trypanosomiasis, *T. gambiense, T. rhodesiense*	Tsetse fly	Humans, wild game	Africa, Central and South America	African trypanosomiasis: 'chancre', fever, 'sleeping sickness' American trypanosomiasis (Chagas' disease): fever, hepatosplenomegaly, lymphadenopathy

incubation period of 1–3 months. Patients often have a temperature pattern characterized by twice-daily peaks. The term 'kala azar' (= black fever) is derived from the discoloration of the skin that is sometimes seen. It is possible to culture the parasite (Fig. 55.1) but this requires specialist expertise and the diagnosis is usually made on the basis of histology (Fig. 55.2) and serology

After routine investigations fail to lead to a diagnosis, George undergoes a liver biopsy that on histological examination reveals amastigotes (non-flagellated forms) of *Leishmania donovani*. An antibody titre of >256 to *L. donovani* is present in a sample of serum (referred to a

national reference laboratory) taken in the out-patients, confirming a diagnosis of visceral leishmaniasis.

Q How is visceral leishmaniasis acquired?

A Leishmaniasis is contracted through a bite from the sandfly. The disease may be cutaneous, mucosal (see Table 55.1), or visceral. These conditions are endemic in Africa, the Middle East, and parts of the Mediterranean, Asia, and South America. Congenital acquisition or transmission by infected blood has been described but is very rare. *L. donovani*, the cause of visceral leishmaniasis, exists in the flagellated form in the sandfly and, following transmission to the human host, reverts to the non-flagellated form when disseminated throughout the reticuloendothelial system. The haematological features (anaemia, neutropenia, and thrombocytopenia) are due to hypersplenism.

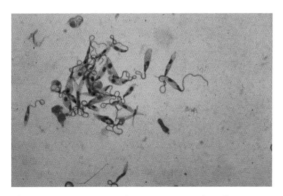

Fig. 55.1 Giemsa stain of promastigotes of *Leishmania* spp. from laboratory culture.

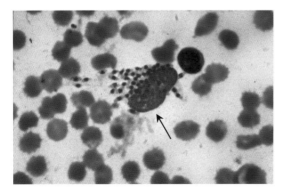

Fig. 55.2 Kala azar (visceral leishmaniasis) diagnosed by the presence of Leishman–Donovan bodies in bone marrow cell (arrow).

Table 55.1 **Leishmaniasis (non-visceral)**

Cutaneous

- Caused by *Leishmania tropica*, *L. aethiopica* (both found in Africa and Asia), and *L. braziliensis* (found in Latin America). Transmitted by a bite from the sandfly. Dogs and rodents are the reservoir
- Characterized by shallow skin ulcers with circular well-defined edges, nodules, and satellite papules
- Differential diagnosis includes leprosy, cutaneous tuberculosis, fungal infection, syphilis, or other spirochaete infections such as yaws
- Diagnosis confirmed by amastigotes in Giemsa-stained smears from lesions, culture after prolonged incubation using specialist media, and serology

Mucosal

- Caused by *L. braziliensis*
- Occurs in 2–3% of cutaneous disease, with epistaxis due to nasal mucosal involvement and lesions on the lips, tongue, and larynx

Q What is the treatment of choice?

A Pentavalent antimony compounds such as sodium stibogluconate are the mainstay of treatment. Amphotericin B, especially in the liposomal form, is increasingly used to treat leishmaniasis.

George is started on sodium stibogluconate. His fever subsides after 10 days, and over the next couple of weeks there is a rise in his haemoglobin and his liver and spleen become smaller as detected clinically and by ultrasound examination.

Q What serious complications may follow visceral leishmaniasis?

A Splenic rupture and haemorrhage, and secondary bacterial or viral infection—which may be overwhelming because of impaired immune responses due to hypersplenism—are major life-threatening complications.

Résumé for undergraduates

Leishmaniasis is an important infection in tropical areas of the world and must therefore be included in the differential diagnosis of fever in the patient recently returned from abroad (although malaria and typhoid fever would be more common). A specimen for histology and blood for serology are important in confirming a diagnosis of visceral leishmaniasis.

Summary: Leishmaniasis

Presentation

Fever, anaemia, hepatosplenomegaly, lymphadenopathy (visceral), or skin ulcers/nodules (cutaneous). History of sandfly bite not always present

Diagnosis

Tissue biopsy (liver, spleen, lymph node, skin, as appropriate), culture (specialized technique), and serology

Management

Pentavalent antimony compounds or amphotericin B and treatment of complications, e.g. plastic surgery for skin deformities, transfusion for severe anaemia

Case 56 Dilip, a 45-year-old motor mechanic with diabetes and renal failure

Dilip, a 45-year-old motor mechanic, has had insulin-dependent diabetes since the age of 17. Over the past 3 years, his renal function has deteriorated. After referral to the renal physicians, appropriate investigations confirm a diagnosis of diabetic nephropathy and that renal dialysis is now indicated.

Q What microbiological investigations should the renal physicians perform when Dilip is referred to them?

A All patients entering a dialysis unit should be screened for urinary tract infection with an mid-stream urine (MSU) sample and for blood-borne virus (BBV) infections. Such patients are likely to undergo extensive invasive procedures over a long period of time, and therefore represent an infection risk to health-care workers performing those manipulations. Furthermore, haemodialysis machines are a potential source of patient-to-patient spread of blood-borne infection, and well-documented outbreaks of hepatitis B and non-A, non-B hepatitis (now known as hepatitis C) have occurred on dialysis units, some with alarmingly high mortality rates. Dilip should therefore be tested for evidence of hepatitis B and C (HBV and HCV, respectively) and human immunodeficiency virus (HIV) infections after appropriate explanation and counselling, (see Case 38) prior to entry to the dialysis unit.

Dilip's results are: anti-HIV-negative; hepatitis B surface antigen (HBsAg)-negative; anti-HCV-negative.

Q What prophylactic measure should now be offered to Dilip?

A He should be offered a course of hepatitis B vaccine, with the aim of inducing protective levels of anti-HBsAg (see Case 28). Individuals who are immunosuppressed, or who have chronic underlying disease, are less likely to make an antibody response to this vaccine, so Dilip should be offered vaccine as soon as it becomes clear that his renal function is deteriorating and that he may therefore eventually require dialysis. He should be given vaccine containing twice the recommended antigen dose, another measure designed to increase the response rate amongst this group of patients.

Q What other measures can be taken to reduce the risk of nosocomial transmission of these blood-borne viral infections on a renal unit?

A These include:

- Optimal infection control practice should be rigorously adhered to (e.g. hand-washing, careful disposal of sharps)
- Use once-only disposable materials wherever possible, including component parts of dialysis machines
- Carriers of HBV should not be allowed to perform invasive procedures on the unit
- All staff on the unit should be protected from HBV infection by vaccination
- All patients entering the unit should be screened for HBV, HCV, and HIV infection. Such screening should be repeated at intervals (e.g. every 3 months) to ensure no that new infections are introduced into the unit, and to provide assurance that spread of infection is not occurring on the unit
- All patients should be vaccinated against HBV
- The management of a new patient arriving on a unit, discovered to be a carrier of any of these viruses, is problematic. Ideally, there should be dedicated dialysis machines on the unit that are used only for these patients. Recent reports of spread of HCV infection within dialysis units suggest spread is associated with being dialysed in the same room at the same time as an HCV-infected patient, rather than being the next patient on a dialysis machine used on an infected patient. Thus, BBV-infected patients

should be dialysed in a suitable isolation facility.

After 2 years of haemodialysis, a donor kidney becomes available for Dilip.

Q What microbiological investigations should be performed on donor and recipient immediately prior to transplantation?

A Donor serum should be tested for evidence of chronic carriage of HBV, HCV, and HIV. There is also a potential risk of transmission of syphilis, so donor sera should be tested to exclude this. Donor organs from HBV or HIV carriers are *not* acceptable for use, as the risks associated with transmission of those infections to the recipient outweigh the potential benefits of the transplantation. The situation with HCV is less clear at present. Recipient serum should also be sent for the same tests, unless by chance screening has been performed recently.

Q What other virological screening assays should be considered?

A Cytomegalovirus (CMV) can be transmitted by organ transplantation, and the immune status of both donor and recipient to CMV should be determined. The immune status of the recipient to varicella-zoster virus (VZV) should also be determined.

Q Why is it necessary to know the VZV immune status of the recipient?

A All transplant recipients are immuno-suppressed, and are therefore at risk of serious consequences of infection with organisms that are otherwise relatively innocuous in immuno-competent hosts. Thus, if a recipient is known to be susceptible to VZV infection and is exposed to someone with chicken pox, passive immunization with varicella-zoster immune globulin is indicated, with the aim of attenuating a possible attack of chickenpox.

On looking through Dilip's medical records, you note that viral serology was performed 3 months ago, when he presented with a febrile illness. Amongst other results you find the fol-lowing: CMV complement fixation test (CFT) <16 (i.e. negative); VZV CFT <16.

Q Does this mean that Dilip has never been exposed to either CMV or VZV?

A No. Complement-fixing antibodies (IgM, and certain subclasses of IgG) appear early during acute infection, and tend to disappear over the following few months. Thus, detection of such antibodies by means of a CFT is a useful approach to diagnosis of recent infection. However, much more sensitive assays (e.g. enzyme-linked immunosorbent assay (ELISA), latex agglutination) should be employed if immune status is being sought.

You receive the following results from Dilip and the kidney donor:

- Donor: anti-CMV (by ELISA), positive
- Dilip: anti-CMV (by ELISA), negative; anti-VZV (by ELISA): positive

Q How do you interpret these results?

A The donor has had prior exposure to CMV, whilst Dilip has not. Dilip has been infected with VZV in the past. He is therefore not at risk of acquiring primary VZV infection (i.e. chickenpox), but he may suffer from reactivation of his own latent VZV, i.e. shingles or zoster (see Case 7).

Q Do the CMV results mean that Dilip is in a high-risk or low-risk group for acquisition of serious CMV disease posttransplantation?

A As a seronegative recipient of a kidney from a seropositive donor, Dilip is at high risk of CMV disease. CMV, like VZV, belongs to the herpesvirus family and exhibits the phenomenon of latency (see Case 4). The donor has been infected with CMV in the past. Thus, CMV will be present within the donor in a latent state and may be transmitted in renal tissue.

Q What categories of CMV infection may occur in a recipient of a solid organ transplant?

A The possibilities are:

1. primary—seronegative recipient of organ from seropositive donor

2. secondary
- reinfection—seropositive recipient of organ from seropositive donor
- reactivation—seropositive recipient of organ from seronegative or -positive donor

Primary infection carries the greatest risk of symptomatic disease.

Dilip receives a kidney transplant and is put on a standard immunosuppressive regimen. The transplant is successful, and Dilip is discharged after 2 weeks with a functioning kidney. He returns for regular follow-up. Seven weeks after the operation he presents with general malaise, and is noted to be febrile (38.5°C). There are no localizing signs.

Q What is your differential diagnosis, and what investigations should you initiate?

A Dilip should be admitted to hospital and investigated thoroughly. Whilst there is a long list of causes of a febrile illness without localizing signs, you must consider particularly: (1) bacterial infection (e.g. urinary or respiratory tract infection, septicaemia); (2) a rejection episode; and (3) CMV infection. *Correct diagnosis is crucial.* If this is a rejection episode, you would increase the immunosuppression whilst, if this is acute CMV, you would attempt to decrease the immunosuppression, to allow Dilip's own immune response to overcome the infection. You would begin by ordering a range of simple investigations such as full blood count, urea and electrolytes, liver function tests, chest X-ray, and septic screen (MSU, sputum, blood cultures).

You receive the following results:
- Hb, 9.7 g/dl
- white cell count, 3.2×10^9/l
- differential: polymorphonuclear leucocytes (PMNLs), 30%; lymphocytes, 65%; monocytes, 5%
- urea and electrolytes, normal
- alanine aminotransferase (ALT), 75 IU/l (normal range, up to 50 IU/l)

- bilirubin, alkaline phosphatase, gamma-glutamyl transferase—within normal ranges
- chest X-ray, normal
- MSU, no growth
- sputum, commensals only
- blood cultures (after 48 hours), no growth

Q How do you interpret these results?

A The absence of a neutrophil response and failure to isolate a pathogen from a patient with no history of recent antibiotics are against an acute bacterial infection. The normal renal function makes an acute rejection episode unlikely. The marrow suppression, particularly of the white cells, together with the biochemical evidence of hepatitis (raised ALT) are typical features of primary CMV infection.

Q In general, how may CMV infection be acquired?

A CMV may be acquired by:
- *Mother to baby*, giving rise to congenital CMV infection (see Case 64)
- *Close contact with small children*. CMV-infected infants excrete CMV in saliva and urine for many months if not years. Spread of infection, e.g. within a day-care centre, can therefore occur through contamination of the environment
- *Sexual transmission*. Virus may be present in saliva and in genital tract secretions
- *Blood transfusion and transplantation*. The likely route in Dilip's case, as he has received a kidney from a seropositive donor

Q In general, what are the consequences of CMV infection?

A These depend on the age and immune status of the patient (see Table 56.1).

Q How would you confirm that Dilip has a primary CMV infection?

A Given the potential seriousness of Dilip's illness, you would ask the laboratory to perform a *rapid diagnostic technique* for the diagnosis of CMV

Table 56.1 Consequences of CMV infection

In fetus and neonate

- Congenital CMV infection (see Case 64)

In immunocompetent individuals

- Asymptomatic—the vast majority
- Infectious mononucleosis syndrome (see Case 15)

In immunosuppressed individuals

- Multisystem disease may arise from primary *or* secondary infection
- In HIV infection (see Case 51)
- In solid organ transplant recipients, fever, marrow suppression, and hepatitis are common; in bone marrow transplant recipients, pneumonitis is a particularly feared life-threatening complication

infection. There are a number of such techniques available, and individual laboratories will differ as to which one they can offer.

1. *Detection of early antigen fluorescent foci* (the DEAFF test; see Fig. 56.1). Although CMV-infected cells may remain morphologically normal for many days, they will nevertheless be expressing viral antigens on the cell surface.

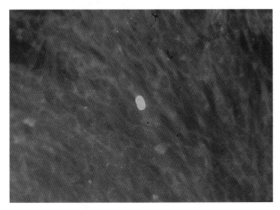

Fig. 56.1 DEAFF test. A single nucleus is seen fluorescing in a cell sheet that is morphologically normal.

Thus, after inoculation of patient material into cell culture, the presence of virus may be seen 24–48 hours later by staining the cells with fluorescent-labelled monoclonal antibodies directed against viral antigens expressed early in the replicative cycle of CMV (the so-called early antigens)

2. *Direct CMV antigen detection*. Here, peripheral blood cells taken directly from the patient are stained with appropriately labelled monoclonal antibodies, to detect CMV antigen expression occurring in vivo

3. *CMV genome detection*. The advent of polymerase chain reaction (PCR) assays means that the presence of the DNA genome (or RNA transcripts derived therefrom) of CMV in peripheral blood can now be demonstrated. Many laboratories have now adopted these molecular diagnostic assays, which are thereby replacing (1) and (2) above

Note that routine tissue culture, which is the standard assay for demonstration of CMV, is inappropriate here, as it may take up to 4 weeks for the virus to produce a cytopathic effect.

Q Why is it important to demonstrate CMV in peripheral blood rather than, say, a urine sample?

A Excretion of CMV in urine is a common finding, especially in immunosuppressed individuals, and may occur in the absence of disease. The presence of replicating CMV in peripheral blood correlates much better with CMV-induced disease.

Q How would you manage Dilip's CMV infection?

A You would reduce his immunosuppression, although this will require careful monitoring of his renal function. There are also anti-CMV drugs available, such as ganciclovir. This drug, however, has toxic side-effects, principally on the bone marrow, causing yet further suppression of white cell production. Foscarnet and cidofovir are also effective anti-CMV agents, but are nephrotoxic.

After a stormy 3 weeks, Dilip recovers from his CMV infection, with his transplanted kidney intact.

Q Could Dilip's severe CMV-induced disease have been prevented?

A Yes, or at least attenuated. As Dilip was known to be a CMV-seronegative recipient of a sero-positive kidney and therefore at increased risk of serious CMV disease, he should have been offered some form of prophylaxis. A number of prophylactic regimens have been shown to reduce the risk of serious CMV infection in recipients of both solid organs and of bone marrow. These include:

- prophylactic aciclovir. Whilst aciclovir has very little anti-CMV effect *in vitro*, trials have nevertheless demonstrated efficacy of this drug if given prophylactically to patients at risk of CMV infection. Valaciclovir is a prodrug of aciclovir with better oral absorption

- prophylactic ganciclovir. Oral absorption of this drug is poor. Valganciclovir is a prodrug with better oral absorption

- administration of CMV hyperimmune globulin, i.e. passive immunization

An alternative to prophylaxis is to monitor transplant recipients very carefully for evidence of active CMV replication, e.g. by weekly surveillance blood sampling using molecular diagnostic techniques. As soon as there is evidence of CMV infection, pre-emptive therapy with ganciclovir can be started, i.e. before the patient becomes ill.

Résumé for undergraduates

Patients entering a dialysis unit should be screened for evidence of blood-borne virus infection (HBV, HCV, HIV). Transplant recipients are at risk of severe CMV infection, which may present as multisystem disease with fever, leucopenia, hepatitis, or pneumonitis (life-threatening). Prevention of post-transplant CMV infection involves use of anti-CMV prophylaxis, posttransplant surveillance for evidence of infection, and treatment when indicated.

Summary: CMV infection in a solid organ transplant recipient

Presentation
Multisystem disease with fever, leucopenia, hepatitis; pneumonitis is life-threatening

Diagnosis
Rapid diagnostic techniques on clinically relevant samples, i.e. DEAFF test, antigen or genome detection on blood sample

Management
Prophylaxis and/or surveillance monitoring for infection for high-risk patients; pre-emptive therapy at earliest sign of infection; reduce immunosuppression if possible.

Case 57 Dr Woolley suffers a needlestick injury

Dr Woolley, a senior house physician, is in the accident and emergency department, dealing with Phil, a 25-year-old gardener who has presented as an emergency case with vomiting and diarrhoea. She performs a routine venupuncture with a syringe and needle and, just as she is attempting to resheathe the needle, prior to transferring it to the sharps bin across the corridor from her cubicle, her bleep goes off, causing her to jerk suddenly. Unfortunately, she jabs the needle into the pulp of her left forefinger. Upset, she rinses the finger under cold running water, but notices that the puncture site oozes blood.

Q What should Dr Woolley do next (assuming that, in the meantime, the needle has now been adequately disposed of!)?

A Dr Woolley has suffered a needlestick, or sharps, injury. She should report this to the appropriate responsible body within the hospital, as soon as is practicable. Precisely who deals with needlestick injuries will vary between hospitals, and possibly also within hospitals at different times of day or night. Possibilities will include the infection control team, the microbiology department, or the occupational health department.

Q What mistakes did Dr Woolley make that resulted in an increased risk of a needlestick injury?

A Firstly, needles should never be resheathed. Resheathing of needles is the single most likely precipitant cause of reported sharps injuries. Dr Woolley would claim that she was doing this as she could hardly walk across the A & E department with a bare needle on her way to the sharps bin—which highlights the second breakdown in procedure. Sharps bins should be conveniently placed close to where venepunctures, or any other invasive procedures, are to be performed, thus obviating the need to carry dirty needles around in search of a safe disposal place.

Q Was Dr Woolley's needlestick injury therefore avoidable?

A Yes. However, despite intensive efforts at education and training, and introduction of appropriate safety procedures, such injuries remain all too common. Accidents do happen. Staff and students should therefore know what procedures should be followed in the unfortunate event of one occurring.

Q What is the most important risk associated with a needlestick injury?

A If the patient whose blood contaminates the needle (referred to as the source, or donor, as opposed to Dr Woolley, who is the recipient) is infected with a blood-borne virus, then there is a significant risk of transmission of infection from the donor to the recipient.

Q Which viruses are blood-borne?

A In the UK, the phrase 'blood-borne viruses' (BBV) refers to hepatitis B virus (HBV), hepatitis C virus (HCV), and human immunodeficiency virus (HIV), viruses that are continuously present in the peripheral blood of chronically infected patients. Many other viruses may be present within peripheral blood, but for most this viraemic stage is transient, e.g. for 24 hours only at a specific stage in the incubation period.

Q What are the risks of transmission of HBV, HCV, and HIV via a needlestick injury?

A These are:

- HBV: 1 in 3 needlesticks from a known HBeAg-positive source (see Case 28 for an explanation of HBeAg positivity) will result in transmission
- HCV: 1 in 30 needlesticks will transmit
- HIV: 1 in 300 needlesticks will transmit

However, there are other factors that influence the chances of transmission in a given incident. Risk of HIV transmission (and, by implication, the hepatitis viruses) is clearly associated with deep injury, visible blood on the device that caused the injury, injury with a needle that had been in an artery or vein from the source patient, and terminal HIV-related illness in the source patients.

Dr Woolley contacts her occupational health department and explains the circumstances of her accident.

Q What is the next step in the management of this incident?

A The first action to be taken is to assess, as far as is possible, the likelihood that Dr Woolley is at risk of acquisition of a blood-borne virus (risk assessment). This clearly depends on whether or not Phil, the donor, is or is likely to be infected with any of the relevant viruses. Someone, not Dr Woolley, should interview Phil and ask about risk factors for BBV infection, e.g. history of injecting drug use, sexual history, medical history (including jaundice), and so on (see Case 28 for risk factors for HBV and HCV infection, and Case 38 for HIV infection). Permission should be sought from Phil to test for evidence of current BBV infection.

Q What tests would the laboratory perform to assess whether Phil is infected with a BBV?

A The test for HIV infection is to look for antibodies to the virus, i.e. anti-HIV. For HBV infection, the test is to look for HBsAg (hepatitis B surface antigen). For HCV infection, the simplest test is to look for anti-HCV, although it must be borne in mind that around 20% of anti-HCV positive individuals are not viraemic, and therefore are not a transmission risk (see Case 29). Needlestick injuries generate considerable anxiety, and most laboratories would be willing, if asked, to perform these tests urgently.

Q Are there any interventions that might reduce the risk of Dr Woolley acquiring: (a) HBV; (b) HCV; and (c) HIV infection, as a result of this incident?

A It depends on the virus.

(a) Yes. With appropriate management, the risk of Dr Woolley acquiring HBV infection as a

result of this incident should be reduced to almost zero, even if Phil turned out to be an HBeAg-positive HBV carrier. Dr Woolley should already have received a course of hepatitis B vaccine (most likely before entering medical school). She should therefore be asked about this, and whether or not she responded to the vaccine adequately. If she was a good responder (>100 mIU/ml), then her vaccine-induced immunity should protect her, although she should in any case be offered a booster dose of vaccine. If she has not been vaccinated, or was a non- or suboptimal responder to vaccine, then she should be offered passive immunization with hepatitis B immunoglobulin (see Fig. 57.1), and either a booster dose of the vaccine or a full accelerated course of vaccination (i.e. 0, 1, 2, and 12 months).

(b) No. At present, there is no vaccine for HCV, and no preparation of antibodies to HCV available for passive immunization. However, recent data suggest that treatment of acute HCV infection (with interferon-alpha) has a very high chance (>90%) of achieving viral clearance. Thus, Dr Woolley should be tested at appropriate intervals to determine whether or not she acquires HCV infection. If the tests become positive, then she should be offered antiviral therapy as soon as possible.

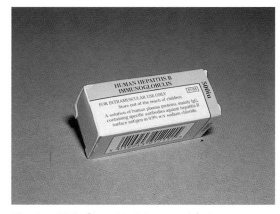

Fig. 57.1 Vial of hepatitis B immunoglobulin.

(c) Yes. Post-exposure prophylaxis (PEP) with antiretroviral drugs may reduce the risk of acquisition of HIV infection. However, the decision to use PEP, and with precisely which drugs, is not straightforward. The principles of PEP are:

- it should be started as soon as possible after the incident—even if, at that stage, the risk of HIV transmission is not certain
- it should consist of combination therapy—two- or three-drug regimens may be recommended according to the perceived degree of risk
- choice of drugs will depend on the donor's prior exposure to antiretrovirals (and hence the possibility of transmission of drug-resistant virus) and the circumstances of the recipient (e.g. certain antiretrovirals are contraindicated in pregnancy)

PEP is a four-week course of drugs; recipients will require considerable support to maintain compliance, especially if they experience drug-related toxicities. The potential benefit of PEP has to be weighed against possible adverse effects—all antiretrovirals are toxic, and there have been severe drug-related illness associated with the use of PEP, including acute hepatic failure necessitating liver transplantation.

Phil is interviewed. He admits to having experimented with injectable drugs 8 years previously on a small number of occasions, but is otherwise fit and well (apart from his gastro-enteritis). He agrees to be tested for evidence of BBV. Dr Woolley knows she had a good response to hepatitis B vaccine. After some discussion, taking into account the low prevalence of HIV infection amongst injecting drug users in this locality, she decides against HIV-PEP.

Q Is there anything else to be done at this stage?

A Yes. It is always a good idea to take a baseline serum sample from the needlestick recipient, for storage in the laboratory. If anything untoward does happen later (e.g. a sample taken 12 weeks later is found to be anti-HCV positive), then the baseline sample can be tested, in order to demonstrate that the recipient wasn't already HCV-infected at the time of the incident. This has important implications for provision of compensation for an occupationally acquired disease.

Three days later, the laboratory reports on Phil's serum: HBsAg-negative; anti-HCV-negative; anti-HIV-negative. Dr Woolley heaves a huge sigh of relief and vows never again to try to resheathe needles. Some time later, she again contacts occupational health, as she was splashed with blood from a patient bleeding profusely from a cut hand.

Q Is Dr Woolley at risk of acquisition of a BBV from such an exposure?

A Possibly. Intact skin provides an effective barrier against most viruses, and certainly against HBV, HCV, and HIV. There are no recorded instances of transmission of any of these viruses following such an exposure. However, the same is not true for non-intact skin. Breaks in the skin may arise through cuts or abrasions, or through a chronic inflammatory process such as dermatitis. Transmission of BBV through splashes on non-intact skin have been reported. Hence the advice to cover up any cuts, or other surface imperfections before any potential exposures to blood or bodily fluids. Blood splashes in the mouth or eye may also transmit infection. Mucosal surfaces are non-keratinized, and therefore are not a barrier to virus infection. However, the risk of transmission through either of the above routes is likely to be much less than from a percutaneous injury such as a needlestick.

Q The above scenario describes a health-care worker (HCW) at risk of BBV infection from one of her patients. Is it possible that patients may be at risk of BBV infection from their HCWs?

A Yes, unfortunately there are circumstances in which the blood of an HCW may come into contact with an open wound of a patient, e.g. if a surgeon cuts their finger whilst operating, their blood may come into contact with the patient's blood. If the surgeon is infected with a BBV, then infection can be transmitted to the patient. Procedures in which this may happen are collectively referred to as 'exposure-prone procedures' or EPPs. If the HCW happens to be infected with a BBV, then the patient is at risk of acquiring that infection. There are plenty of documented cases of HCW-to-patient transmission of BBVs.

Q Is there anything that can be done to reduce the risk of HCW-to-patient transfer of infection?

A Yes. Firstly, if a known incident occurs, then the patient should be managed as a recipient of a needlestick injury, i.e. the need for prophylaxis against HBV or HIV should be assessed, and appropriate monitoring instituted for development of HCV infection.

In addition, the Department of Health in the UK has issued strict guidelines to regulate the activities of HCWs who are infected with a BBV, in terms of their fitness to practise EPPs. Some of these are fairly complex, but in essence:

- An HCW who is known to be infected with HIV is *not* allowed to perform any EPPs

- An HCW who is known to be a carrier of HBV is *only* allowed to perform EPPs if he/she is *not* HBeAg-positive *and* has a low HBV DNA

- An HCW who is known to be chronically infected with HCV is *not* allowed to perform EPPs.

The construction and implementation of these guidelines is fraught with difficult moral and ethical dilemmas. They exist to protect patients, but have to be balanced against the rights of HCWs, and the degree of risk that BBV-infected HCWs pose to their patients. Any HCW who is restricted by the guidelines can appeal against them to the United Kingdom Advisory Panel (UKAP). In the light of these guidelines, it would be inadvisable for any student who knows he/she is infected with HBV, HCV, or HIV, to consider a career that would involve EPPs (e.g. surgery, obstetrics and gynaecology). There are plenty of alternative careers in medicine in which being infected with a BBV poses no risk at all to the patient.

Summary: Needlestick injuries

Risk

Needlestick injuries may result in transmission of HBV (1/3), HCV (1/30), HIV (1/300)

Management

- Perform risk assessment, including testing of source patient if possible; obtain baseline serum from recipient

- For HBV options include: administration of HBIg; booster dose of HBV vaccine; accelerated course of HBV vaccine (e.g. 0, 1, 2 months)

- For HCV, monitor recipient for evidence of HCV infection. If positive, offer antiviral therapy

- For HIV, consider post-exposure prophylaxis with antiretroviral drugs

Self-assessment

1. Which of the following statements are correct?
   (a) HIV post-exposure prophylaxis should be offered to all recipients of needlestick injuries
   (b) All recipients of needlestick injuries should be offered hepatitis B immunoglobulin
   (c) All health-care workers who are anti-HCV-positive are banned from performing exposure-prone procedures (EPPs)
   (d) A baseline serum sample should be taken from all recipients of needlestick injuries
   (e) Blood splashes on to intact skin do not carry a risk of transmission of blood-borne viruses

2. Which one of the following statements is correct?
   (a) Needles should be resheathed before disposal in a sharps bin
   (b) HCV infection can be transmitted from a surgeon to a patient during operation
   (c) Exposure-prone procedures (EPPs) are those where the operator may come into contact with the patient's blood
   (d) Recipients of needlestick injuries should have their anti-HBs levels measured at the time of the incident
   (e) BBV transmission via needlestick injuries is more likely to occur from health-care worker to patient rather than from patient to health-care worker

3. Which one of the following is not an AIDS-defining illness in an HIV-infected patient?
   (a) Chronic diarrhoea due to cryptosporidiosis
   (b) CMV retinitis
   (c) Tuberculosis

(d) Oral candidiasis
(e) Carcinoma of the uterine cervix

4. Which one of the following statements regarding the use of antiretroviral therapy is true?
   (a) All antiretroviral regimens must include a protease inhibitor (PI)
   (b) Monitoring of the efficacy of antiretroviral drug therapy is by measurement of the CD4 count
   (c) The development of diabetes mellitus is a recognized complication of HAART
   (d) All HIV-infected patients should be treated with HAART
   (e) Patients with a CD4 count of >500/mm^3 and a low viral load can be treated initially with zidovudine alone

5. Which one of the following statements regarding CMV infection in transplant recipients is not true?
   (a) Renal transplant recipients at highest risk of serious CMV disease are those who were CMV-seronegative pretransplant, and received a kidney from a seropositive donor
   (b) Bone marrow transplant recipients at highest risk of serious CMV disease are those who were CMV-seronegative pretransplant, and received marrow from a seropositive donor
   (c) CMV infection is far more common than CMV disease posttransplantation
   (d) In a renal transplant recipient, identification of CMV replication in a peripheral blood sample is a worse prognostic marker than identification of CMV in a urine sample
   (e) Manifestations of CMV disease in a renal transplant recipient may include fever, leucopenia, and abnormal liver function

6. Screening of a patient prior to solid organ transplantation should include all but which *one* of the following?

(a) A test for anti-HIV

(b) A test for anti-HCV

(c) A test for anti-CMV

(d) A test for anti-VZV

(e) A test for anti-HBs

7. Which *one* of the following is *not* recognized as a life-threatening complication of malaria?

(a) Acute heart failure

(b) Disseminated intravascular coagulation

(c) Cerebral involvement

(d) Acute renal failure

(e) Hypoglycaemia

8. Which of the following statements regarding malaria are true?

(a) Malaria is spread by bites of anopheline mosquitos of either sex

(b) *P. falciparum* does not have an exo-erythrocytic liver stage in its life cycle

(c) Malaria may occur in a traveller despite complete adherence to antimalarial prophylaxis

(d) The absence of typical tertian fevers makes a diagnosis of falciparum malaria unlikely

(e) Malaria should be considered in the differential diagnosis of fever in a traveller for up to a year after his/her return from abroad

9. Which of the following bacteria is the most common cause of bacteraemia or bloodstream infection?

(a) *Staphylococcus saprophyticus*

(b) *E. coli*

(c) *Neisseria meningitidis*

(d) Beta-haemolytic streptococcus group A (*Strep. pyogenes*)

(e) *Pseudomonas aeruginosa*

10. Which antibiotic regimen is most appropriate to treat bacteraemia or bloodstream infection secondary to urinary infection before the results of culture and susceptibility tests are available?

(a) Clarithromycin and tetracycline

(b) Nitrofurantoin

(c) Gentamicin and ampicillin

(d) Flucloxacillin and metronidazole

(e) Vancomycin

11. Which one of the following is a significant risk factor for the development of systemic candida infection such as candidaemia?

(a) Recent broad-spectrum antibiotics

(b) Candida isolated from environmental sources

(c) Enteral nutrition

(d) Asymptomatic HIV infection

(e) A diet of natural yogurt three times daily

12. Of what is *Aspergillus fumigatus* a recognized cause?

(a) Encephalitis

(b) Endocarditis

(c) Pneumonia

(d) Cholangitis

(e) Hepatitis

13. Which laboratory test result may suggest a diagnosis of infective endocarditis?

(a) Thrombocytopaenia

(b) Elevated creatinine

(c) Raised alkaline phosphatase

(d) Abnormal complement profile

(e) Elevated cardiac enzymes

14. Why is an aminoglycoside antibiotic usually administered with a penicillin antibiotic to treat infective endocarditis?

(a) It can be administered once daily

(b) It acts synergistically with the penicillin to enhance bacterial killing

(c) It provides Gram-negative cover

(d) Regular blood levels, which are routine with aminoglycosides, facilitate monitoring of responses to therapy

(e) These agents penentrate deep in to endocardial and myocardial tissue

15. What is the most likely explanation for a false-negative tuberculous skin test, e.g. Mantoux, Heaf?

(a) Patient on antituberculous treatment

(b) Overwhelming infection with tuberculosis, e.g. miliary tuberculosis

(c) Previously treated tuberculosis over 10 years ago

(d) Concurrent lobar pneumonia

(e) Previously received BCG

16. After contact with a patient with 'open' or infectious tuberculosis, chemoprophylaxis is most likely to be administered to which one of the following?

(a) Elderly females

(b) Patients with asthma

(c) Neonates

(d) Patients who have not received BCG

(e) Patients who have recently had a myocardial infaction

17. A skin test may be useful in the diagnosis of which infection?

(a) Legionellosis

(b) Infectious mononucleosis

(c) Toxoplasmosis

(d) Histoplasmosis

(e) *Pneumocystis carinii* pneumonia

18. Which of these is a well recognized complication of Q fever?

(a) Severe septic shock

(b) Infective endocarditis

(c) Brain abscess

(d) Severe coagulopathy

(e) Bronchiectasis

19. Which vaccine is most specifically recommended following splenectomy?

(a) *Haemophilus influenzae* type b

(b) Hepatitis B

(c) Tetanus

(d) Hepatitis A

(e) Combined mumps, measles, and rubella (MMR)

20. Which antibiotic, when used in combination, is useful in the treatment of bone and joint infection caused by staphylococci?

(a) Erythromycin

(b) Fusidic acid

(c) Gentamicin

(d) Mupirocin

(e) Metronidazole

CHAPTER 7

Pregnancy and the neonate

SECTION 7
Pregnancy and the neonate

Case 58 Irritability, feeding difficulties, and hypoxia in Sarah just after birth

After a 3-day pyrexial illness in her mother, Sarah is born by vaginal delivery at 30 weeks and weighs 1.8 kg. She is transferred to the special care baby unit (SCBU) for observation, but on day 4 she becomes irritable, difficult to feed, and hypoxic, requiring intubation and ventilation. Biochemical investigations exclude a metabolic cause such as hypoglycaemia, and there is no clinical or other evidence of congenital abnormality or intraventricular haemorrhage.

Q What microbiological investigations should be carried out to exclude infection?

A Non-specific signs such as those described are compatible with neonatal infection, and the presence of risk factors such as maternal pyrexia or prolonged rupture of membranes makes infection likely. A septic screen that includes two sets of blood cultures, cerebrospinal fluid (CSF), urine, and respiratory secretions for bacterial culture should therefore be carried out. A throat swab in viral transport medium, faeces, and CSF should also be sent for virological studies, as enteroviruses can cause severe neonatal infection.

Q How may neonatal bacterial infection be classified?

A Early-onset infection is defined as occurring during the first 3–4 days of life and is usually caused by pathogens acquired during passage down the birth canal, during traumatic delivery, or immediately following a Caesarean section. Late-onset infection presents 5 days after delivery or later, and is usually due to pathogens acquired from the mother, staff, or occasionally from inadequately cleaned or decontaminated equipment. The most frequently implicated bacteria are listed in Table 58.1.

Blood cultures, urine, CSF, and respiratory secretions are taken and sent to the microbiology laboratory. Sarah is started on intravenous (IV) penicillin and gentamicin to cover streptococcal and Gram-negative infection pending the results of investigations. The following day it is reported that Gram-positive bacilli are seen in a Gram film from all of the blood culture bottles.

Q What is the most likely pathogen?

A Significant bacteraemia and not contamination is likely, as all the bottles are positive (see Case 47). The Gram film findings in the setting of a premature neonate with systemic infection is very suggestive of listeriosis (infection caused by *L. monocytogenes*; see Table 58.2 and Fig. 58.1), but the subsequent culture results will exclude infection due to other Gram-positive bacilli such as *Clostridium* spp. or *Bacillus* spp.

Q What are the clinical features of listeriosis associated with pregnancy?

Table 58.1 Bacterial pathogens important in the neonate

Neonatal bacterial pathogen	Special features
β-haemolytic streptococci group B (*S. agalactiae*) (see also Case 5)	Usually acquired from mother's vagina and accounts for 43% of early-onset neonatal sepsis, including bacteraemia, meningitis (see Case 41), and pneumonia
Coliforms, including *E. coli*	Similar spectrum of disease to that of group B streptococci. Outbreaks of multiresistant *Klebsiella pneumoniae* in neonatal units occasionally occur
Listeria monocytogenes	Recognized cause of serious infection in the neonate and mother
Pseudomonas spp.	*P. aeruginosa* (see Case 22) causes ventilator-associated pneumonia, and other species are implicated in the premature neonate
Staphylococcus aureus	May cause localized (skin pustules, conjunctivitis, infected umbilical cord) or systemic (bacteraemia, pneumonia, osteomyelitis) infection and the scalded skin syndrome (see Case 9)
Staphylococcus epidermidis	Intravascular catheter-associated bacteraemia (see Case 35) and, occasionally, meningitis if congenital abnormality present or if CSF shunt required later
Neisseria gonorrhoeae	Ophthalmia neonatorum (conjunctivitis) from mother (see Case 61)
Chlamydia trachomatis	Inclusion conjunctivitis during first week and pneumonia in second to third weeks of life (see Case 61)

Table 58.2 *Listeria monocytogenes*

- Short Gram-positive bacilli with tumbling motility at 25°C, slightly haemolytic on blood agar. There are at least six other species, e.g. *L. ivanovii*, but these are rarely implicated in human disease
- Transmission (see Fig. 58.1) is by ingestion of contaminated foodstuffs (see Case 23 and Fig. 58.2), mother to baby, or contact with, for example, resuscitation equipment
- A haemolysin, listeriolysin O, is a potential virulence factor but, in non-pregnant patients, impaired cell-mediated immunity (such as also occurs in patients with lymphoma or diabetes mellitus) is a more important predisposing factor to infection

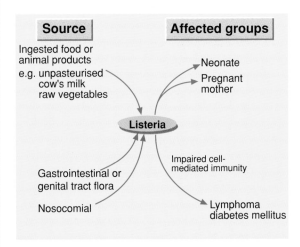

Fig. 58.1 Sources of and at-risk patients for listeriosis.

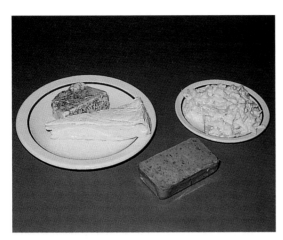

Fig. 58.2 Foods (soft cheese, coleslaw, paté) associated with listeriosis.

A Four clinical syndromes are described:

- abortion: maternal flu-like illness during the last 4–5 months of the pregnancy, with loss of the fetus

- maternal infection: flu-like illness just before delivery, with rigors, myalgia, and pharyngitis. Early-onset infection in the neonate may follow

- early-onset neonatal infection: intrauterine acquisition of listeria due to haematogenous spread to the placenta. May present acutely with pneumonia, bacteraemia, diarrhoea, and meningitis or, occasionally, subclinically

- late-onset neonatal infection: acquired during passage down the birth canal, especially in premature babies, or may be acquired from a nosocomial source. Presents from the fourth to fifth day onwards with meningitis and bacteraemia. Mother is usually well

The IV penicillin is changed to ampicillin, the gentamicin continued (believed to act synergistically with the ampicillin), and serum assays of gentamicin are carried out every other day. *L. monocytogenes* is isolated from blood cultures but the CSF is sterile. Sarah gradually improves over the next 3 days, is discharged from the SCBU after a further 4 days, and ultimately goes home to be followed up in the community and at the paediatric outpatients.

Q Is *L. monocytogenes* part of the normal flora of the pregnant woman?

A Yes. Listeria may be detected in the faeces of 30–40% of pregnant women (and many non-pregnant individuals), but is often intermittent or transient.

Q Does maternal carriage predict the development of listeriosis?

A No. Asymptomatic rather than symptomatic carriage is the norm, and systemic maternal infection may not be associated with a positive faeces sample. Isolation from blood cultures or CSF is the only reliable means of diagnosing maternal and neonatal listeriosis, but amniotic fluid or placenta should be cultured when abortions occur, or when listeria infection is suspected at delivery. Reliable serological tests are not available to diagnose listeriosis.

Q Which is more common, sporadic infection due to *L. monocytogenes* or clusters of cases/epidemic infection?

A Most cases are sporadic and no source is usually ever identified. It is true, however, that there was an increase in cases, approaching epidemic proportions, during the late 1980s in the UK, which may have been related to the increased consumption of contaminated foods such as soft cheeses and paté (see Fig. 58.2). Localized outbreaks have also been described associated with animals (e.g. sheep) and in hospitals where transmission has occurred via hand contact with contaminated equipment (e.g. thermometers).

Q Is listeriosis associated with recurrent abortions?

A This is a controversial point. A study conducted in the 1960s suggested that listeriosis caused recurrent abortions in some women, but this has not been confirmed in further clinical studies. If listeriosis is a cause, experience suggests that it is quite uncommon and accounts for a very small proportion of recurrent abortions.

Q What advice should be given to pregnant women about avoiding infection due to *L. monocytogenes*?

A Pregnant women and immunocompromised patients at risk should avoid certain foods, e.g. soft ripened cheeses (brie, camembert), all types of paté, cooked–chilled meals, and ready-to-eat poultry unless thoroughly reheated. Patients should also be advised about good hygiene in the storage and preparation of foods, such as keeping food for as short a time as possible, ensuring the refrigerator is working properly, storing cooked foods separately from raw foods, discarding left-over reheated food, and, finally, observing the reheating and standing times when using a microwave oven.

Résumé for undergraduate students

Listeriosis, which is caused by *Listeria monocytogenes*, an opportunist pathogen, is not common but remains an important cause of meningitis in the immunocompromised patient, e.g. patient with Hodgkin's lymphoma, and meningitis/blood-stream infection in the neonate and pregnant mother. Ampicillin needs to be added to the empirical treatment of the above conditions if listeriosis is likely and those at risk need to be advised to avoid foodstuffs that pose a risk such as soft cheeses.

Summary: Listeriosis

Presentation

Unexplained fever or meningitis in a pregnant woman, neonate, or immunocompromised patient

Diagnosis

Isolation of *L. monocytogenes* from blood, CSF, or birth products

Management

Avoidance of at-risk foods such as soft cheeses. Ampicillin with gentamicin is the treatment of choice

Case 59 Deborah, 23 years old and 12 weeks pregnant, develops a rash

Deborah, 23 years old and 12 weeks pregnant, presents to the antenatal clinic with a 1-day history of fever and a diffuse erythematous rash on the face and trunk (see Fig. 59.1). She has also noticed some swelling of her wrists.

Q Which infectious diseases need to be considered in the differential diagnosis?

A Whilst there are a number of non-infectious causes of a rash and arthralgia (e.g. a connective tissue disorder such as systemic lupus erythematosus, a drug, or other allergy), the important diagnoses to confirm or refute in this case are acute rubella virus and acute parvovirus B19 infections.

Deborah gives a history of rubella vaccination as a teenager. This is her first pregnancy. She remembers looking after her neighbour's son 2–3 weeks ago, the day before he developed a rash. On examination, Deborah's rash is maculo-

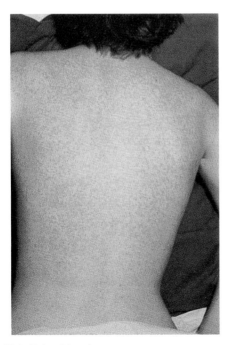

Fig. 59.1 Deborah's rash.

papular, most noticeable on the face but also present on the trunk. There is no lymphadenopathy. There is bilateral swelling and tenderness of the carpal and metacarpal joints.

Q What investigations should be carried out?

A Rubella and parvovirus serology. The history of rubella vaccination is *not* sufficient to rule out a diagnosis of acute primary rubella infection. A percentage of individuals may not respond to the vaccine, or vaccine may have been incorrectly stored, resulting in vaccine failure, with the patient remaining susceptible to rubella. Although there may be features in an individual case more suggestive of parvovirus than rubella infection or vice versa (e.g. the parvovirus rash characteristically waxes and wanes, cervical adenopathy is more likely in rubella), a clinical diagnosis cannot be relied upon, and thus both serologies should be performed.

Q For each of the following rubella serology results (1)–(4), assign the most appropriate interpretation (a)–(c).

1. Rubella IgG negative, IgM negative
2. Rubella IgG negative, IgM positive
3. Rubella IgG positive (>50 IU/ml), IgM positive
4. Rubella IgG positive (>50 IU/ml), IgM negative
   (a) Evidence of rubella infection in the past
   (b) No evidence of rubella infection at any time
   (c) Evidence of recent rubella infection

A Correct interpretation of these results requires an understanding of the differences between IgG and IgM immune responses. Figure 59.2 shows the evolution of an immune response following infection with a virus. As can be seen, the IgM response appears marginally sooner than the IgG, but is only transient, whereas the IgG response persists, usually for life.

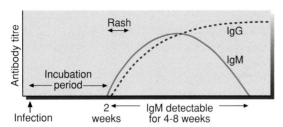

Fig. 59.2 Antibody response in primary rubella infection.

Thus, the correct answers are:

1. Rubella IgG negative, IgM negative. (b) No evidence of rubella infection at any time. Note that, if this is the result from Deborah's serum, then the laboratory will also add a comment along the lines of 'Please send repeat sample in 5 days time.'

Explanation. Despite her history of rubella vaccination, Deborah's serum contains no rubella-specific IgG. She is therefore not immune to rubella and is susceptible to infection. Note that antibody may not appear until a day or two *after* the rash, so it is still possible that Deborah is suffering an acute rubella infection. To resolve this, a repeat serum sample, taken 5 days or later after appearance of the rash, must be tested. If that serum is also seronegative, then Deborah's current illness is not rubella. She should be advised to have rubella vaccination post-partum.

2. Rubella IgG negative, IgM positive. (c) Evidence of recent rubella infection. The lab report on Deborah's serum would therefore say 'Suggests acute rubella. Please send second sample for confirmation.'

Explanation. The IgM response appears slightly earlier than IgG, and therefore this combination of results is possible, if somewhat unusual. The implication is that the patient is suffering an attack of acute rubella. However, given the significance of that diagnosis in a pregnant woman (see below), and the ever-present possibility of laboratory error, this must be confirmed by testing a repeat sample taken a few days later, demonstrating continued presence of the IgM and IgG seroconversion. Some laboratories may only report the negative IgG

result on the first specimen, deferring the IgM testing until a second sample is available.

3. Rubella IgG positive (>50 IU/ml), IgM positive. (c) Evidence of recent rubella infection. The lab report would read 'These results strongly suggest acute rubella infection. Please send second sample for confirmation.'

Explanation. For reasons given in 2, it is wise to seek a repeat sample, which may enable demonstration of a rising IgG titre, and will allay any doubts over possible laboratory errors.

4. Rubella IgG positive (>50 IU/ml), IgM negative. (a) Evidence of rubella infection in the past

Explanation. As there is no IgM present, Deborah has not suffered a recent attack of rubella. The presence of IgG indicates that she has been exposed to this virus in the past, either the wild-type or vaccine (or both). This IgG further indicates that she is immune to rubella. Some laboratories would still ask for a second sample, just to confirm this.

Q Why is the diagnosis of maternal rubella infection in pregnancy so important?

A Rubella virus may cross the placenta and infect the developing fetus, resulting in the congenital rubella syndrome.

Q What are the main features of the congenital rubella syndrome?

A A wide range of abnormalities have been reported. The common ones include:

- general: growth retardation
- cardiac: patent ductus, pulmonary artery stenosis
- eye: cataract, retinopathy, microphthalmia
- ear: sensorineural deafness
- central nervous system (CNS): encephalitis, mental retardation

Q In a pregnant woman with rubella, what single factor influences the risk of development and the severity of the congenital rubella syndrome?

A The *stage in pregnancy* at which the rubella infection is acquired. Thus, the risk of congenital rubella syndrome from maternal infection in the first few weeks of pregnancy is almost 100%, whilst maternal rubella in the third trimester carries no risk.

Gestation	Risk	Clinical features
0–8 weeks	90–100%	Multiple defects, cardiac/eye/CNS
8–12 weeks	80–90%	Multiple defects, cardiac/eye/CNS
12–18 weeks	Declining to 0%	Deafness, mental retardation
> 18 weeks	Rare (<1%)	Deafness

Q How may rubella be prevented?

A By use of a live attenuated vaccine. In 1988, the UK changed from a strategy of vaccinating only women of childbearing age to that of universal vaccination in the second year of life (in combination with measles and mumps; MMR). This has the advantage of interrupting the circulation of rubella virus in the community, rubella being predominantly a disease of childhood, and therefore dramatically reducing the risk of a susceptible pregnant woman coming into contact with rubella.

Q If Deborah's serology had indicated a recent rubella infection, how would you manage her?

A The only alternatives for Deborah are to continue with the pregnancy, with the attendant risk of her baby having the congenital rubella syndrome, or to have a termination. The management of a case of acute rubella in a pregnant woman thus involves informed discussion with the patient and her partner as to the risk and likely consequences of fetal infection, before a decision whether or not to continue with the pregnancy is made.

Q How would your management of Deborah differ if she had presented with only a history of contact with a rash, being herself completely asymptomatic?

A This is, in fact, a considerably more common clinical scenario—a pregnant woman giving a history of contact. Once again, rubella serology should be requested. The principles of interpretation of the results are similar to those in the case illustrated above, but the time-scale of sampling may differ. For instance, for a patient found to be seronegative on first sampling, a repeat sample taken 4 weeks after exposure would be requested. Whilst the incubation period between infection and production of antibodies is usually 2–3 weeks (see Fig. 59.2), in rare instances, this may be delayed as long as 4 weeks.

In fact, the following results are received on Deborah's serum: rubella IgG-positive, IgM-negative; parvovirus B19 IgM-positive; parvovirus B19 DNA-positive

Q How do you interpret these results?

A The rubella results indicate that Deborah is immune to rubella. The presence of IgM directed against parvovirus B19 indicates a recent infection with this virus. This is confirmed by the finding of parvovirus B19 DNA. Through the use of MMR, rubella virus infection in pregnancy is now very uncommon in the UK, and a pregnant woman with a rash is far more likely to have an acute parvovirus infection, as is the case here.

Q What are the clinical manifestations of acute parvovirus B19 infection?

A Most infections are asymptomatic, but a variety of syndromes may follow acute infection:

- in children, infection may result in the slapped cheek syndrome, also known as fifth disease or erythema infectiosum (see Fig. 59.3)

- in adults, a non-specific maculopapular rash may arise and, most often in females, there may be painful (arthralgia) or frankly swollen (arthritis) joints. The joint manifestations can be polyarticular and severe, mimicking early rheumatoid arthritis. Parvovirus arthritis is self-limiting, but may take months to resolve

- in patients with underlying chronic haemolytic anaemia, parvovirus infection can result in an aplastic crisis and, in immunosuppressed patients, chronic infection with associated chronic marrow suppression may occur. The pathogenesis of these complications is

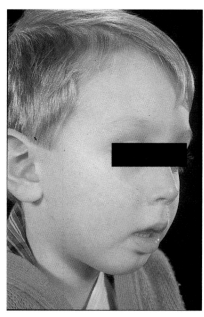

Fig. 59.3 A child with erythema infectiosum, showing the typical malar redness.

discussed for postgraduates in more detail in Case 67

The consequences of parvovirus infection in pregnancy are discussed below.

Q What effects may parvovirus B19 infection have in pregnancy?

A Although maternal parvovirus infection may be clinically indistinguishable from rubella (both may present with a rash with or without lymphadenopathy; both viruses are arthritogenic, especially in adult females) and both viruses may cross the placenta and infect the fetus, the consequences to the fetus are very different. Parvovirus B19 infects bone marrow precursor cells (see Case 67), resulting in a temporary cessation of marrow production. Maternal infection in the first 20 weeks of pregnancy is associated with:

- an increased risk of spontaneous termination of the pregnancy

- if the maternal infection occurs between 9 and 20 weeks, then fetal heart failure secondary to parvovirus-induced fetal anaemia may result in presentation with hydrops fetalis

- there are no reports of congenital malformations in babies from those pregnancies that survive

Women who are more than 20 weeks pregnant when they acquire parvovirus infection can be reassured that the likelihood of any adverse events arising from this are extremely small.

For those students still confused by the various combinations of results given in this case, the essential messages are that, if a pregnant woman reports contact with a rash, or develops a rash herself, then you *must* consider the possibilities of acute rubella or parvovirus infections. It is always advisable to send an initial serum sample, together with clear clinical details to ensure that the laboratory will perform the most appropriate tests. Repeat testing is also often required. If in any doubt, discuss the interpretation of results and management with the local virologist or microbiologist!

Summary: Rash in pregnancy

Diagnoses
To exclude: rubella, parvovirus infection

Investigations
One or more serum samples for rubella and parvovirus serology

Complications
Congenital rubella syndrome: risk depends on stage of pregnancy; parvovirus: risk of miscarriage or hydrops fetalis

Prevention
Rubella vaccination; no vaccine for parvovirus

Case 60 **Kate, a 23-year-old pregnant physiotherapist**

Kate, a 23-year-old physiotherapist, arrives at the antenatal clinic, 12 weeks into her first pregnancy. During this routine consultation, the midwife explains to Kate that she will need to give a blood sample for some routine tests.

Q What blood tests should be performed on all antenatal women?

A Apart from standard haematological tests—full blood count, blood group—all antenatal women in the UK should be screened for rubella, syphilis, hepatitis B virus (HBV), and human immuno-deficiency virus (HIV) status.

Q What kind of syphilis test is performed on antenatal sera, and why?

A An enzyme-linked immunosorbent assay (ELISA) test for antibodies against *T. pallidum*. The purpose is to identify women who may have active syphilis. Infection can be passed from mother to baby, resulting in congenital syphilis. This is preventable by identifying infected mothers and treating appropriately with penicillin.

Q What kind of rubella test is performed on antenatal sera, and why?

A The test detects IgG antibody against rubella virus, i.e. a marker of past infection or vaccination, which will provide immunity should there be any subsequent exposure to the virus during the pregnancy. With the use of rubella vaccine, initially for all girls aged 11 and over and, since 1988, as part of the MMR vaccine administered to all 12–18 month old children, the vast majority of women of child-bearing age in the UK are rubella-immune and, indeed, rubella itself is a very rare disease. The biggest risk group is now immigrant women who come from countries where rubella vaccination is not routine, and who may have been exposed to infection in their own country early in pregnancy. For women who are found to be antibody-negative, efforts should be made to ad-minister rubella vaccine in the post-partum period, such that they will be immune in future pregnancies. The consequences of rubella infection during pregnancy are discussed in Case 59.

Q What kind of hepatitis B test is performed on antenatal sera, and why?

A The test is for hepatitis B virus surface antigen (HBsAg; see Case 28). Women who are chronic carriers of HBV (and therefore HBsAg-positive) may pass infection on to their babies—on a worldwide basis, such vertical transmission is by far the most important route of spread of HBV. By taking appropriate action (discussed below), vertical transmission of HBV is largely preventable.

Q What are the possible consequences, should a neonate acquire HBV infection from his/her mother?

A Neonates exposed to HBV are far more likely to become chronically infected themselves than are older children or adults. This is because of the immature state of the neonatal immune system, which cannot mount a sufficient response to eliminate the infection.

The potential consequences of chronic infection in a neonate are essentially the same as for an adult who becomes chronically infected (i.e. chronic inflammatory hepatitis, cirrhosis, and hepatocellular carcinoma; see Fig. 28.3, Case 28). However, there are two important consequences of chronic infection that apply particularly to neonates. Firstly, the result of chronic infection of baby girls is that, when they become of child-bearing age, they stand a high chance of passing their infection on to their offspring, who in turn will become chronically infected. Such generation-to-generation transmission of HBV is an extremely efficient way for the virus to maintain itself within a population and, in countries where vertical transmission is the major mode of spread, over 20% of the population may be HBV carriers. Secondly, the young age of infection (i.e. day 1) means that the long-term, life-threatening complications of infection will appear in individuals aged around 20–30 years old. This imposes major health and economic burdens in those countries where vertical transmission is common, as people are struck down at what should be the most productive period of their lives. Thus, prevention of vertical transmission of HBV is a highly desirable intervention.

It transpires that Kate is HBsAg-positive. She believes one of her earlier sexual partners was a drug addict, but he is unavailable for testing and there is no history of any other risk factors for HBV infection.

Q What further action should now be taken?

A There are a number of issues to be considered: the effect of HBV infection on Kate herself; the possibility of vertical transmission; the possibility of transmission of infection to other close contacts, particularly her husband.

All women, discovered by antenatal screening to be infected with HBV, should be referred to an appropriate specialist for further investigation. This should include follow-up and testing of all sexual and family contacts. Sexual partners and children who have not already been infected with HBV should be offered vaccination.

Q What further tests should be performed on Kate?

A A repeat sample should be sent to the laboratory to confirm her HBsAg positivity, and to determine her HBeAg/anti-HBe status (see Case 28 for explanation of e/anti-e markers). The 'e' status of carrier mothers is a major determinant of the risk of vertical transmission. Babies of HBeAg-positive mothers have about a 90% chance of infection, compared to only 25–30% for babies of anti-HBe-positive mothers.

Q What action can be taken to reduce the risk of HBV infection of Kate's baby?

A Two interventions have been proven, in large-scale clinical trials, to reduce vertical transmission

of HBV—passive immunization of the neonate (i.e. a single dose of hepatitis B immunoglobulin given as soon as possible after birth) and active immunization (the first dose given as soon as possible after birth, followed by doses at 1, 2, and 12 months of age). Passive immunization alone reduces the risk of transmission by about 70%; active immunization alone reduces the risk of transmission by about 70%. Combined passive/active immunisation reduces the risk of transmission by around 90%.

Thus, ideally, babies of HBV carrier mothers should be given a dose of HBIg in one thigh, and the first dose of HBV vaccine in the other thigh, as soon as possible after birth (and definitely within 48 hours). However, HBIg is in fairly short supply, and current UK policy is therefore designed to offer this only to those babies at highest risk of infection, i.e. those whose mothers who are anti-HBe-negative. Hence the need to assess Kate's e/anti-e status.

Kate, also shown to be HBeAg positive, delivers a healthy baby girl. HBIg and vaccine are administered by the hospital midwives, and mother and baby go home 2 days later.

Q Is there anything further to be done?

A Yes. It may seem obvious, but steps must be taken to ensure that Kate's baby receives the follow-up doses of HBV vaccine. Several audits of the management of such babies in the late 1990s showed that an alarming number failed to receive all the recommended doses. There are many potential reasons for this. Many babies are from ethnic minority groups, for whom English is not their first language, and those mothers may not understand the need to take their babies for further injections. There needs to be excellent communication between the hospital-based care team and the family's primary care team, with specific designation of responsibility for achieving subsequent vaccination doses.

Q Should Kate be discouraged from breast-feeding her baby?

A No. Breast-feeding does not increase the risk of mother-to-baby transmission of HBV and, from a virological viewpoint, HBV infection is not a contraindication to breast-feeding.

Q What kind of HIV test is performed on antenatal sera, and why?

A The test is for the presence of anti-HIV. Although antibodies are only a marker of past infection, the fact that anyone who has ever been infected with HIV is always infected with HIV (i.e. the clearance rate of infection is 0%) means that the presence of anti-HIV indicates current infection with the virus. The reason for antenatal anti-HIV screening is in order to identify pregnancies where there is a risk of vertical transmission of HIV, so that appropriate measures may be taken to reduce that risk (see below).

Q What are the possible routes of infection of a fetus/neonate with HIV?

A Theoretically, for any virus that exists in the maternal bloodstream, there are three potential times and routes of transmission:

- antenatally—through transplacental spread
- perinatally—through exposure to an infected birth canal and/or maternal blood at the time of birth
- postnatally—through infected breast-milk

For HIV, whilst transmission through all three routes is possible, it is believed that most babies become infected perinatally.

Q If no intervention is offered, what are the chances of the baby of an HIV-infected mother becoming infected?

A Overall, about 15–25% of babies of HIV-infected mothers acquire infection.

Q What factors influence the rate of vertical transmission of HIV?

A The risk is dependent on the stage of HIV infection in the mother. The lower the maternal CD4 count, and the higher the maternal viral load, then the greater the risk of transmission. Thus, although an overall rate is quoted above, this does vary significantly in different countries—in Africa the rate is of the order of 25%; in Europe, it is much closer to 15%.

Q What possible interventions are there to reduce the risk of HIV infection of babies of carrier mothers?

A The interventions most likely to influence vertical HIV transmission are:

- antiretroviral therapy of the mother
- antiretroviral therapy of the baby
- delivery by Caesarean section
- avoidance of breast-feeding

The use of antiretroviral drugs in pregnancy is complicated. All drugs have a potential for toxic side-effects, and this worry is compounded in pregnancy by the possibility of fetal damage. Management of antiretroviral therapy in pregnancy should therefore be supervised by a physician/obstetrician with appropriate experience. The British HIV Association (BHIVA) regularly publish up-to-date extensive recommendations on this topic.

The beneficial effects of Caesarean section (CS) are dependent on this being undertaken as a planned elective procedure—i.e. it is not sufficient to allow an HIV-infected woman to go into labour and then perform the CS.

HIV is excreted in breast milk and, overall, breast-feeding just about doubles the risk of vertical transmission. In developed countries, recommendation to avoid breast-feeding is not controversial, as there are safe and effective alternatives. However, in other countries, this is not a straightforward issue. Denial of the benefits of breast milk may carry a greater risk to the baby than that of acquiring HIV infection.

With active management of HIV-infected pregnancies, neonatal HIV infection is almost an entirely preventable disease—large studies in the USA have reported infection rates of < 1% with the use of antiretroviral therapy, elective CS, and non-breast-feeding.

Q Should the babies of HIV-carrier mothers be tested for the presence of anti-HIV in a peripheral blood sample taken shortly after birth?

A No, this will not be helpful in determining whether or not an individual baby has acquired

HIV infection from his/her mother, as maternal antibodies will have crossed the placenta. Thus, the presence of anti-HIV at or near birth in the neonate is not evidence of infection.

Q How, therefore, would you determine whether the baby of an HIV-carrier mother had acquired HIV infection or not?

A You would test for the presence of virus itself in the baby's blood. This is done using very sensitive genome amplification assays. It is recommended that such babies are tested at 0, 1, 3, and 6 months after birth to confirm the presence or absence of HIV infection. Serological diagnosis of infection can only be made routinely by demonstrating the persistence of anti-HIV antibodies after 18 months of age.

Q What is the risk of mother infected with hepatitis C virus (HCV) passing this infection on to her baby?

A Most studies have indicated a transmission rate of around 5%. The risk is higher in mothers who are co-infected with HIV, presumably because the HCV viral load in such individuals is much higher.

Q Why, then, is a test for HCV infection not included in the routine battery of tests performed on antenatal sera?

A Because at present there is no proven intervention that will affect the basal rate of transmission.

Thus, if no action can be taken as a result of performing a test, there is no rationale for performing the test in the first place.

Q Should HCV-infected mothers be discouraged from breast-feeding?

A No. There are ample data to demonstrate that the risk of neonatal HCV infection is not affected by breast-feeding, unless the mother is co-infected with HIV, in which case she will already have been discouraged from breast-feeding because of the risk of HIV transmission.

Summary: Blood-borne viruses in pregnancy

Diagnosis

All antenatal sera should be screened for HBsAg and anti-HIV, but not anti-HCV

Management

- HBV-infected mother. Assess HBeAg/anti-HBe status of mother. Prophylaxis to baby consists of vaccine ± HBIg. Follow up mother, family, and sexual contacts—vaccinate as necessary

- HIV-infected mother. Antiretroviral therapy to mother and baby; deliver by elective Caesarean section; avoid breast-feeding

- HCV-infected mother. No intervention

Case 61 A sticky eye in Daniel, 5 days old

You are called to the postnatal ward to see baby Daniel. Daniel was born 6 days ago, by vaginal delivery after an uneventful labour, and discharged from hospital 48 hours later. His Apgar scores were 9 at one minute and 10 at 5 minutes. His mother, Susan, has brought him back to the postnatal ward, as she has noticed that his left eye is red and swollen and he is not opening it. He has been breast-feeding without difficulty, and is otherwise well. On examination, his left eye is indeed swollen (see Fig. 61.1), with beads of thin yellowish liquid exuding on to his cheek. On pulling apart the eyelids, there is a thin film of whitish exudate over the cornea and the conjunctivae are reddened. The right eye shows similar, but less marked changes. There are no other abnormal physical signs.

Q What is the clinical diagnosis?

A The signs are those of acute conjunctivitis. In a young baby this condition is known as ophthalmia neonatorum.

Q What are the common causes of ophthalmia neonatorum?

A These are:

1. Infection (see Table 61.1)

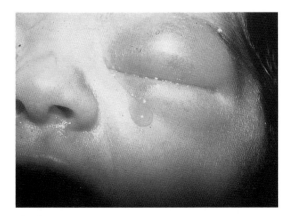

Fig. 61.1 Daniel's eye.

Table 61.1 Infectious causes of ophthalmia neonatorum
Chlamydia trachomatis
• Strains D–K (i.e. the same strains as those responsible for genital infection)
• Onset 5–14 days after birth
• Follicular keratoconjunctivitis
Neisseria gonorrhoeae
• Onset on first or second day of life
• Severe purulent conjunctivitis
Staphylococcus aureus
• Onset 5–10 days after birth
• Known as 'sticky eye'
• May be associated with outbreak of staphylococcal sepsis on maternity ward
Other causes include *Streptococcus pneumoniae*, *Haemophilus influenzae*, herpes simplex virus

2. Chemical irritation. This was common when it was standard practice to use ocular silver nitrate prophylaxis against *N. gonorrhoeae*, but such prophylaxis is not indicated today. The disease was self-limiting, occurring within the first 24 hours and lasting 1 or 2 days

Q What investigations should be performed?

A A conjunctival smear should be Gram-stained. In acute bacterial conjunctivitis, large numbers of neutrophils are seen. Bacteria may be present within or outside leucocytes. Gonococci may be seen as intracellular Gram-negative diplococci. One smear should be stained for chlamydial basophilic intracytoplasmic inclusion bodies in epithelial cells (using Giemsa, or fluorescent antibody stains). Swabs should be taken for culture of *C. trachomatis*, *N. gonorrhoeae*, other bacteria, and herpes simplex virus (HSV). Note that each swab must be placed in an appropriate transport medium (e.g. Amies charcoal for *N. gonorrhoeae*, chlamydial and viral transport medium for *C. trachomatis* and HSV, respectively) before transport to the laboratory. A more modern approach to diagnosis is via genome detection using molecular amplification techniques, which have the advantage of being relatively rapid and not requiring viable organisms to reach the laboratory.

Q What is the treatment of choice?

A Definitive treatment will depend on the results of the above investigations, but the most likely diagnosis in a 6 day-old baby with follicular conjunctivitis is chlamydia infection, and presumptive therapy with oral erythromycin should be started after collection of the swab. Systemic tetracycline should never be administered to an infant or child because of its effect on teeth and bones. Thus, systemic erythromycin is preferred for severe infection, and also to prevent the development of chlamydia pneumonia. Suspected gonococcal conjunctivitis must also be treated promptly with systemic benzylpenicillin or a suitable alternative (e.g. a cephalosporin) if penicillin-resistant strains are present, as corneal ulceration and perforation may occur. Chloramphenicol ointment for the treatment of other bacteria is appropriate only if chlamydia and gonorrhoeal infections have been ruled out.

Q Should any further investigations be performed?

A Yes. The pathogenesis of gonococcal and chlamydial ophthalmia neonatorum involves acquisition of the relevant organism during passage of the baby through the birth canal. If either of these organisms is confirmed in Daniel's eye, then his mother should be counselled, screened, and treated appropriately, as should her sexual contacts (see Case 36).

Q What other eye disease is caused by *C. trachomatis*?

A Trachoma is caused by *C. trachomatis* strains A–C. This is endemic in Africa and the Middle East. Organisms are spread between patients by hands, leading to a chronic follicular keratoconjunctivitis. In overcrowded and unhygienic conditions, secondary bacterial infection is a common complication. Scarring of the cornea occurs, leading to blindness, of which trachoma is the most common infectious cause in the world.

Résumé for undergraduates

Ophthalmia neonatorum (sticky eye in a neonate) is most probably caused by infection with *Neisseria gonorrhoeae*, *Chlaymdia trachomatis*, or *Staphylococcus aureus*. A conjunctival smear should be Gram-stained, and appropriate therapy commenced (e.g. systemic benzylpenicillin for *N. gonorrhoeae*, oral erythromycin for *C. trachomatis*). Appropriate testing of the baby's mother and her contact(s) should be instituted if either of these two organisms is identified as the cause.

Summary: Ophthalmia neonatorum

Presentation
Acute purulent conjunctivitis within 14 days of birth

Pathogenesis
Acquisition of *N. gonorrhoeae*, or *C. trachomatis* infection on passage through birth canal; nosocomial acquisition of *S. aureus* on maternity ward

Management
Identification of causative organism by appropriately stained smears and culture; prompt topical or systemic antibiotics; treatment of mother and her sexual contacts for chlamydial infection, gonorrhoea

Case 62 Lily, 12 weeks pregnant, whose son has developed chickenpox

Lily, a 30-year-old mother of two, attends your surgery because her 8-year-old son has chickenpox (see Case 7). She mentions that she is 12 weeks pregnant.

Q Is this situation of concern?

A Yes. You have a pregnant woman who has been exposed to chickenpox. If Lily is susceptible to varicella-zoster virus (VZV) infection, then she may herself suffer an attack of chickenpox during this pregnancy, which may have consequences for herself and her fetus.

Q What are the complications of chickenpox in pregnancy?

A There are possible adverse effects for both *the mother*:

- chickenpox pneumonia. This, the most common life-threatening complication of primary VZV infection, is more likely to occur in an adult than in a child, and is also more likely in a pregnant, rather than a non-pregnant woman, with an incidence in some studies as high as 10%

and for *her baby*:

- congenital varicella syndrome (see Fig. 62.1, Box 62.1). This rare complication arises in

> ### Box 62.1 The congenital varicella syndrome
>
> - Skin loss and scarring; usually unilateral, segmented
> - Hypoplasia of limb bud development; rudimentary digits
> - CNS: cortical, cerebellar atrophy; microcephaly
> - Eye: microphthalmia; chorioretinitis; cataracts
> - General: intrauterine growth retardation; psychomotor retardation

1–2% of cases of maternal chickenpox in the first 20 weeks of pregnancy. Virus crosses the placenta and infects the fetus.

- herpes zoster in infancy. If the maternal infection is after 20 weeks of pregnancy, then the only potential problem for the offspring is that he/she may develop herpes zoster in early childhood. This proves that virus can indeed cross the placenta.

- neonatal chickenpox. If the maternal infection occurs at the end of pregnancy, then there is a risk that the baby will be born before the mother has had time to mount an immune response and to transfer immunity, in the form of antibodies, across the placenta. The baby will therefore be at risk of developing neonatal chickenpox, which carries a high morbidity and mortality.

Q How should you manage Lily?

A You need to determine whether or not she is at risk of primary VZV infection.

Q How can you ascertain whether she is susceptible to VZV infection?

A The simplest method is to ask her—or her parents, if possible—whether she has ever had chickenpox. The features of chickenpox are sufficiently distinctive that a clinical diagnosis is usually correct, and therefore a past history of

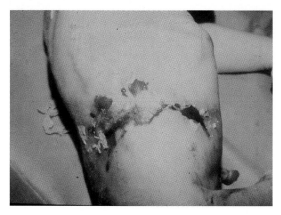

Fig. 62.1 Varicella embryopathy, unilateral skin scarring.

chickenpox correlates very well with the presence of antibodies to VZV. Thus, if the answer is 'yes', you can reassure Lily that she is immune from an attack of chickenpox, and no further action need be taken.

Q What if the answer is 'no' or 'don't know'?

A You should check her immune status by sending a serum sample to be tested for the presence or absence of anti-VZV antibodies. Of women *without* a personal history of chickenpox, 80% are nevertheless anti-VZV positive, and therefore immune.

Lily is not aware that she has had chickenpox in the past. You send a serum sample off for determination of her immune status to VZV, and the result is negative (i.e. no anti-VZV detected).

Q How do you proceed now?

A You would offer her varicella-zoster immune globulin (VZIg, given intramuscularly). This is an example of passive immunization—the VZIg will provide Lily with antibodies to VZV made by someone else. The reason for doing this is that, should she acquire infection from her known exposure, the VZIg will *attenuate* (but not prevent) the attack of chickenpox, thereby reducing the risk that she will suffer from chickenpox pneumonia. There is also evidence that VZIg reduces the risk of transplacental spread of virus, and hence of the congenital varicella syndrome. The VZIg needs to be administered within 10 days after the potential exposure to virus.

Q What is the management of a pregnant woman who has contact with someone with herpes zoster (i.e. shingles)?

A Although a patient with shingles excretes considerably less virus into his/her surroundings than a patient with chickenpox, he/she is still infectious—the vesicles contain virus in high titre. Consequently, the management is the same as for exposure to chickenpox, which is summarized in diagrammatic form in Fig. 62.2.

Milly, the next patient in your antenatal clinic, gives a history of a recent contact with a child with chickenpox (chickenpox is very common!). Unfortunately, she did not think to

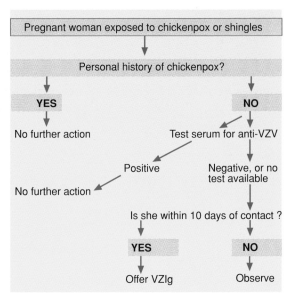

Fig. 62.2 Algorithm for management of exposure to VZV in pregnancy.

tell you about this at the time, and she now presents with a typical chickenpox rash. She is 37 weeks pregnant.

Q Is it worth offering her a dose of VZIg?

A No. VZIg given at this stage will have no effect on the course of her illness.

Q How should she be managed?

A The first worry is that she may develop chickenpox pneumonia. You would therefore observe her carefully over the next few days and, if there were any cause for concern, you would refer her to hospital for further investigation and treatment. Whilst aciclovir and its derivatives are not licensed for use in pregnancy, they may nevertheless be potentially life-saving drugs in this situation and, thus far, they have an excellent safety record.

Milly remains reasonably well, but 3 days after the onset of her rash she goes into labour, and delivers a healthy baby girl.

Q Is there anything to be concerned about in this situation?

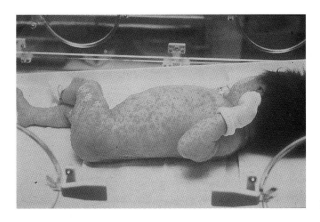

Fig. 62.3 Baby with neonatal varicella.

A Yes, very much so. You should be worried that Milly may have gone into labour before she has had time to pass on any protective antibodies to her fetus. Her baby has been potentially exposed to the virus *in utero* at the time of maternal viraemia (which occurs a couple of days before appearance of the rash) and will also be exposed to virus peri- and postnatally. In the absence of protective maternal antibodies, the baby would therefore be at considerable risk of neonatal varicella (see Fig. 62.3) which has a high mortality.

Q How long does it take for mothers with chickenpox to develop antibodies that can cross the placenta?

A Up to 7 days after onset of the maternal rash. Thus, all babies born 7 days (or later) after development of the maternal rash will have detectable anti-VZV in their serum, and are not at risk of life-threatening neonatal varicella. The risk period, therefore, is for babies born within 7 days of onset of the maternal rash, as these babies may be anti-VZV negative.

Q How would you manage Milly and her baby?

A Milly's baby should be given VZIg immediately after birth, once again with the intention of *attenuating* the severity of infection. Some authorities also recommend giving the baby prophylactic high-dose aciclovir orally in addition to VZIg. Separation of mother and baby at birth is not recommended, as there is no evidence that this reduces the risk of neonatal disease.

Note that the same rationale applies to mothers who develop chickenpox *after* their baby is born. By definition, they cannot have passed any protective immunity to their offspring, who are therefore at risk of acquiring infection. Babies up to the age of 30 days are at risk of developing chickenpox with the same high morbidity and mortality of neonatal chickenpox, and should at least be offered VZIg prophylaxis.

Tilly, a third patient in your antenatal clinic, gives a history of a painful blistering rash on one side of her trunk for the past 4 days. On examination, the rash has the typical appearance of herpes zoster. She is 16 weeks pregnant.

Q Is her fetus at any risk?

A No. Herpes zoster is the manifestation of secondary, or reactivated VZV infection. Tilly will therefore be anti-VZV positive, and antibodies will cross the placenta and protect her fetus. Also, in shingles, viraemia is very short-lived, thus reducing the chance of virus reaching and crossing the placenta.

Résumé for undergraduates

Maternal chickenpox in pregnancy is associated with an increased risk of varicella pneumonia. If in the first 20 weeks of pregnancy, the fetus may acquire the congenital varicella syndrome, characterized by skin scarring and impaired limb bud development. If the maternal infection is late in pregnancy, the baby may be at risk of neonatal varicella, and may therefore need varicella immunoglobulin (VZIg). Management of a pregnant woman in contact with chickenpox or shingles requires assessment of her immune status and possible use of VZIg.

Summary: Chickenpox in pregnancy

Risks

Maternal pneumonia; varicella embryopathy; neonatal chickenpox

Management

- Pregnant woman in contact with chickenpox or shingles. Check VZV immune status; if negative, offer VZIg

- Pregnant woman with chickenpox. Aciclovir for pneumonia; if within 7 days of labour, VZIg to neonate

Case 63 Mrs Fisher, 25 years old, pregnant, and with a history of genital herpes

Mrs Fisher thinks she may be pregnant for the first time. She is 25 years old. Her last menstrual period was 6 weeks ago, and a 'kit pregnancy test' from the chemist's was positive. She had an attack of genital herpes when she was 17, and she suffers from occasional recurrent attacks, about every 6 months. She has heard that this can be very dangerous for her baby and is therefore worried.

Q What is the serious complication of maternal genital herpes in pregnancy?

A Neonatal herpes simplex infection, arising from passage of the neonate through an infected birth canal.

Q Why is neonatal herpes such a feared disease?

A The clinical features of neonatal herpes simplex infection are listed in Table 63.1. Neonates are unable to control the spread of HSV infection, presumably owing to their immunological immaturity. Involvement of internal organs is common and life-threatening, and many of the survivors suffer long-term damage. The advent of potent antiviral agents, e.g. aciclovir, has not led to a significant improvement in mortality and morbidity, presumably because by the time antiviral therapy is instituted much of the damage has already been done.

Q By what routes may a neonate acquire HSV infection?

A The most obvious route is via passage through an infected maternal birth canal, and this does indeed account for about 90% of cases of neonatal herpes. However, the source of neonatal infection is not always the mother. A small minority of babies with neonatal herpes acquire their infection postnatally (rather than perinatally) from a non-maternal source, e.g. from being kissed by a father,

Table 63.1 Neonatal herpes simplex infection

- Incidence: UK, 1/70 000 births, USA, 1/10 000 births
- Presents around 8–12 days after delivery, with non-specific signs, e.g. poor feeding, weight loss, fever
- Infection is restricted to skin, mouth, or eyes in only 15–25% of cases
- Spread in the other 65–75% may involve multiple organs, e.g. liver, adrenals, brain, and may occur in the absence of skin lesions, making diagnosis difficult
- Mortality is 70–90% in disseminated disease
- Long-term morbidity includes severe developmental impairment

grandparent, or even, heaven forfend, a health-care worker, with a cold-sore.

Q What types of maternal genital herpes infection are there?

A HSV is a herpesvirus, and therefore exhibits latency. Thus, maternal infection may be primary or secondary (primary and secondary infections in relation to herpesviruses are explained in Case 4).

Q Which type of maternal infection carries the greatest risk of giving rise to neonatal herpes?

A Most babies with neonatal herpes acquire infection from mothers undergoing a primary genital HSV infection late in pregnancy. There are two likely reasons for this. Firstly, the amount of virus present in the genital tract will be vastly greater in a primary infection, where local spread may be extensive, as opposed to a recurrent infection, which is usually very localized. Secondly, mothers with recurrent infections will have antibodies that can cross the placenta, and there is evidence that this passive transfer of HSV-specific immunity is important in protecting the neonate from serious neonatal herpes.

Q Is genital HSV infection always symptomatic?

A No, in fact very much the opposite. The development of serological assays that can distinguish between antibodies to HSV-1 and -2 has demonstrated that many more people are anti-HSV-2-positive than give a history of genital herpes. Thus, although symptomatic primary genital HSV infection is a very dramatic and debilitating disease (see Case 37), the majority of primary genital HSV infections are asymptomatic. Furthermore, in patients with latent genital HSV infection, asymptomatic reactivation and excretion of virus occur much more frequently than does symptomatic recurrent disease.

Q In those babies with neonatal herpes acquired from their mothers, should you expect there to be a maternal history of genital herpes?

A No. Hopefully you answered this correctly having read the previous several questions. Most infected babies arise from mothers undergoing primary infection and so, by definition, they will not have a personal history of previous genital herpes. In addition, their primary attack is itself more likely than not to be asymptomatic.

Mrs Fisher has heard that she will have to have swabs taken at regular intervals towards the end of her pregnancy to see if she is having a recurrent attack, and that, if any of these swabs are positive, she will have to undergo a Caesarean section, rather than be allowed a normal delivery.

Q Is this statement true?

A No. This is an outdated strategy devised before the natural history of neonatal herpes was fully understood, when it was believed that most cases arose from mothers with asymptomatic recurrent infections. Whilst it is true that asymptomatic recurrences do occur, they are of low titre, very transient, and carry a very low risk of inducing neonatal herpes, as the babies of such mothers are

protected by maternal antibody. This policy resulted, in years gone by, in unnecessary Caesarean sections, whilst having no effect at all in preventing neonatal HSV. The practice of surveillance cultures should be abandoned.

Q What strategies could be devised to try and reduce the incidence of neonatal herpes infection?

A For all of the reasons outlined above, it is extremely difficult to devise strategies for reducing the incidence of neonatal herpes. The 'at risk' mother is one who has had no prior genital HSV infection, but who may be exposed to an infected sexual partner. Serological screening for antibodies to HSV-2 may have a role, but even a strategy based on that is likely to be ineffective, as the percentage of genital infections that are due to HSV-1 rather than HSV-2 has dramatically increased with the introduction of safe sex practices.

Q How, therefore, would you manage Mrs Fisher?

A Strongly reassure her that her baby will be at very low risk of neonatal herpes. From a virological point of view, the only possible intervention would be to offer delivery by Caesarean section if she has a clinically evident recurrence at the time of labour. Visible lesions contain much higher titres of virus than are shed from the cervix during an asymptomatic attack, and thus the risk of transmission of infection is considerably greater. The only proviso to this advice is if the membranes have been ruptured for a considerable time (e.g. more than 6 hours), in which case Caesarean section may not reduce the risk of transmission of infection.

There are a number of myths and misconceptions surrounding the subject of prevention of neonatal herpes infection. Such information as is known with certainty is as follows.

- A history of genital herpes is an unreliable guide as to which women are genitally infected with HSV

- Surveillance cultures during pregnancy do not predict which women will be excreting virus asymptomatically during delivery

- Asymptomatic excretion of virus during labour in such women poses little risk to their neonates
- Most babies with neonatal herpes do *not* have mothers (or fathers) with a history of genital herpes
- If herpetic lesions are visible when a woman presents in labour, *regardless of her personal history in relation to genital herpes*, she should be delivered by Caesarean section.

Résumé for undergraduates

Neonatal herpes has an awful prognosis as virus is usually internally disseminated, whether or not there are external skin lesions. Babies may acquire neonatal infection following passage through an infected birth canal or postnatally, e.g. from contact with a cold sore. Most maternal infections giving rise to infected babies are primary infections acquired in the second half of pregnancy.

Summary: Genital herpes in pregnancy

Risk

Neonatal herpes simplex infection, which has high morbidity and mortality

Maternal genital HSV infections

- Primary: high risk of neonatal infection; Caesarean section advisable
- Recurrent: low risk; Caesarean section only indicated if visible lesions present during labour

Case 64 An unexpected blood count from Mrs Archer, 16 weeks pregnant

Mrs Archer attends for a routine antenatal appointment. By dates she is 16 weeks pregnant. Her history and physical examination are unremarkable, and she is on no regular medication. She is a nurse on one of the paediatric wards at the local hospital. You carry out the usual routine antenatal investigations, including a full blood count. Four days later you receive the following report from the haematology laboratory.

Full blood count:

Haemoglobin (Hb), 11.6 g/dl

White cell count 11.0×10^9/l, including 5% large unclassifiable cells (LUC)

Differential white cell count and film:

Neutrophils, 44%

Lymphocytes, 45%

Monocytes, 6%

LUC, 5%

Atypical mononuclear cells seen. ?recent virus infection

Q How do you interpret these results, and what should you do now?

A These results are something of a surprise. You discuss the findings with the haematologist. The large unclassifiable cells (LUC) are cells that, on the basis of size and nuclear staining, do not fall into the groups of white blood cells that the automated counter is able to recognize. The high LUC count prompted a film to be made and examined, revealing the atypical mononuclear cells (see Case 15). These cells may appear during many acute viral infections, but are most often seen in cases of infectious mononucleosis (IM), or glandular fever.

You thus need to consider the differential diagnosis of acute IM (see Case 15):

- Epstein–Barr virus (EBV)
- cytomegalovirus (CMV)
- *Toxoplasma gondii*
- acute HIV seroconverting illness

You ask Mrs Archer to return to the clinic, explaining that one of her blood tests is abnormal and that you need to take some more blood for further investigation.

Q What tests should you order to determine the cause of Mrs Archer's illness?

A Monospot or Paul Bunnell tests are useful in the diagnosis of EBV infection (these tests are explained in Case 15). Serum should also be sent for CMV and toxoplasma serology. Anti-HIV testing will not be helpful at this point (see Case 38), but Mrs Archer should be asked about possible risk factors for HIV infection.

You receive the following results: monospot, negative; toxoplasma latex test, <16; CMV titre 256 (by complement fixation test (CFT)).

Q How do you interpret these?

A The negative monospot result decreases the likelihood of this being EBV infection, although a minority of cases (5–10%) may be negative by both this and the Paul Bunnell test. If no other diagnosis is reached, then EBV-specific serology should be requested (see Case 15).

The toxoplasma latex test is a screening assay for the presence of antibodies to toxoplasma. The titre here is less than 16, which means that there is no evidence that Mrs Archer has ever been infected with this agent. Had this result been positive, then a toxoplasma-specific IgM test should be requested, to determine whether the infection is recent or not.

The CMV CFT result indicates the presence of large amounts of complement-fixing antibody against this virus.

Q Does the CMV result confirm a recent CMV infection?

A No. The serological ways in which recent infection with a given virus can be confirmed are:

- demonstration of the presence of virus-specific IgM
- demonstration of a rise in antibody titre in two separate samples taken a few days apart

The CFT does not distinguish between IgG and IgM, both of which may fix complement. An assay for the detection of IgM anti-CMV should therefore be performed. It may also be possible to demonstrate a rise in IgG titre as the laboratory may have received an earlier sample from Mrs Archer for rubella and syphilis serology at around 12 weeks of pregnancy.

On consultation with the laboratory, further tests are initiated, and you receive the following results.

Sample 1 (12 weeks): CMV CFT <16

Sample 2 (16 weeks):

    CMV CFT, 256

    CMV IgM-positive (strong reaction)

Indicates recent infection with CMV

Q What type of CMV infection do I think this is?

A CMV is a herpesvirus and thus exhibits latency. It is therefore possible to undergo both primary and secondary (reactivation or re-infection) infections (these are explained in Case 4) with CMV. As Mrs Archer has progressed from being antibody-negative to antibody-positive, i.e. she has sero-converted to CMV, in addition to which she has generated a strong IgM response, it is highly likely that she has undergone a primary infection.

Q What are the risks to Mrs Archer and her fetus of a CMV infection during pregnancy?

A The virus may cross the placenta, and infect the fetus. The baby will then be born congenitally infected with CMV (see Table 64.1). The chances of this happening during a primary CMV infection are around 40–50%.

Table 64.1 Congenital CMV infection

- The most common congenital infection: 1 in 300 births in the UK. May arise as a result of maternal primary or secondary CMV infection, both of which are usually asymptomatic
- Damage to the fetus may arise during any trimester of pregnancy (unlike congenital rubella infection)
- Diagnosis is by detection of IgM anti-CMV in cord blood, or by isolation of CMV from a neonatal throat swab or urine sample in the first 3 weeks of life

---

Q Is it possible to determine whether, in Mrs Archer's case, the virus has crossed the placenta?

A Yes. The presence of virus can be sought in amniotic fluid obtained by amniocentesis. After 20 weeks of pregnancy, it is also possible to detect IgM anti-CMV in cord blood obtained by cordocentesis. These techniques are extremely specific, but their sensitivity, although high, is not 100%. Thus a positive result is indicative of transplacental transmission, but a negative result, whilst making it less likely, doesn't necessarily rule it out. These techniques carry a small, but finite, risk to the mother and the pregnancy.

Q What are the possible consequences to the fetus of congenital CMV infection?

A Of all babies congenitally infected with CMV:

- 80–85% are normal at birth, and develop normally
- 5–10% are symptomatic at birth, with cytomegalic inclusion disease (see Table 64.2)
- 5–10% have no abnormalities at birth, but damage becomes apparent on follow-up, e.g. hearing defects (uni- or bilateral), impaired intellectual performance, poor motor skills

Note. As evidenced by the above statistics, the majority of *infected* babies are not *affected*—this is a very important distinction to make.

Q How are you going to counsel Mrs Archer?

Table 64.2 **Clinical features of cytomegalic inclusion disease**

In utero

- Intrauterine growth retardation

At birth

- CNS: microcephaly, encephalitis, seizures, apnoea, focal neurological signs
- Outside the CNS: hepatitis, hepatosplenomegaly, thrombocytopenia, pneumonitis, myocarditis

On follow-up

- 20% mortality during infancy
- Survivors have significant morbidity that may be:
  - (a) severe, e.g. mental retardation, blindness, deafness
  - (b) mild, e.g. defects in perceptual skills, learning disability

A She has suffered an asymptomatic primary CMV infection in pregnancy. There is a 40–50% chance that this infection will have crossed the placenta and infected her fetus. She may wish to undergo amniocentesis for prenatal diagnosis (detection of CMV in amniotic fluid). If there is evidence of transplacental transmission, the outcomes of congenital infection, and their statistical likelihood, are outlined above. There is no evidence that treatment of Mrs Archer with anti-CMV drugs (ganciclovir, foscarnet) would have any effect on the outcome—both drugs are toxic and are not indicated in pregnancy. Mrs Archer may wish to continue with the pregnancy, in the knowledge of the risks of fetal damage, or opt for a termination. This decision is one that can only be taken by the patient following consultation with her partner, her GP, and her obstetrician.

Q How would you devise a strategy for the prevention of congenital CMV infection?

A This is difficult. There is currently no vaccine available to prevent CMV infection. Both primary and secondary CMV infections are almost invariably asymptomatic (as was the case with Mrs Archer). Thus, diagnosis of maternal infection would necessitate diagnostic screening during pregnancy. In the UK, screening all antenatal sera for the presence of anti-CMV is not indicated because:

- serious congenital infection may arise from both maternal primary and secondary CMV infections (i.e. in women initially seronegative or seropositive)
- avoidance of sources of CMV infection (small children, sexual partners) by seronegative women is not practicable

However, contrary views have been expressed in the USA, where maternal secondary CMV infection is believed to pose very little risk to the fetus. Thus, efforts are made to identify seronegative women and counsel them about avoidance of CMV infection.

Q Should Mrs Archer's baby receive antiviral treatment if it is shown to be congenitally infected with CMV?

A There are limited data suggesting that long-term ganciclovir therapy of *symptomatic* congenitally CMV-infected babies may prevent further sensorineural hearing loss. However, for babies who are asymptomatic at birth, there is no way of distinguishing the small proportion of those babies who will develop CMV-related problems from the vast majority who will not, and the currently available anti-CMV agents are too toxic to be administered to all those babies.

Q Mrs Archer was working on a paediatric ward. Do you think that a nurse on such a ward who becomes pregnant should be moved to a different working environment?

A No. This is another controversial topic. Certain groups of workers are more likely to be exposed to CMV at work, including health-care workers looking after children and immunosuppressed patients, as both of these patient groups are significant excretors of CMV. Nursery and child day-care workers are similarly at risk. However, the significance of such occupational exposure is unclear, as women may be exposed to CMV during pregnancy from their (and other) children and their sexual partners. Congenital CMV infection is no more common in the occupational groups mentioned above. Thus, a nurse in this setting does not need to be moved. She should, however, be reminded to be scrupulous in hand-washing, which is the key to the prevention of hospital-acquired infection.

Q What infections in pregnancy may give rise to congenital abnormalities?

A These include:

- Rubella (Case 59)
- CMV (see above)
- Toxoplasmosis (see Box 64.1)
- Varicella-zoster virus (Case 62)
- Syphilis (Case 36)

In addition, a number of virus infections can be transmitted vertically (i.e. from mother to baby), e.g. hepatitis B virus (Case 28), hepatitis C virus (Case 29), HIV (Case 38), HTLV-1 (Case 66). Whilst these infections are clinically important to the baby, they do not give rise to congenital abnormalities.

Q What is toxoplasmosis, and how may it be acquired?

A Infection with the protozoan parasite, *Toxoplasma gondii*. The definitive host of this organism is any member of the cat family that becomes infected by eating tissues of infected prey and sheds oocysts in faeces. Oocysts may infect intermediate hosts, e.g. sheep, pigs, cattle, humans, within whom a parasitaemia is followed by invasion of organs and tissues, and the formation of tissue cysts. Humans may become infected by four routes:

- ingestion of oocysts from soil or water contaminated with cat faeces
- ingestion of viable tissue cysts in raw or undercooked meat, or in milk from infected intermediate hosts
- transplantation of organs containing tissue cysts
- transplacental transmission from a mother who is acutely infected

---

Box 64.1 Clinical features of toxoplasmosis

Presentation

Acute infection, acquired postnatally

- May be asymptomatic
- Fever, malaise, myalgia
- Lymphadenopathy—usually cervical; may be one isolated enlarged node that may persist for months
- Glandular-fever-like illness (see Case 15)

In the immunosuppressed

- Reactivation of latent tissue cysts may occur, with manifestations dependent on the site of reactivation
- Encephalitis (see Table 51.1 in Case 51)
- Myocarditis

Congenital infection (varied manifestations)

- Asymptomatic (the majority)
- Non-specific symptoms, e.g. intrauterine growth retardation, hepatosplenomegaly
- Severe disease, with hydrocephalus, intracranial calcification, retinochoroiditis (the 'classic triad'); extensive internal organ involvement (liver, heart, lungs)
- Ocular complications—retinochoroiditis; may not present until many years after birth; due to reactivation of retinal cysts

Diagnosis

- Serology—a rise in antibody titre and the presence of specific IgM
- Antigen or genome detection techniques are available in reference laboratories
- Tissue histology

Treatment

- Immunocompetent hosts—therapy usually not indicated
- Immunosuppressed hosts—sulphadiazine and pyrimethamine, with folinic acid replacement; clindamycin is an alternative
- In pregnancy—spiramycin, a macrolide similar to erythromycin
- Congenital infection—specific therapy should be given during the first year of life in order to reduce the incidence of late ocular sequelae

Q What are the clinical features of toxoplasmosis?

A These vary with the age and immune status of the host (see Box 64.1). There is some controversy as to whether acute infection may be associated with retinochoroiditis, or whether the latter is always due to reactivation of retinal cysts acquired *in utero*.

Q How may congenital toxoplasmosis be prevented?

A Pregnant women should be educated as to the routes of transmission of the organism, and given clear advice as to how to reduce the risk of infection:

- avoid cleaning out cat litter trays. Otherwise, use gloves, and wash hands afterwards
- wear gloves when gardening, and wash hands afterwards
- do not eat raw/undercooked meat or unpasteurized milk. Wash hands after handling raw meat

There is currently no antenatal screening programme in the UK to identify toxoplasma-seronegative pregnant women. Re-testing seronegative women at intervals during pregnancy would allow identification of cases of acute infection (through seroconversion), which could then be managed appropriately. Such programmes do exist in other countries.

Résumé for undergraduates

CMV is the most common cause of congenital infection in the UK, affecting about 1 in 300 babies. 5–10% of babies have severe disease evident at birth; 5–10% are normal at birth but defects become apparent during development. The remaining 80–85% are normal at birth and develop normally. Toxoplasmosis may also be transmitted vertically and give rise to fetal damage.

Summary: Congenital CMV

Incidence

The most common congenital infection: 1 in 300 babies infected

Clinical features

Cytomegalic inclusion disease (5–10%); normal at birth, defects evident later (5–10%); normal at birth, normal development (80–85%)

Pathogenesis

Transplacental transmission of virus from maternal primary or secondary CMV infections that are usually asymptomatic

Diagnosis

IgM in cord blood; culture of CMV from throat or urine within 3 weeks of birth

Self-assessment

1. Which one of the following statements regarding screening in pregnancy is not true?

  (a) All antenatal sera should be screened for the presence of antibodies to *T. pallidum*

  (b) All antenatal sera should be screened for the presence of IgG anti-rubella antibodies

  (c) All antenatal sera should be screened for the presence of HBsAg

  (d) All antenatal sera should be screened for the presence of antibodies to HCV

  (e) All antenatal sera should be screened for the presence of antibodies to HIV

2. Which of the following statements are correct?

  (a) Vertical transmission of HBV can be reduced by vaccination of the neonate

  (b) Women found to be non-immune to rubella should be vaccinated in early pregnancy

  (c) Vertical transmission of HIV can be reduced by elective Caesarean section

  (d) HIV-infected mothers should be advised not to breast-feed

  (e) HBV-infected mothers should be advised not to breast-feed

3. Which of the following statements regarding HIV-infection in pregnancy is *not* true?

  (a) HIV is excreted in breast milk

  (b) Without intervention, the risk of vertical transmission of HIV infection from carrier mothers is of the order of 20%

  (c) The risk of vertical transmission of HIV infection can be reduced by antiretroviral therapy given during pregnancy, parturition, and postnatally to the offspring

  (d) Diagnosis of vertical transmission of HIV is routinely performed by testing cord blood for the presence of anti-HIV

  (e) Screening for HIV infection in antenatal sera is performed by testing for the presence of antibodies to the virus

4. Which one of the following organisms is not associated with the development of ophthalmia neonatorum?

  (a) *Chlamydia trachomatis*

  (b) *Staphylococcus aureus*

  (c) *Neisseria gonorrhoea*

  (d) Adenovirus

  (e) *Haemophilus influenzae*

5. Which of the following is appropriate for the treatment of ophthalmia neonatorum due to chlamydia infection?

  (a) Systemic penicillin

  (b) Topical erythromycin

  (c) Systemic erythromycin

  (d) Systemic gentamicin

  (e) Topical fusidic acid

6. Which one of the following statements regarding rubella in pregnancy is not correct?

  (a) Rubella-specific IgM is often present at the onset of rash

  (b) Rubella-specific IgM rarely persists for more than 8 weeks after natural infection

  (c) A pregnant woman found to lack IgG antibodies to rubella should be offered immediate vaccination

  (d) Maternal rubella infection after 20 weeks of pregnancy carries no risk of congenital rubella

  (e) Babies with congenital rubella may have multiple organ damage

7. Which of the following is not a recognized complication of maternal parvovirus infection in pregnancy?

  (a) Fetal cataracts

  (b) Spontaneous miscarriage

(c) Fetal hydrops

(d) Maternal polyarthritis

(e) Maternal rash

8. Which one of the following statements regarding varicella-zoster virus infection in pregnancy is *not* true?

(a) The most common life-threatening maternal complication of chickenpox in pregnancy is pneumonia

(b) Maternal chickenpox may be acquired by contact with a person with shingles

(c) Transplacental transfer of VZ virus only occurs if maternal infection is in the first half of pregnancy

(d) Neonates whose mothers develop chickenpox in the week after delivery should be given zoster immune globulin (ZIg) prophylaxis

(e) Unilateral failure of limb-bud development is a feature of the varicella embryopathy syndrome

9. Which of the following statements concerning varicella-zoster virus infection are true?

(a) Varicella-zoster virus (VZV) contains a DNA genome and belongs to the family Herpesviridae

(b) The congenital varicella syndrome has only been described in the offspring of mothers who develop chickenpox in the first half of pregnancy

(c) The absence of a history of chickenpox correlates well with the absence of antibodies to VZV in women of child-bearing age

(d) Women who develop chickenpox in the first half of their pregnancies should be given varicella-zoster immunoglobulin in order to reduce the risk of varicella pneumonia

(e) A neonate whose mother develops herpes zoster (shingles) 1 week after delivery is at risk of developing neonatal chickenpox and should be given varicella-zoster immunoglobulin

10. Which *one* of the following statements regarding HSV infection is *not* true?

(a) Primary genital herpes infections due to HSV-2 have a higher recurrence rate than those due to HSV-1

(b) Aciclovir treatment of genital herpes infection does not prevent latent infection of the lumbosacral ganglia

(c) More than 50% of mothers of infants with neonatal infection have a history of previous or current genital herpes

(d) Clinical features of neonatal herpes include the occurrence of disseminated infection in the absence of skin lesions

(e) The source of infection of babies with neonatal herpes may not be the mother

11. Match the disease manifestations in a fetus or neonate with the most likely infectious cause.

(a)	Encephalitis	(i)	CMV
(b)	Unilateral skin scarring	(ii)	HSV
(c)	Cataracts	(iii)	VZV
(d)	Fetal heart failure	(iv)	Rubella
(e)	Hepatosplenomegaly	(v)	Parvovirus

12. Which *one* of the following statements regarding CMV infection is *not* true?

(a) CMV belongs to the herpesvirus family

(b) The site of latency of CMV is the B lymphocyte

(c) CMV is the most common cause of congenital infection is this country

(d) CMV gives rise to multisystem disease in immunocompromised hosts

(e) CMV is commonly present in the salivary glands

13. Which *one* of the following statements regarding CMV infection is *not* true?

(a) CMV infection can be transmitted by blood and blood products

(b) The majority of babies with congenital CMV infection have evidence of disease at birth

(c) CMV is demonstrable in 0.3 to 1.5% of neonates in the UK

(d) CMV infection in a pregnant woman is almost always asymptomatic

(e) CMV infection may cause neonatal jaundice

14. Which of the following is the most common cause of neonatal bacteraemia?

(a) *Streptococcus pneumoniae*

(b) *Pseudomonas aeruginosa*

(c) *Acinetobacter baumannii*

(d) *Staphylococcus aureus*

(e) *Streptococcous agalactiae* (beta-haemolytic streptococcus Group B)

15. Which of the following statements about the epidemiology of listeriosis in the UK is true?

(a) Soft cheeses are almost always the source

(b) Clusters of cases, i.e. 2–3 cases occurring together over a short period, is the most common pattern of illness

(c) All patients have an underlying recognized cause of immunodeficiency, are pregnant, or are neonates

(d) Most cases are sporadic

(e) Environmental investigation of food outlets usually pinpoints a source

8

CHAPTER 8

Miscellaneous

SECTION 8
Miscellaneous

Case 65 David, a 22-year-old student with a swollen testis

David, a 22-year-old medical student, limps gingerly into your surgery. His main complaint is that of a painful, swollen right testis. He was well until 2 days ago, when he felt unable to attend lectures, with non-specific aches and pains, a headache, and a temperature of 37.8°C. He first noticed his testicular swelling this morning, when he woke up feeling sick. He is an active sportsman, but can recall no recent injury or trauma that might account for the swelling. He has no history of sexually transmitted diseases, and has no dysuria or urethral discharge. He has a steady girlfriend, who is well. He has had no serious illnesses in the past. On examination, he has a low-grade fever, but no other abnormal physical signs apart from his right testis, which is about double the size of his left testis, and tender (see Fig. 65.1).

Q What is the diagnosis? Name one infectious cause of this condition.

A David has symptoms and signs of orchitis. The most likely cause, in someone of this age, is mumps virus infection. In a younger patient, the initial diagnosis of a painful swollen testis must be torsion, as this is a surgical emergency, and, although this would be unusual in a 22-year-old, it should still be borne in mind.

On checking David's history, it transpires that he has never received mumps vaccine. You re-examine him, paying particular attention to his face and neck. However, you can find no evidence of salivary gland enlargement, and the orifices of his parotid ducts are not inflamed.

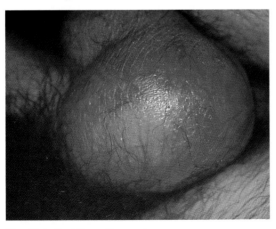

Fig. 65.1 David's swollen testis.

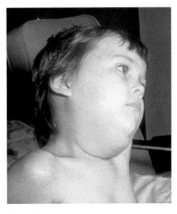

Fig. 65.2 Parotitis.

Table 65.1 **Mumps virus infection**

Asymptomatic seroconversion (i.e. subclinical infection)

Approximately 30% of infections

Prodromal illness

Malaise, myalgia, low-grade fever, for 1–2 days

Parotitis (see Fig. 65.2)

Occurs in 95% of cases of symptomatic disease

Is bilateral in 75% of cases

Glands are swollen and tender, duct orifices red and oedematous

Swelling lasts 4–7 days

Submandibular and sublingual glands occasionally involved

Central nervous system

Meningitis (see Case 41)

   Aseptic meningitis in 5–10% of mumps patients (males > females)

Encephalitis (see Case 42)

   Is due to spread of mumps virus from the meninges into the brain (ie meningoencephalitis)

   About 1 in 6000 cases

   May cause convulsions, focal neurological signs, motor or sensory disorders

Other

   Hearing loss; may occur in absence of meningitis or encephalitis

   Guillain–Barré syndrome (rare)

Orchitis, epididymitis, and oophoritis

20–40% postpubertal males, usually unilateral, 5% postpubertal females

Bilateral orchitis in one-third of cases

Risk of sterility due to testicular atrophy is, however, very small

Oophoritis, presenting with lower abdominal pain, and pelvic tenderness, may cause diagnostic difficulties

Pancreatitis

Usually not severe

Other manifestations

Myocarditis (rare)

Arthritis (rare)

Renal dysfunction (rare)

In a pregnant female—increased risk of abortion

The role of mumps infection as a trigger for juvenile-onset insulin-dependent diabetes mellitus is controversial

Q Do these findings rule out mumps virus infection?

A No. Whilst parotitis is usually the dominant clinical feature of mumps (see Fig. 65.2), any of the associated manifestations of mumps can occur before, simultaneously, or after the parotitis, or even in its complete absence. The pathogenesis of mumps infection includes a viraemic phase, where virus spreads in the bloodstream and can infect many end-organs, giving rise to a number of clinical manifestations (see Table 65.1). Most of the complications are more common in postpubertal patients compared to children.

You reassure Peter that his swollen testis is likely to be due to mumps, and advise bed rest.

Q Are there any investigations you can do to confirm your diagnosis?

A Mumps virus can be grown in tissue culture in the laboratory, from saliva, urine, or cerebrospinal fluid (CSF). The easiest sample to send to the laboratory is urine. Sending an acute serum sample is also good practice.

Peter returns to your surgery 3 days later, with evident parotid gland swelling, confirming your clinical diagnosis. You receive a laboratory report 1 week later stating that mumps virus was isolated from his urine sample.

Q What type of vaccine is available for the prevention of mumps?

A Mumps vaccines contain live attenuated strains of virus, usually combined with live attenuated measles and rubella viruses in the MMR vaccine (see Appendix 2). One potential drawback of the use of such vaccines is that failure to achieve sufficient attenuation may result in the vaccine causing clinical disease. One of the mumps vaccines used in the UK (the Urabe strain), which gave rise to an unacceptably high incidence of vaccine-induced mumps meningitis (about 1/10 000 doses of vaccine), has now been withdrawn.

Q Why is mumps included in the recommended list of childhood vaccinations?

A Most male medical students, when asked this question in an exam, will answer 'because of orchitis', but this is *not* the reason why, in the UK, we aim to vaccinate every single child against mumps (and in any case it is a sexist answer, ignoring as it does the complication of oophoritis). Neither do we do it in order to prevent small children looking like hamsters for a while, with their swollen parotid glands! The correct answer is because of the central nervous system complications of mumps infection, i.e. meningitis and meningoencephalitis. Even though the prognosis of these complications is good, cost–benefit analysis demonstrates that the cost of universal vaccination is more than offset by the savings to be made from reducing hospitalizations due to these particular manifestations of mumps virus infection. The wide range of clinical syndromes and complications associated with mumps virus infection is listed in Table 65.1.

However, there is one cautionary note to be struck when considering mumps vaccination. All of the non-parotitic manifestations of mumps are more common in older patients. Vaccination of a proportion of children may reduce circulating wild-type virus, and therefore more non-immunized children will evade natural infection during their childhood. These individuals remain susceptible to mumps infection as they become older and so, overall, suboptimal vaccination may paradoxically generate an increase in the incidence of mumps complications, as the average age of infection increases.

Summary: Mumps

Clinical features

Parotitis, meningitis, meningoencephalitis, orchitis, oophoritis, pancreatitis

Diagnosis

Clinical; virus isolation from urine, CSF, saliva; serology

Management

Symptomatic

Prevention

Live attenuated vaccine; given to prevent CNS complications

Case 66 Lenny, a 38-year-old Jamaican with a palpable skin rash

Mr Lenny Rowe, a 38-year-old Jamaican man who has lived in the UK for 30 years, is referred to the dermatology clinic because of a skin rash. He first noticed slightly raised patches of itchy skin some months ago. The skin in those patches has recently become further thickened and in the past 2 months discrete nodules have appeared. There is nothing else of note in his history, except that his mother died of 'a blood disorder'. The only abnormal signs on examination are moderately enlarged axillary lymph nodes and several nodules in the skin. Routine investigations reveal a normal haemoglobin and white cell count, but a decreased platelet count of 70×10^9 per ml. A biopsy of a skin nodule is reported as showing a T cell lymphoma.

Q Is there any further diagnostic test that should be performed?

A There is a distinct possibility that this patient may be suffering from adult T-cell leukaemia lymphoma (ATLL; see Table 66.1), which is known to arise from infection with human T-cell lymphotropic virus type 1 (HTLV-1). You should therefore request HTLV-1 serology, and ask for a careful review of his blood film.

Table 66.1 **Adult T-cell leukaemia lymphoma**

- *Epidemiology*. Common in Japan, the Caribbean, Central and South America, equatorial Africa, but rare elsewhere
- *Clinical presentation*. Variable. Acute or chronic leukaemia, or cutaneous lymphoma
- *Malignant cell*. T cell, CD4+ (i.e. helper subset), expresses high levels of the receptor for interleukin-2. Unlike HIV, HTLV-1 does not bind to CD4.
- *Prognosis*. Usually culminates as a highly malignant monoclonal proliferation of T cells

---

Lenny is shown to be anti-HTLV-1-positive. Abnormal white cells with the characteristic morphology (including highly irregular nuclei) shown in Fig. 66.1 are seen in his blood film, which confirms the diagnosis of ATLL.

Q What type of virus is HTLV-1?

A A retrovirus, i.e. it possesses a reverse transcriptase enzyme that enables it to copy its RNA genome

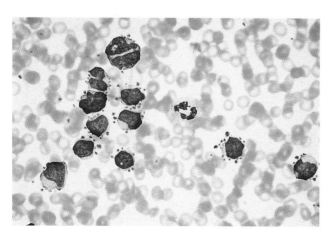

Fig. 66.1 Malignant ATLL cells in peripheral blood.

into DNA. Retroviruses are widespread in nature, but HTLV-1 was the first human retrovirus to be discovered. Other human retroviruses include HTLV-2, and the human immunodeficiency viruses HIV-1 and -2.

Q What is the treatment of ATLL?

A This is difficult and often not successful. First-line therapy is aggressive chemotherapy using standard lymphoma treatment regimens. Azidothymidine (AZT), a reverse transcriptase inhibitor, has not been shown to be of any clinical benefit when used alone in this disease. Use of combination therapy with anti-lymphoma and anti-retroviral drugs together is under investigation.

Lenny is admitted to hospital and a regimen of four chemotherapeutic agents is instituted. Whilst in hospital, he complains of constipation, frequency in passing urine, and an intense thirst. He also becomes noticeably depressed.

Q What complication of ATLL is he suffering from now?

A Constipation, polyuria, polydypsia, and depression are all features of hypercalcaemia, which is frequently present in ATLL. The mechanism of this is unclear, but may be due to the release of cytokines, such as interleukin-1 and T cell growth factor-beta, from the malignant cells, which have osteoclast-activating properties.

Q What is the evidence implicating HTLV-1 as the causative agent of ATLL?

A This includes:

- The epidemiology of HTLV-1 infection exactly parallels that of ATLL (i.e. common in Japan, the Caribbean, South America)
- Patients with ATLL are invariably HTLV-1-seropositive
- Virus can be isolated from malignant ATLL cells. The viral genome is integrated into the chromosomal DNA of the cell

Q How do you think Lenny acquired his infection with HTLV-1?

A The routes of spread of HTLV-1 are:

- vertical (i.e. mother to baby)
- sexual
- blood-borne (e.g. transfusion, intravenous drug abuse)

Lenny's mother died 'of a blood disorder', which may have been a leukaemia, suggesting that he may have acquired his infection from her. This would be entirely compatible with his presentation 38 years later. As with other virus-associated malignancies, ATLL has a long latent period, e.g. 30–40 years.

The exact mode of vertical transmission of HTLV-1 is believed to be postnatally via breast milk, rather than *in utero* or perinatally. Advice to anti-HTLV-1-positive mothers not to breast-feed their babies, plus exclusion of anti-HTLV-1-positive blood from the blood supply, has resulted in a dramatic fall in HTLV-1 seropositivity in Japan. HTLV-1 is highly cell-associated, and thus administration of acellular blood products does not transmit infection. Thus, haemophiliacs are not at risk of infection from their Factor VIII. Blood donor screening for HTLV-1 (and -2) infection is now routine in the UK.

Q Is HTLV-1 infection associated with any other clinical conditions?

A Yes. Tropical spastic paraparesis (TSP), the features of which are outlined in Box 66.1. This syndrome is known in Japan as HTLV-1-associated myelopathy (HAM). TSP has been recognized as a distinct syndrome in the Caribbean for many years, where it is the most common cause of demyelinating disease, i.e. it occurs more frequently than multiple sclerosis. The pathogenesis of TSP is unclear. To date, no major differences between 'leukaemogenic' and 'neurogenic' strains of HTLV-1 have been reported.

Q What is the likelihood of an HTLV-1-infected individual developing ATLL or TSP?

A Only a small minority of HTLV-1-infected individuals will present with ATLL or TSP. The lifetime risk of the former is of the order of 2% in

> ### Box 66.1 Tropical spastic paraparesis
>
> **Epidemiology**
>
> - Mean age of onset 40 years
> - Female:male, 2:1
> - Geographic distribution parallels HTLV-1 seroprevalence
>
> **Clinical features**
>
> - Insidious presentation, stiffness/weakness in one or both legs resulting in spastic paraparesis. Sphincter disturbance and penile impotence are common
> - Cranial nerve and upper limb involvement rare
> - Only minor objective sensory impairment
>
> **Diagnosis**
>
> - Anti-HTLV-1 found in serum and CSF, often in very high titre
>
> **Treatment**
>
> - Steroids of short-term benefit only
>
> **Prognosis**
>
> - 30% patients are bedridden after 10 years; 45% cannot walk unaided by crutches

individuals infected in the first year of life, and of the latter is 0.25%.

Q What diseases are associated with HTLV-2 infection?

A The data implicating HTLV-2 as a cause of disease are much less clear-cut. Neurological disease similar to TSP, large granulocytic cell leukaemia, and cutaneous diseases ranging from eczema to debilitating lymphocytic infiltration of the skin have all been described in HTLV-2-infected individuals. However, the vast majority of such individuals (mostly intravenous drug abusers) do not have any of these manifestations of disease.

Résumé for undergraduates

Human T-cell lymphotropic virus type 1 (HTLV-1) is a retrovirus. Infection with HTLV-1 is common in Japan and the Caribbean. Infection is acquired vertically, sexually, and through blood transfusion, and can give rise to adult T-cell leukaemia lymphoma (ATLL) or tropical spastic paraparesis (TSP), a disease with similarities to multiple sclerosis.

> ### Summary: Human T-cell lymphotropic virus type 1 (HTLV-1) infection
>
> **Routes of spread**
>
> Vertical (breast milk); sexual; blood transfusion
>
> **Geographic distribution**
>
> High prevalence in Japan, Caribbean, South America
>
> **Disease associations**
>
> Adult T-cell leukaemia lymphoma (ATLL); tropical spastic paraparesis (TSP)
>
> **Prevention**
>
> Avoid breast-feeding; screen blood donors in endemic areas

Case 67 Richard, a young man with lethargy and breathlessness

Richard, an 18-year-old student, complains of lethargy and weakness that have become more prominent since he first became ill 3 days ago, with general malaise, a fever, a runny nose, and an irritating cough. Today he has also noticed some shortness of breath after climbing the stairs in his home. He has had no serious illness in the past and is on no regular medication. His mother and sister both suffer from an uncharacterized chronic haemolytic anaemia. On examination, Richard is pale and his resting pulse is 90/min. He has a palpable spleen.

Q What initial investigations would you perform?

A A full blood count and film should be done as this patient has symptoms (lethargy, shortness of breath) and signs (pale, resting tachycardia) of anaemia, with a background of a positive family history.

That afternoon, you receive the following results:

haemoglobin (Hb), 5.0 g/dl; mean corpuscular volume (MCV), 86 fl; no reticulocytes seen

white cell count, 2.2×10^9/l

platelets, 80×10^9/l

Q How do you interpret these results and what would your next investigation be?

A All elements of the blood are below normal values, suggesting bone marrow failure. Examination of a bone marrow aspirate is therefore indicated.

The bone marrow report shows marked erythroid hypoplasia. Granulopoiesis and megakaryopoiesis are active and mildly reduced.

Q Is Richard's family history likely to be relevant to his presentation with acute bone marrow failure?

A Richard was, in fact, investigated as a child, but his haemoglobin was normal at that time, and nothing further was done. However, the history of a 'flu-like illness' followed by bone marrow failure in a patient with a family history of chronic haemolytic anaemia is suggestive of acute infection with parvovirus B19, resulting in an aplastic crisis.

Q How might you confirm your diagnosis?

A At this stage of infection, patients are viraemic, i.e. virus particles are present in their peripheral blood. Electron microscopy of a serum sample may thus reveal these particles. Alternatively, parvovirus DNA can be identified in peripheral blood by hybridization techniques, or using the polymerase chain reaction (PCR) assay.

You observe Richard carefully over the next few days. His haemoglobin, white cell, and platelet counts gradually begin to rise. However, 9 days after his initial presentation, an erythematous maculopapular rash develops on his face, trunk, and limbs, and the next day Richard complains of pain in the small joints of his hands.

Q Do these new symptoms and signs indicate that Richard has acquired a new infection?

A No. Rash and arthralgia/arthritis are well recognized complications of parvovirus infection (see Case 59), arising typically 7–10 days after the viraemic, febrile stage of the illness.

Richard's rash lasts 4 days, and his joint symptoms, initially relieved by paracetamol, also disappear. On follow-up in outpatients 2 weeks later, his full blood count shows an Hb of 11.3 g/dl, a white cell count of 5.4×10^9/l, and a platelet count of 180×10^9/l. Subsequent investigations confirm a diagnosis of chronic haemolytic anaemia due to pyruvate kinase deficiency.

Q What are the pathogenetic mechanisms underlying the various manifestations of parvovirus infection seen in this patient?

A The pathogenesis of parvovirus B19 infection has been studied in healthy adult volunteers, intranasally inoculated with virus. The salient features, illustrated in Fig. 67.1, are:

- a viraemic phase (1 week post-inoculation) associated with a non-specific febrile illness
- infection of bone marrow progenitor cells leading to transient bone marrow arrest
- immune complex manifestations (i.e. rash and joint involvement) evident at 18–21 days, as the IgG antibody response to infection becomes detectable

The effects of the bone marrow arrest are not clinically evident in otherwise healthy individuals. However, in patients with chronic haemolytic anaemia, in whom erythrocytes have a shortened life span, the profound reticulocytopenia may result in the depression of haemoglobin concentrations to critical levels—a so-called aplastic crisis.

Q What is the treatment of an aplastic crisis?

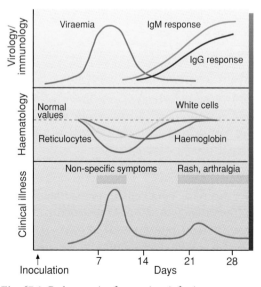

Fig. 67.1 Pathogenesis of parvovirus infection.

A Treatment involves blood transfusion until the bone marrow recovers. Family members with chronic haemolytic anaemia who are seronegative for parvovirus antibody will also be at risk, especially as the index patient will be excreting virus at this stage of his/her illness. Normal human immunoglobulin contains anti-parvovirus antibody and may protect those susceptible individuals.

Immunosuppressed patients (e.g. HIV infection, leukaemics, bone marrow transplant recipients) may fail to eliminate the virus, resulting in chronic infection with consequent chronic anaemia and transfusion dependence. Treatment with intravenous normal human immunoglobulin (which contains anti-parvovirus antibodies) may be successful in eliminating infection.

Q Could Richard's aplastic crisis have been diagnosed by detection of parvovirus-specific IgM in his serum?

A No. The reason for this is evident in Fig. 67.1— the aplastic crisis occurs during the viraemic phase of the illness, before the patient has mounted a detectable immune response. However, specific IgM detection is the mainstay of diagnosis in patients presenting with rash and/or joint manifestations.

Q What diseases are caused by parvovirus B5?

A There is no such virus! The rather clumsy nomenclature of parvovirus B19 arose from the code number of the original serum sample in which it was discovered. Thus there are no parvovirus A or parvovirus B 1–18 viruses.

Résumé for undergraduates

Parvovirus infection causes transient bone marrow arrest, with a drop in red cells, white cells, and platelets. In otherwise normal individuals, these drops are not clinically relevant, but in patients with underlying chronic haemolysis, parvovirus infection can cause an aplastic crisis.

Summary: Human parvovirus B19 infection

Disease associations

Erythema infectiosum, arthritis, aplastic crisis; in pregnancy: miscarriage, hydrops fetalis

Pathogenesis

Manifestations arise from virus infection of rapidly dividing cells in bone marrow and immune complex formation

Diagnosis

Serology; detection of viral DNA

Case 68 Michael, a law student recently returned from Africa with a fever

Michael, a 19-year-old law student, presents to A&E complaining of feverishness, shivering, headache, and generalized aches and pains. He first felt ill 2 days ago, and feels he is getting worse. On direct questioning, he also reports that his throat has become painful since yesterday. He has no relevant past medical history. He has just returned to the UK from abroad and, although on no regular medication, he has been taking malaria prophylaxis. On examination, he is febrile (39°C) and his pharynx is inflamed, but there are no other physical signs.

Q What further history is relevant?

A The information provided thus far is non-specific, and you are faced with a long list of possible differential diagnoses. The first point to clarify is exactly where and when Michael has been on his travels.

Michael took a year out between leaving school and starting law at university. For the past 6 months he has been back-packing around West Africa, returning to England 7 days ago. Apart from some moderate diarrhoea 4 weeks after his arrival in Africa, he was well during the trip and is adamant that he complied with his prescribed malaria prophylaxis throughout. For the last month of his travels, he was in a rural part of Nigeria.

Q What is your differential diagnosis now?

A Malaria must remain high on the list, despite the history of prophylaxis, as this is never 100% effective (see Case 50). Other infections compatible with Michael's presentation include typhoid, typhus, and influenza. However, the history of time spent in rural west Africa immediately before his return to England raises the distinct possibility of lassa fever, which should set the alarm bells ringing!

Table 68.1 Lassa fever

- *Aetiology*: infection with lassa fever virus (an arenavirus)
- *Natural reservoir of infection*: rodents
- *Geographic distribution*: west Africa, e.g. Nigeria, Sierra Leone
- *Incubation period*: 3–21 days
- *Presentation*: insidious onset, fever, malaise, 'flu-like illness'
- *Complications*: hypotension, oliguria, haemorrhage
- *Mortality*: 5–25% in different outbreaks

Q What is lassa fever, and why is the diagnosis of such major importance?

A Lassa is one of a group of diseases known collectively as the viral haemorrhagic fevers (VHF). The key features of lassa fever are listed in Table 68.1. Apart from the associated high mortality, its formidable reputation for person-to-person spread has major management implications.

Q What are the principles of management of a case of VHF such as lassa fever?

A There are strict guidelines issued by the UK Department of Health, which are designed to achieve optimal patient care and minimize the risks of spread of infection. As with any serious medical problem, the most important point to remember is 'if in doubt, ask for help'. Your local infectious diseases physician/medical microbiologist should have access to the national guidelines, and will know how to trigger the correct chain of response. The broad principles of management are:

1 no laboratory work must be carried out on specimens from these patients until a blood film has been examined for the presence of malarial parasites. Malaria is itself a medical

Box 68.1 Viral haemorrhagic fever syndromes

Disease	Causative agent	Clinical features	Geographical distribution	Transmission	Comment
Yellow fever	Yellow fever virus (flavivirus family)	Multisystem disease, with jaundice and haemorrhagic manifestations	Central and S. America, Africa	Mosquito	Preventable by vaccination
Dengue haemorrhagic fever	Dengue viruses (four serotypes, flavivirus family)	Uncomplicated dengue: adults, older children, fever, muscle and joint pain, rash Dengue haemorrhagic fever (DHF): young children, hypovolaemic shock, bleeding, 5% mortality	Pacific islands, Asia, Caribbean	Mosquito	Pathogenesis of DHF unknown
Haemorrhagic disease with renal syndrome	Hantaviruses (bunyavirus family)	Clinical features: vary. Asymptomatic disease; mild (nephropathica endemica, N. Europe); severe (Korean haemorrhagic fever)	China, S.E. Asia, Europe	Rodents	Hantavirus pulmonary syndrome recently described in USA
Ebola and Marburg diseases	Ebola and Marburg viruses (filovirus family)	Outbreaks associated with very high mortality rates (50–90%)	SubSaharan, central and eastern Africa	From monkeys; human-to-human spread	Natural reservoir of these viruses not yet identified

emergency (see Case 50) and statistically is more likely than any viral haemorrhagic fever.

2 the blood film and any other patient samples must be taken with extreme care and rendered safe where possible by immersion in 10% formalin. Strict attention must be paid to the safe disposal of all instruments used in specimen taking and preparation.

3 laboratories undertaking work on any samples from these patients must be notified in advance and must have suitable containment facilities

4 the patient must be transferred to an isolation facility. If there is a strong likelihood of VHF, then the patient must be admitted directly to a designated high-security isolation unit

5 the local consultant for communicable disease control or equivalent must be informed, and through him/her the appropriate surveillance unit (e.g. in the UK the Communicable Disease Surveillance Centre (CDSC)) that holds national responsibility on behalf of the Department of Health

6 if the diagnosis is strongly suspected or confirmed, then close contacts of the patient must be identified and placed under surveillance

CDSC confirms that the area in Nigeria in which Michael was staying is endemic for lassa fever. Repeated blood films are sent to the laboratory, and no malarial parasites are seen. Lassa fever is therefore strongly suspected and Michael is transferred to the nearest high-security isolation unit. The diagnosis is confirmed by identification of virus in clinical material in a laboratory with Category 4 isolation facilities.

Q Is there any antiviral agent available for the treatment of lassa fever?

A Yes. Ribavirin, a nucleoside analogue with a broad antiviral spectrum, is active against the lassa fever virus. It can also be used prophylactically for individuals visiting endemic areas.

Intravenous ribavirin therapy is started. Over the next few days, Michael becomes prostrate, with a high fever, and shows evidence of plasma leakage (facial oedema, pleural effusion, ascites) and bleeding (petechiae on skin and mucous membranes). However, with intensive supportive therapy, his fever subsides after 7 days, and he makes a rapid recovery, although his tiredness persists for many weeks. Happily, no family member, close friend, or health-care worker develops symptoms.

Q What are the other viral haemorrhagic fevers?

A There are a number of virus infections that can produce severe haemorrhagic disease in humans. These viruses belong to a number of different virus families, have distinct geographic distributions, and utilize different modes of spread. The salient features of some of them are listed in Box 68.1.

Résumé for undergraduates

Life-threatening haemorrhagic fevers may arise through infection with a wide range of viruses. Many of these are geographically limited in distribution and a travel history is essential in evaluation of the patient. Patients with suspected VHF and samples derived from them *must* be managed and handled in strict isolation facilities.

Summary: Viral haemorrhagic fevers

Presentation
Febrile illness, followed by hypovolaemic shock and haemorrhage, in a patient with a history of recent travel

Diagnosis
Clinical suspicion; laboratory diagnosis in specialized centres

Management
Exclude malaria; isolation and referral to tropical disease specialist; notify authorities

Case 69 Polyarthralgia in Susan, a 25-year-old

Susan, a 25-year-old woman, has a 5-day history of polyarthralgia involving the toes, fingers, and wrists. Two weeks earlier she had a bout of acute diarrhoea, vomiting, and abdominal pain lasting 6 days for which no microbiological cause was found. There is no history of a skin rash, eye symptoms, or urethral discharge.

Q What are the likely causes of her polyarthralgia?

A The following should be considered:

* connective tissue diseases, such as rheumatoid arthritis, may present as described above. Subsequent episodes and a positive rheumatoid factor will confirm the diagnosis
* viral arthritis, due to rubella (see Case 59) or parvovirus (see Case 67) should be considered. A history of exposure, the presence of a characteristic rash, or vaccination history (rubella) may help in diagnosis. Other viruses less commonly implicated in arthralgia include Epstein–Barr virus, mumps, enteroviruses, e.g. echoviruses, adenoviruses, and acute hepatitis B infection (when arthralgia is an immune complex-mediated phenomenon)
* enteropathic arthropathies, associated with Crohn's disease and ulcerative colitis. This usually involves the larger joints of the lower limbs and recurrent gastrointestinal symptoms are likely
* psoriasis-associated joint disease, which characteristically affects the sacroiliac joint. The presence of characteristic skin lesions suggests the diagnosis
* septic arthritis, due to *Staphylococcus aureus*, streptococci, etc., may be accompanied by risk factors such as trauma, previous joint disease, or immunosuppression, and affects one or at most two joints. The absence of systemic symptoms such as fever and arthritis makes the diagnosis less likely here

* Reactive arthropathies, which may follow gastroenteritis due to *Salmonella*, *Shigella*, *Campylobacter*, and *Yersinia*. The history of a diarrhoeal illness makes this possible here
* Reiter's disease, in which skin lesions occur in 50% of cases and in which urethritis and conjunctivitis are also present. A similar syndrome of urethritis, conjunctivitis, and arthritis may follow the oculogenital form of infection with *Chlamydia trachomatis* (see Case 61)

Q Which gastrointestinal pathogen is likely to have been responsible here?

A Probably one of three, i.e. *Campylobacter*, *Salmonella*, and *Shigella*. These are routinely sought in stool samples by most microbiology laboratories using selective (e.g. desoxycholate-citrate agar for *Shigella*) and enrichment (e.g. selenite broth for *Salmonella*) techniques. *Yersinia* species (see Table 69.1) cause gastroenteritis less commonly and are not routinely sought in clinical specimens but may be implicated in reactive arthropathy.

Q How may yersiniosis be diagnosed?

A Attempts to isolate these bacteria from faeces are hampered by slow growth, and cold enrichment or selective agar media are required. *Yersinia* spp. may occasionally be recovered from lymph nodes taken at

---

Table 69.1 *Yersinia* species

* *Y. enterocolitica* and *Y. pseudotuberculosis* are Gram-negative motile non-lactose-fermenting rods
* May survive and replicate at 4°C
* Reservoirs include domestic (Fig. 69.1), agricultural, and and aquatic environments, and wild animals
* *Y. pestis*, the aetiological cause of human plague, is a worldwide zoonotic infection transmitted by flea bites

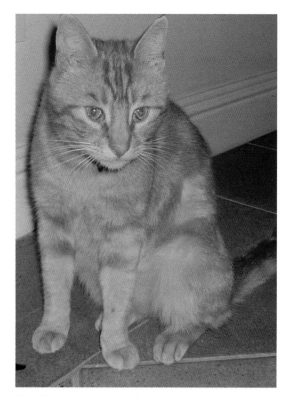

Fig. 69.1 Domestic animals, a possible reservoir of *Yersinia* spp.

laparotomy when associated with intraabdominal pathology. Synovial effusions are usually sterile in the presence of polymorphonuclear cells. Paired sera, 10–14 days apart, may confirm a diagnosis by showing a rise in antibodies, but sera should be appropriately absorbed to prevent cross-reaction with other bacteria, including *Salmonella*, and *Yersinia* serology is usually confined to regional or reference laboratories. A reactive polyarthralgia is seen in 10–30% of adults following infection with *Y. enterocolitica* and is related to the presence of HLA-B27.

Susan's faeces are negative on culture for *Campylobacter*, *Shigella*, *Salmonella*, and *Yersinia*, and blood cultures are sterile. Serum taken from her confirms that she has been vaccinated against or been infected with rubella in the past, is negative for antibodies to parvovirus, and she has no markers for a connective

tissue disorder. A repeat serum sample taken 2 weeks later shows a rise in antibody titre to *Y. enterocolitica* from 1 in 32 in the first specimen to 1 in 512, confirming a diagnosis of reactive arthritis due to yersiniosis.

Q What other clinical conditions are associated with *Yersinia*?

A A number of conditions of unconfirmed aetiology have been associated with *Yersinia* but the most widely recognized of these are:

- gastroenteritis, clinically indistinguishable from that due to many other causes but often accompanied by blood and mucus
- mesenteric adenitis/terminal ileitis, often indistinguishable from appendicitis. Usually due to *Y. pseudotuberculosis*
- bacteraemia/bloodstream infection, especially in immunocompromised patients or those with liver disease, including those with iron overload, e.g. thalassaemia, requiring frequent transfusions
- erythema nodosum
- plague (*Y. pestis*)

Q How is yersiniosis treated?

A Many of the various forms of yersiniosis are self-limiting and it is not clear whether antimicrobial chemotherapy significantly alters the natural history. Exceptions to this include systemic infection such as bacteraemia or deep-seated infection such as liver abscesses or osteomyelitis. *Y. enterocolitica* is usually resistant to penicillin, ampicillin, and many of the cephalosporins. Trimethoprim, a tetracycline, or, more recently, a fluoroquinolone such as ciprofloxacin, are preferred. Bacteraemic infection is probably best treated with a combination of one of the above plus an aminoglycoside such as gentamicin.

Résumé for undergraduate students

Yersinia spp. are not common bacterial pathogens but may occasionally be relevant in the patient with diarrhoea, arthritis, and abdominal pain. Specialist laboratory culture techniques are required in the laboratory and so close liaison is required to confirm a diagnosis.

Summary: Yersiniosis

Presentation
Variable, but includes gastroenteritis, arthralgia, abdominal pain

Diagnosis
Culture of faeces, joint fluid, etc. Rise in antibodies

Management
Often self-limiting. Antibiotics such as tetracyclines, trimethoprim, or a quinolone

Case 70 Problems on Friday afternoon for a senior house officer

Virginia, a recently appointed senior house officer in health care of the elderly is called to see an 84-year-old man with vomiting and diarrhoea at 3 p.m. on Friday, 13th August! Cedric has been an inpatient for 2 weeks for assessment of increasing immobility and treatment of a mild chest infection. He has been vomiting since earlier that day, and in the last 3 hours has passed two watery stools. He appears mildly dehydrated; Virginia takes blood to check his urea and electrolytes and he is started on intravenous (IV) normal saline. One of the nurses remarks that Cedric is the fourth patient on the ward with diarrhoea and vomiting occurring over the last 48 hours.

Q What should Virginia do first?

A She should ascertain the nature of the symptoms of the other patients to determine whether they are similar to those of Cedric, and again treat dehydration if present. If they appear similar and there are no identifiable reasons why these patients should have gastrointestinal symptoms, e.g. laxative use, diverticular disease, or recent antibiotics, it seems very likely that there is an outbreak of gastroenteritis on the ward.

Q Who should she contact now?

A After informing and discussing the problem with a senior colleague, preferably the consultant in health care of the elderly, she should inform the hospital infection control team, i.e. the infection control doctor (most likely a consultant microbiologist) and infection control nurses, to ensure that early control measures may be implemented.

The infection control team visit the ward that afternoon and investigate the outbreak in conjunction with the medical and nursing staff. It transpires that, over the previous 5 days, seven patients have developed gastrointestinal symptoms and two staff nurses and a physiotherapist have gone off work with similar symptoms (see Fig. 70.1). Vomiting, sometimes projectile in character, has almost always been the initial symptom and this has usually been followed by moderate to severe diarrhoea for 2–3 days. Abdominal pain has not been a prominent symptom. Only two patients are or have been on antibiotics in the preceding couple of weeks, and no obvious food source is implicated. Sadly, no specimens from patients or staff have been sent to microbiology to confirm a diagnosis.

Q What is the likely aetiological cause of the outbreak?

A The occurrence of this outbreak on a health care of the elderly ward, the short and generally mild nature of the symptoms, and the absence of an obvious food source all point to a viral aetiology such as that caused by noroviruses, previously referred to as small round structured viruses (SRSV), causing winter vomiting disease. Other causes such as *Salmonella*, *Shigella*, and *Campylobacter* must be excluded by stool culture and, because antibiotic-associated diarrhoea caused by *Clostridium difficile* (see Case 33) is more common in the elderly (Cedric had a recent respiratory infection for which he most probably received antibiotics), cytotoxin analysis (indicating *C. difficile* disease) should also be requested when faeces samples are submitted to the microbiology laboratory.

Q How may a viral aetiology be confirmed?

A Elecron microscopy of a fresh sample of faeces taken early in the course of the illness (i.e. in the first 24 hours) may confirm the presence of noroviruses such as Norwalk virus (see Case 24), the cause of winter vomiting disease, but the sensitivity from microscopy is only about 50%. Diagnosis by antigen detection (ELISA) or polymerase chain reaction (PCR) is superior and is becomimg the investigation of choice. In the elderly, noroviruses are the most likely viral aetiology, as rotavirus, astrovirus, calici-

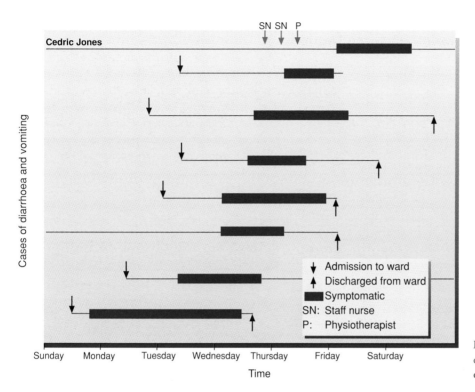

Fig. 70.1 Time course of the outbreak.

virus, and adenovirus (types 40 and 41; see Case 24) are less common in this setting and are more commonly implicated in childhood diarrhoea. Isolation of noroviruses from tissue culture has never been achieved.

Q What measures should be taken to control spread?

A Symptomatic patients should be nursed in isolation cubicles with their own toilet facilities. As ever, hand-washing is the single most important infection control measure. Staff movement to other wards should be restricted, and those who have symptoms must not work, as they are a potential source of further spread. Symptomatic patients should not be transferred to other wards or institutions because of the risk of spreading the outbreak to these areas. Affected patients or staff are considered non-infectious when they have been asymptomatic for 48–72 hours. Asymptomatic patients should also not be transferred to other institutions until 48 hours or more after the last symptomatic case has elapsed, because they might be incubating the infection.

PCR of faeces is carried out on Saturday morning and reveals noroviruses in five stool specimens. There are only two isolation cubicles on the ward, however, and by Monday eight patients are symptomatic and a further two members of staff have gone off ill; another ward is by now also affected. One of the patients, Doris, is visited by her son who is the local MP and, in passing, he remarks that he is surprised at the décor and conditions of the ward, which are poor, especially the absence of carpets in the ward areas.

Q What alternative is there to nursing patients in isolation cubicles?

A During outbreaks there may be insufficient isolation cubicles in which to care for all affected patients. If this is the case, cohort nursing—that is, nursing affected patients in the same part of the ward together, using the same nursing staff—is recommended. Thus, physical separation of patients with symptoms from those without, together with restriction of the movements of nursing and other staff contacts, will help reduce the chances of spread.

Q Why does the ward have tiled floors instead of carpets?

A Tiled floors are in general easy to clean and in particular are not damaged by commonly used surface disinfectants. Carpets, however, are difficult to keep clean, do not usually withstand the use of surface disinfectants such as hypochlorite, and, if stained, are unsightly. Furthermore, dust accumulating in carpets may be a potential source of spread of some hospital pathogens, such as methicillin-resistant *Staphylococcus aureus* (MRSA; see Case 54). Therefore, carpets should not be fitted in clinical areas.

Q For how long is the outbreak likely to continue?

A Nosocomial outbreaks of gastroenteritis due to noroviruses can 'rumble' on for some weeks, and may spread to involve further wards and clinical areas. This is because these agents are very infectious and aerosol spread derived from projectile vomiting results in secondary cases. Attempts to limit spread may be hampered by inadequate isolation facilities, poor communications, and a failure to close wards to admissions and discharges early on.

Cedric makes a speedy recovery from his illness but the outbreak spreads to involve a further three general medical and health care of the elderly wards, resulting in considerable disruption of clinical services and additional expense.

Résumé for undergraduate students

Hospital-acquired diarrhoea is increasingly common and is most commonly caused by a *C. difficile* toxin induced by antibiotics, and viruses such as noroviruses. Viral casues, although usually mild and short in duration, can result in large outbreaks with significant disruption, and close liaison with the infection control team is essential to rapidly control spread.

Summary: Nosocomial diarrhoea

Presentation

A cluster of patients with diarrhoea and vomiting, acquired in hospital, with evidence of spread (viral gastroenteritis), a point source (food-borne *Salmonella*), or common exposure to antibiotics (*C. difficile*)

Diagnosis

Clinical presentation; culture for conventional bacterial pathogens; PCR, antigen detection, or electron microscopy of stools for viruses; and toxin detection for *C. difficile*

Management

Fluid replacement and isolation or cohort nursing of symptomatic patients, with scrupulous hand-washing to prevent spread. Staff with symptoms should not continue to work

Self-assessment

1. Which one of the following statements regarding human T-cell lymphotropic virus (HTLV-I) is not true?

(a) Seroprevalence studies indicate that infection with this virus is unevenly spread throughout the world

(b) The CD4 molecule acts as a receptor on susceptible cells

(c) Infection is a risk factor for the development of tropical spastic parapesis

(d) Infection can be spread vertically via breast milk

(e) The virus belongs to the retroviridae family of viruses

2. Which one of the following statements regarding adult T-cell leukaemia/lymphoma (ATLL) is not true?

(a) Lymphomatous infiltration of the skin may be the presenting feature

(b) The lifetime risk of development of ATLL in an individual known to be anti-HTLV-1-positive is of the order of 50%

(c) DNA copies of the HTLV-1 genome are found in the malignant cells

(d) Hypercalcaemia is a well-recognized complication of disease

(e) Reverse transcriptase inhibitors, e.g. azidothymidine, are ineffective in treatment of ATLL

3. Which one of the following statements regarding mumps virus infection is not true?

(a) Mumps meningitis may occur in the absence of parotitis

(b) Most complications of mumps virus infection are more common in post-pubertal individuals

(c) Mumps virus is not present in the brain tissue of patients with mumps encephalitis

(d) Mumps can be prevented by the prophylactic use of a live attenuated viral vaccine

(e) The CSF pleocytosis associated with mumps virus infection is predominantly due to mononuclear cells

4. Which of the following is not a well-recognized complication of mumps virus infection?

(a) Pancreatitis

(b) Meningitis

(c) Nerve deafness

(d) Pelvic inflammatory disease

(e) Parotitis

5. Which one of the following viruses is not a cause of viral haemorrhagic fever?

(a) Ebola virus

(b) Lassa fever virus

(c) Yellow fever virus

(d) Marburg virus

(e) Ross river virus

6. Which one of the following statements concerning lassa fever is untrue?

(a) The natural reservoir of lassa fever virus is a rodent

(b) Infection may occur in patients recently returned from South America

(c) Ribavirin is useful in treatment

(d) Isolation of all cases is recommended

(e) Mortality is less than that arising from Marburg virus infection

7. Which one of the following is not a well recognized consequence of acute parvovirus B19 infection?

(a) Exanthem subitum

(b) Erythema infectiosum

(c) Slapped cheek syndrome

(d) Spontaneous miscarriage

(e) Aplastic crisis

8. In relation to the pathogenesis of parvovirus B19 infection, which one of the following statements is correct?

(a) Skin rash arises at the time of viraemia

(b) Parvovirus may be detected in a blood sample at the time of presentation with arthritis

(c) Parvovirus arthritis is more common in males than females

(d) Aplastic crises may occur in patients with sickle cell anaemia

(e) Chronic parvovirus infection may occur in immunocompetent individuals infected in childhood

9. Which one of the following is a well recognized cause of reactive arthritis?

(a) *Staphylococcus aureus*

(b) *Campylobacter jejuni*

(c) *Staphylococcus epidermidis*

(d) *Streptococcus pneumoniae*

(e) *Pseudomonas aeruginosa*

10. *Yersinia* species are well recognized causes of which one of the following?

(a) Terminal ileitis

(b) Pyelonephritis

(c) Diverticulitis

(d) Hepatitis

(e) Ascending cholangitis

11. Which laboratory tests are appropriate in confirming a viral cause of gastroenteritis?

(a) Serology

(b) Viral culture

(c) Polymerase chain reaction (PCR)

(d) Direct antigen detection

(e) Electron microscopy

12. Which one of the following measures is most useful in helping contain a nosocomial or hospital-acquired outbreak of viral gastroenteritis?

(a) Buying in food for all patients and staff

(b) Restricting admissions to patients less than 50 years of age

(c) Restricting staff movement to other wards

(d) Prohibiting discharges of patients home

(e) Reducing the number of nurses on the ward to prevent staff transmission

Appendices

Rational use of the microbiological laboratory

General

Sensible and rational use of the laboratory helps confirm infection, guides treatment by providing susceptibility results, assists in the control of infection in the hospital and in the community, and provides important epidemiological information to guide future public health strategies.

- Specimens should be taken *before* the start of antimicrobial chemotherapy, especially if the infection is life-threatening, e.g. bacteraemia.

- Specimens and accompanying request forms, including those submitted electronically, should include name, age, full clinical details, and whether the patient is on antibiotics.

- If there is likely to be a delay, specimens should be refrigerated. Blood cultures, however, should be placed in an incubator.

- The laboratory should be contacted in advance for vital or difficult to repeat specimens, e.g. joint aspirates, cerebrospinal fluid (CSF), especially if taken out of hours.

- The results from bacteriological investigations are usually available within 24–48 hours and positive blood or CSF results will usually be 'phoned in'.

- Most laboratories provide a standard range of tests. However, some of the specialized or sophisticated tests or assays need to be forwarded to reference laboratories.

- If in doubt about diagnosis, treatment, prevention, or control of infection, *ring up and ask*!

Genitourinary tract investigation

Urine

- Urine culture, i.e. a midstream urine (MSU) specimen, is not always essential in the management of uncomplicated urinary infection/cystitis except in children and pregnant women.

- An early morning large-volume specimen is required for the investigation of tuberculosis.

Genital

- Cervical and urethral rather than vaginal swabs are required to confirm infection with *Neisseria gonorrhoeae* or *Chlamydia trachomatis*. Urine is also suitable for PCR.

- Candidosis, trichomonas infection, and anaerobic vaginosis are diagnosed with a vaginal swab.

- Vesicle fluid or a swab in viral transport medium is needed to diagnose genital herpes; serology is not helpful here.

- A serum sample is appropriate to exclude syphilis, hepatitis B, and HIV disease when assessing a patient for sexually transmitted disease.

Gastrointestinal and abdominal investigations

Faeces

- 2–3 consecutive daily specimens are required to exclude salmonella, shigella, campylobacter, and especially protozoan (e.g. *Giardia*) infections.

- Details of travel abroad should be supplied to ensure appropriate investigations, e.g. for cholera, and of recent antibiotics to exclude *Clostridium difficile* disease.

- In the investigation of possible viral gastro-enteritis, it is essential that a faecal sample is sent *as early as possible* in the course of the illness.

Intraabdominal

- Pus or tissue is preferable to a swab in diagnosing infection, especially that due to anaerobes.

- Fresh fluid from external drains rather than fluid in drainage bags, which may be contaminated or stale, should be sent for culture.

Skin investigations

- Wound swabs are only indicated if there is clinical evidence of local (e.g. erythema) or systemic (e.g. pyrexia) infection and should not be taken routinely postoperatively.

- Pus, if present even in small volumes, is superior to a swab in isolating the cause of wound infection.

- Blood cultures should always be taken in patients with cellulitis or erysipelas as β-haemolytic streptococci may not be recovered from superficial swabs and the presence of bacteraemia has therapeutic and prognostic implications.

- Skin scrapings from the edge, not the centre, of lesions, placed in a sterile container or between two glass slides; nails or hairs should be taken to isolate the aetiological agent of dermato-phyte infections.

- Skin rashes due to viral illnesses may require laboratory investigation, e.g. serology.

- In vesicular disease, vesicle fluid should be sent for viral culture or dried on to a glass slide for subsequent electron microscopy.

Respiratory tract investigations

Upper

- Most 'viral-type illnesses' do not require laboratory confirmation.

- A throat swab may be indicated to confirm or exclude streptococcal tonsillitis, but if diphtheria is suspected (e.g. recently returned from the developing world where vaccination is not widespread) *the laboratory must be informed* to ensure appropriate culture methods are used.

- A pernasal rather than a nasopharyngeal swab is required to confirm a diagnosis of whooping cough (pertussis).

Lower

- Mucoid sputum (i.e. saliva) rarely if ever reflects pathology in the lung parenchyma.

- Bronchoscopy specimens, e.g. bronchoalveolar lavage are preferable when microbiologically confirming the aetiology of pneumonia, especially if atypical (e.g. *Chlamydia* spp.) or occurring in the immunocompromised patient where opportunist pathogens such as *Pneumocystis carinii* or *M. tuberculosis* are important.

- Three consecutive early morning sputa should be taken when investigating possible tuberculosis. Phone to request an urgent Ziehl–Neelsen stain if patient is gravely ill or 'open' tuberculosis suspected.

- A nasopharyngeal aspirate for antigen detection is the optimal approach for the diagnosis of viral bronchiolitis or pneumonia in infants and small children. In adults, a throat swab in viral transport medium may be useful in the diagnosis of influenza.

- Paired serum samples to detect a rise in antibodies to influenza and other causes of infection, e.g. *Legionella*, should also be taken; this approach is also useful in the investigation of atypical pneumonia. Urine is also useful for legionella antigen detection.

Neurological investigations

- A sample of CSF and blood cultures are the basic investigations in the diagnosis of bacterial meningitis. Polymerase chain reaction (PCR) of the CSF and blood (EDTA bottle) are especially useful in diagnosing meningococal meningitis if the patient has already received antibiotics. Microscopy of purpuric spots to detect Gram-negative diplococci is also diagnostic

- CSF, a throat swab in viral transport medium, faeces (enteroviruses), and urine (mumps) for viral culture with paired sera are recommended to confirm viral meningitis.

- The diagnosis of herpes encephalitis is best made by neurological imaging techniques or by brain biopsy, although the latter is much less common with the availability of computerized tomography (CT) and magnetic resonance imaging (MRI) scans. Investigation of CSF using PCR is now the microbiological diagnostic test of choice for herpes encephalitis but is only performed in reference laboratories.

Investigations of systemic disease

- Two sets of blood cultures (at least three if infective endocarditis suspected) are required in diagnosing bacteraemia. Details of time and site of venepuncture, clinical features, and proposed antibiotic treatment should be supplied with the specimens.

- A number of thick and thin blood smears are necessary to diagnose malaria in a pyrexial patient recently returned from an endemic area.

- A single high titre (e.g. >1/256 for legionellosis), demonstration of a fourfold or greater rise in titre (e.g. <1/16 rising to 1/128 for mycoplasma), or a positive IgM (e.g. rubella) are required for serological confirmation of infection.

- Tissue specimens may be required to definitely diagnose certain infections, e.g. invasive pulmonary aspergillosis, cytomegalovirus infection of the intestine, cutaneous leishmaniasis.

APPENDIX 2

Immunization against infectious diseases (UK recommendations)

Please note. The recommendations and schedules that follow are those pertaining to the UK. They will be similar, but not necessarily identical, to the guidelines issued in many countries with a similar population profile

Further details can be found in *Immunisation against Infectious Disease* issued by the Department of Health, the Welsh Office, the Scottish Office Department of Health, the Department of Health, Social Services and Public Safety, Northern Ireland, Her Majesty's Stationary Office, London.

Active immunization (i.e. induction of protective host immune response)

Routine universal vaccines

Vaccine	Organism	Nature of vaccine	Primary course	Booster
D/T/P	Diphtheria	Toxoid	3 doses at 2, 3, 4 months	Pre-school
	Tetanus	Toxoid		Pre-school and 14–15 years
	Pertussis	Acellular		Pre-school
Hib	*Haemophilus influenzae*, type b	Conjugated capsular antigen	3 doses at 2, 3, 4 months	
Men	Meningo group C	Conjugated oligosaccheride	3 doses at 2, 3, 4 months	
Polio	Poliovirus	Live attenuated (Sabin)	3 doses at 2, 3, 4 months	Pre-school and 14–15 years
MMR	Measles	Live attenuated	12–15 months	Pre-school
	Mumps	Live attenuated		
	Rubella	Live attenuated		
BCG	Tuberculosis	Live attenuated	10–14 years; neonatal if high-risk community	

Vaccines for at-risk groups only

Hepatitis B virus

Nature of vaccine

Hepatitis B surface antigen, i.e. subunit vaccine

Course of vaccination

For newborn: 4 doses; at 0, 1, 2, and 12 months

For all others: 3 doses; at 0, 1, 6 months

Booster

Requirement for booster dose in known responder is controversial; current practice is for a single booster at 5 years; earlier if anti-HBs response suboptimal

Target groups

Babies of HBV carrier mothers (may also require HBIg; see Case 60)

Parenteral drug misusers

Individuals who change sexual partners frequently

Sexual and close family contacts of a case or carrier

Prisoners

Patients with chronic renal failure (see Case 56)

Recipients of blood/blood products, e.g. haemophiliacs, dialysis patients

Health-care workers* (HCWs; because of risk of occupational exposure)

* For HCWs, anti-HBs response should be checked 2 months after last dose. Non-responders may not be fully protected.

Influenza

Nature of vaccine

Killed, purified surface proteins (H and N proteins)

Contents revised yearly to account for changes in circulating virus

Currently must contain A/H1N1, A/H3N2, and B strains

Course of vaccination

One dose in early winter

Booster

Repeat vaccine annually

Target groups

1. All individuals over the age of 65

2. Adults and children (> 6 months) with:
   chronic respiratory disease, including asthma
   chronic heart disease
   chronic renal disease
   diabetes mellitus and other endocrine disorders
   immunosuppression due to disease or treatment

3. Residents of facilities where rapid spread may follow introduction of infection: nursing homes old people's home

---

Pneumococcus

	Vaccine a	Vaccine b
Nature of vaccine	Capsular polysaccharide from 23 serotypes.	Conjugate vaccine covering 7 serotypes.
	Not effective in children <2 years	Used in children >2 months
Course of vaccination	One dose	Depends on age
Booster	Repeat after 5–10 years	Not known
Target groups (patients with)	1. All those over 65 years of age as with influenza vaccine	Children, 2–24 months, at risk (see 2–4, vaccine a)
	2. Splenic dysfunction, e.g. splenectomy, sickle cell disease	
	3. Chronic disease, e.g. diabetes mellitus; lung, heart, renal disease	
	4. Immunosuppression, e.g. HIV infection	

Varicella

Nature of vaccine

Live attenuated

Course of vaccination

Single dose

Booster

Not indicated at present

Target groups

Immunosuppressed children*

Non-immune health care workers at occupational risk

* Vaccine is not licensed in UK at present for immunosuppressed children; it is available on a named-patient basis.

Anthrax

Nature of vaccine

Sterile filtrate from culture of *B. anthracis*

Course of vaccination

Four doses at 0, 3, 6, and 32 weeks

Booster

Annual reinforcing dose recommended

Target groups

Workers at risk of exposure to the disease

Rabies*

Nature of vaccine

Whole virus grown in human diploid cells and killed

Course of vaccination

Three doses at 0, 7, 28 days

Booster

Every 2–3 years if still at risk

Target groups

Occupationally exposed individuals

* This is pre-exposure prophylaxis; for post-exposure use of vaccine see Case 45.

Hepatitis A

Nature of vaccine

Whole virus grown in human diploid cells and killed

Course of vaccination

Single dose provides protection for 1 year

Booster

Recommended at 6–12 months after initial dose. Provides immunity for at least 10 years

Target groups

Travellers to areas of moderate or high HAV endemicity; patients with chronic liver disease; occupationally exposed e.g. sewage workers; homosexual males; injecting drug users

Vaccines primarily for foreign travel

- Vaccines include rabies, yellow fever, Japanese encephalitis, tick-borne encephalitis, cholera, typhoid, and meningococcal meningitis.
- The exact requirements depend on destination, planned activities, level of sanitation.
- Seek expert advice on current indications and administration protocols.

Passive immunization (i.e. administration of pre-formed antibodies)

Human normal immunoglobulin (HNIg)

- Derived from normal blood donors; contains antibodies to viruses currently prevalent in the general population.
- Prophylaxis against hepatitis A (but this is better provided by active vaccination).
- Protection of immunosuppressed children exposed to measles.

Hepatitis B immunoglobulin (HBIg)

- Derived from blood donors with high titres of anti-HBs.
- Provides immediate protection against HBV infection.
- Can be administered simultaneously with vaccine.

- Should be given as soon as possible after exposure to HBV, including:
  (a) infants of high-risk carrier mothers (i.e. those who are not anti-HBe positive);
  (b) individuals with high-risk needlestick injury (post-exposure prophylaxis).

Human rabies immunoglobulin (HRIg)

- Derived from vaccinees with high-titre anti-rabies antibodies.
- Given as post-exposure prophylaxis if high-risk exposure.
- Half of dose is infiltrated around the wound; remainder given intramuscularly.

Varicella-zoster immunoglobulin (VZIg)

- Derived from individuals recently recovered from zoster
- Given to seronegative individuals, at high risk of severe disease, after exposure to VZV, i.e.:
  (a) pregnant women;
  (b) neonates of non-immune mothers, or whose mother develops chickenpox within the period 7 days prior to birth to 30 days thereafter;
  (c) immunosuppressed patients.

Tetanus immunoglobulin

Given within 24 hours to unvaccinated individuals or those whose immune status is unknown following a wound:

- with a significant degree of devitalized tissue;
- puncture-type with contact with soil or manure;
- with clinical evidence of sepsis.

Some of the more commonly used antimicrobial agents

Commonly used antibacterial agents

Agent	Spectrum/activity	Main uses	Comment/side-effects
Penicillins			
Benzylpenicillin	Streptococci, *Neisseria*, spirochaetes	Streptococcal cellulitis, pneumococcal infections, gonorrhoea, meningococcal infections, syphilis	Parenteral administration only; cheap
Ampicillin	Broad-spectrum but many bacteria have become resistant	UTI, RTI	Amoxycillin has same activity but better pharmacokinetics; cheap
Flucloxacillin	Staphylococci as resistant to staphylococcal β-lactamase	Methicillin-sensitive staphylococcal infections; the agent of choice	Cheap
Piperacillin/ azlocillin	Gram-negative bacilli including *Pseudomonas* spp.	Hospital infections such as bacteraemia/bloodstream infections	Parenteral administration only; being replaced by combinations with β-lactam inhibitors
Cephalosporins			
Cephradine/ cephalexin	Broad-spectrum but many hospital bacteria resistant	UTI; soft tissue infections	Cheap
Cefuroxime	Broad-spectrum but better cover against Gram-negative bacilli	UTI; RTI; surgical prophylaxis	
Cefoxatime	Good cover against Gram-negative bacilli but not against *Ps. aeruginosa*	Hospital infections such as bloodstream infections, pneumonia, abdominal sepsis	Risk factor for VRE, MRSA, and *Cl. difficile*; parenteral administration only
Ceftazidime	Like cefoxatime but active against *Ps. aeruginosa*	Pseudomonal infections in hospital and in patients with cystic fibrosis	More expensive; risk factor for VRE, MRSA, and *Cl. difficile*; parenteral administration only

Commonly used antibacterial agents (*cont'd*)

Agent	Spectrum/activity	Main uses	Comment/side-effects
Cefixime	Broad-spectrum but not against *Ps. aeruginosa*	RTI and soft tissue infections in hospital and community	More expensive; can be administered orally
Cefpirome	Like ceftazidime but more stable against β-lactamases	Second-line agent for serious hospital infection, e.g. RTI	Parenteral administration only
Other β-lactam agents			
Co-amoxyclav (amoxycillin + clavulanic acid)	Broad-spectrum including anaerobes	UTI; RTI; soft tissue infections; treatment and prophylaxis of surgical abdominal infections	Replacing ampicillin/ amoxycillin in many situations
Piperacillin/ tazobactam	Broad-spectrum including anaerobes, *Ps. aeruginosa*; stable against many β-lactamases	Second-line agent for more complicated hospital infections	Expensive; parenteral administration only
Meropenem	Broad-spectrum including anaerobes, *Ps. aeruginosa*	Second-/third-line agent for difficult hospital infections	Good CNS penetration; parenteral administration only
Aztreonam	Active against Gram-negative bacteria only	Alternative to amino-glycosides in hospital	Not commonly used; parenteral administration only
Aminoglycosides			
Gentamicin, tobramycin, amikacin, netilimicin	Gram-negative bacilli; no activity against anaerobes or against staphylococci and streptococci unless used in combination with other agents	Serious Gram-negative infections, e.g. bacteraemia, endocarditis, neutropenic fever	Parenteral administration; renal and ototoxicity; regular levels essential
Macrolides			
Erythromycin	Staphylococci, streptococci, mycoplasma, chlamydia, legionella	RTI; soft tissue infection in patients allergic to penicillin; STD	GIT intolerance common
Clarithromycin, azithromycin	As with erythromycin but better activity against Gram-negative bacilli including *H. influenzae*	As with erythromycin	More expensive but probably better tolerated
Quinolones			
Nalidixic acid	Gram-negative bacilli except *Ps. aeruginosa*	UTI only	Cheap

Commonly used antibacterial agents (*cont'd*)

Agent	Spectrum/activity	Main uses	Comment/side-effects
Ciprofloxacin	Gram negative bacilli, including *Ps. aeruginosa*; little activity against staphylococci and streptococci	Complicated UTI; bacteraemia; complicated hospital-acquired pneumonia; some GIT infections such as typhoid fever	May affect growing cartilage
Ofloxacin	Similar to ciprofloxacin but more active against chlamydia and staphylococci/ streptococci	Second-line agent for community-acquired pneumonia; STD (chlamydia and gonorrhoea)	As for ciprofloxacin
Levofloxacin/ moxifloxacin	Enhanced activity against staphylococci/streptococci but less active against *Ps. aeruginosa*	Second- or third-line agents for pneumonia	As for ciprofloxacin
Miscellaneous agents			
Nitrofurantoin	Gram-negative bacteria but not *Ps. aeruginosa*	UTI	Cheap; nausea not infrequent
Trimethoprim	Gram-negative bacilli; some activity against streptococci and staphylococci; with sulphamethoxazole (co-trimoxazole) active against *Pneumocystis carinii*	UTI; RTI; pneumocystis pneumonia	Allergy, skin reactions, especially with co-trimoxazole
Tetracyclines	Staphylococci/streptococci, chlamydia, rickettsiae, brucella	Q fever; brucellosis; chlamydial diseases; atypical pneumonia	Contraindicated in pregnancy and childhood due to effects on growing bones and teeth
Vancomycin/ teicoplanin	Gram-positive bacteria only; not active against Gram-negative bacilli	MRSA infections; infection in patients allergic to penicillin (e.g. endocarditis); second-line agent for *Cl. difficile* (vancomycin)	Parenteral except to treat *Cl. difficile*; regular levels required with vancomycin
Clindamycin	Staphylococci/streptococci anaerobes	Soft tissue infections; gangrene unresponsive to penicillins	Diarrhoea due to *Cl. difficile*
Rifampicin	Mycobacteria; the meningococcus, staphylococci	Tuberculosis (in combination); meningococcal prophylaxis; complicated staphylococcal infections (in combination), e.g. device-related	Induces liver enzymes

Commonly used antibacterial agents (*cont'd*)

Agent	Spectrum/activity	Main uses	Comment/side-effects
Fusidic acid	Staphylococci	Bone and joint infections (in combination)	Cholestatic jaundice especially if given parenterally
Linezolid	Mainly against Gram-positive bacteria such as staphylococci/streptococci	Second-line agent to treat MRSA; also to treat VRE	Monoamine oxidase inhibitors reactions; low platelets; new agent, still being assessed
Metronidazole	Anaerobes; protozoa	Treatment and prophylaxis of surgical infections; also treatment of giardiasis, amoebiasis, trichomonal infections	'Antabuse-type' reaction with alcohol; neuropathy if prolonged use

Abbreviations: UTI, urinary tract infections; RTI, respiratory tract infections; VRE, vancomycin-resistant enterococci; MRSA, methicillin-resistant *Staphylococcus aureus*; CNS, central nervous system; GIT, gastro-intestinal tract; STD, sexually transmitted diseases.

Commonly used antifungal agents

Agent	Spectrum/activity	Main uses	Comment/side-effects
Polyenes			
Nystatin	Most fungi	Oral and genital candidiasis	Largely replaced by other agents which are easier to administer
Amphotericin B	Most fungi; dermatophytes less sensitive	Candidaemia; cryptococcal and aspergillus infection	Parenteral administration only; electrolyte disturbances; renal impairment
Liposomal amphotericin B	As for amphotericin B	As for amphotericin B	Expensive; better tolerated
Imidazoles			
Miconazole/ clotrimazole	Most fungi	Mucosal and cutaneous; mycoses	Poor absorption from gut
Ketoconazole	Poor activity against aspergillus	Second-line agent for superficial and cutaneous mycoses	Hepatitis (1:10 000) and gynaecomastia
Itraconazole	Most fungi	Second-line agent for prophylaxis and treatment of systemic mycoses	Oral and intravenous administration only
Fluconazole	Most fungi except aspergillus	Candidaemia; cryptococcal infection	Some candida species resistant
Voriconazole	Most fungi	Second-line agent for systemic mycosis	Relatively new agent; still being assessed
Other agents			
Griseofulvin	Dermatophytes	Hair and nail dermatophyte infection	3 weeks or more required to build up levels in keratin
Capsofungin	Most fungi	Alternative to amphotericin B	New agent but appears very safe
Flucytosine (5-FC)	Yeasts only	Cryptococcal meningitis and candidaemia, with amphotericin B; UTI (can be used alone)	Bone marrow suppression; regular serum levels required
Terbinafine	Dermatophytes	Skin, hair, and nail mycoses but not those caused by candida	Dermatophyte infection

Abbreviation: UTI, urinary tract infection.

Commonly used antiprotozoal and antihelminth agents

Agent	Spectrum/activity	Main uses	Comment/side-effects
Antimalarials			
Quinine	All 4 plasmodium species	Treatment of complicated or resistant falciparum malaria	Cardiac arrhythmias
Chloroquine	Hepatic phases	Treatment and prophylaxis of falciparum malaria	Retinopathy occasionally; many strains resistant
Pyrimethamine	Active against plasmodia and toxoplasma	Treatment and prophylaxis of malaria and toxoplasma	Bone marrow depression if glucose-6-phosphate dehydrogenase deficient
Other agents			
Metronidazole (see also antibacterials)	Flagellates, amoebae	Giardiasis; amoebiasis; trichomonas vaginitis	'Antabuse-like' reaction with alcohol; neuropathy if prolonged use
Sodium stibogluconate	*Leishmania* spp.	Visceral, cutaneous, mucosal leishmaniasis and kala azar	Anaphylaxis; renal and hepatic toxicity
Praziquantal	Trematodes and cestodes	Schistosomiasis; tapeworms; liver and lung fluke	Diarrhoea
Mebendazole	Broad-spectrum antihelminthic agent	Hookworm, roundworm, threadworm and whipworm infestations	Teratogenic

Commonly used antiviral drugs

Agent	Main therapeutic uses	Comments	Side-effects
Agents active against herpes simplex (HSV) and varicella zoster (VZV) viruses			
Aciclovir	Primary HSV (mucosal, keratitis); recurrent HSV (prophylaxis); herpes encephalitis; disseminated disease; primary and recurrent VZV infection	Nucleoside analogue DNA synthesis inhibitor; also available as valaciclovir, a valyl ester with better oral absorption	Remarkably non-toxic
Famciclovir	As for aciclovir	Nucleoside analogue DNA synthesis inhibitor; oral prodrug of penciclovir	Remarkably non-toxic
Agents active against cytomegalovirus (CMV)			
Ganciclovir	Prophylaxis and treatment of CMV infections in immunocompromised patients	Nucleoside analogue related to aciclovir but much better activity against CMV; also available as valganciclovir, an oral prodrug	Quite toxic, particularly to bone marrow
Cidofovir	Treatment of CMV retinitis	Nucleotide analogue (i.e. already monophosphorylated) DNA synthesis inhibitor	Nephrotoxic; must give in combination with probenecid
Foscarnet	Prophylaxis and treatment of CMV infections; aciclovir-resistant HSV	Sodium phosphonoformate, a pyrophosphate analogue; DNA synthesis inhibitor; active against herpesviruses	Nephrotoxic
Agents active against human immunodeficiency virus (HIV) I: reverse transcriptase inhibitors (RTIs)			
Nucleoside analogue RTIs			
Zidovudine (AZT)			Bone marrow toxicity (macrocytic anaemia)
Zalcitabine (ddC)			Neuropathy; pancreatitis
Didanosine (ddI)			Neuropathy; pancreatitis
Stavudine (d4T)			Neuropathy; pancreatitis
Lamivudine (3TC)		Also has activity versus hepatitis B virus (HBV)	
Abacavir			Hypersensitivity reactions
Tenofovir		Nucleotide analogue (i.e. already monophosphorylated)	Nephrotoxic
Non-nucleoside analogue RTIs			
Efavirenz			Rash
Nevirapine			Rash including Stevens–Johnson syndrome

Commonly used antiviral drugs (*cont'd*)

Agent	Main therapeutic uses	Comments	Side-effects
Agents active against human immunodeficiency virus (HIV) II: protease inhibitors			
Amprenavir, Indinavir, Lopinavir, Nelfinavir, Ritonavir, Saquinavir			Interference with lipid metabolism, including lipodystrophy, hyperlipidaemia, insulin resistance, hyperglycaemia
Agents active against human immunodeficiency virus (HIV) III: fusion inhibitors			
Enfuvirtide		Newly licensed agent; not much experience with this in the UK yet	
Agents active against viral hepatitis			
Interferon-alpha	Treatment of chronic HBV infection (action believed to be immuno-modulatory); chronic HCV infection (in combination with ribavirin)	Multifunctional agent; has antiviral and immuno-modulatory activity; very broad-spectrum *in vitro* activity	'Flu-like illness'; bone marrow suppression; depression; autoimmunity
Lamvivudine	Chronic HBV infection	Reverse transcriptase inhibitor (see under HIV above)	
Ribavirin	Chronic HCV infection (given in conjunction with interferon-alpha); also used in respiratory syncytial virus (RSV; see below), lassa fever	Broad-spectrum antiviral	Haemolytic anaemia
Adefovir	Treatment of chronic HBV infection	Nucleotide analogue (as per cidofovir, tenofovir)	Newly licensed agent; may be nephrotoxic
Agents active against influenza			
Amantadine	Treatment and prevention of influenza A virus infection	Only active against influenza A virus	CNS stimulation, confusion, agitation, especially in the elderly
Zanamivir, oseltamivir	Treatment and prevention of severe influenza virus infection	Neuraminidase inhibitors; active against all influenza viruses	
Agents active against respiratory syncytial virus (RSV)			
Ribavirin	Treatment of severe RSV infection in high-risk patients; may be useful in severe acute respiratory syndrome (SARS)	Needs to be administered by nebulizer	

APPENDIX 4

Notifiable diseases (United Kingdom)

Diseases notifiable under the Public Health (Control of Disease) Act 1984, and the Public Health (Infectious Diseases) Regulations 1988.

- Acute encephalitis
- Acute poliomyelitis
- Anthrax
- Cholera
- Diphtheria
- Food poisoning
- Leprosy
- Leptospirosis
- Malaria
- Measles
- Meningitis
- Meningococcal septicaemia (without meningitis)
- Mumps
- Ophthalmia neonatorum

- Paratyphoid fever
- Plague
- Rabies
- Relapsing fever
- Rubella
- Scarlet fever
- Smallpox
- Tetanus
- Tuberculosis
- Typhoid fever
- Typhus
- Viral haemorrhagic fever (VHF)*
- Viral hepatitis
- Whooping cough
- Yellow fever

* This means Argentine VHF (Junin), Bolivian VHF (Machupo), Chikungunya VHF, Congo/Crimean VHF, dengue fever, Ebola virus disease, haemorrhagic fever with renal syndrome (Hantaan), Kyanasur Forest disease, Lassa fever, Marburg disease, Omsk VHF, and Rift Valley disease.

Outline of the subject matter of each case

Outline of the subject matter of each case

Section 1 Skin and mucous membranes

Section 2 Respiratory tract

Section 3 Gastrointestinal tract

Section 4 Genitourinary tract

Section 5 Central nervous system

Section 6 Systemic infections

Case 47 Bloodstream infections/septicaemia; *Escherichia coli*; septic shock

Case 48 Systemic candidiasis; opportunist mycoses

Case 49 Infective endocarditis

Case 50 Malaria

Case 51 Human immunodeficiency virus (HIV) infection; AIDS; cytomegalovirus (CMV); cerebral toxoplasmosis; pneumocystis pneumonia; cryptococcal meningitis; *Mycobacterium avium* complex disease; progressive multifocal leucoencephalopathy (PML); cryptosporidiosis; Kaposi's sarcoma

Case 52 Tuberculosis; atypical mycobacteria

Case 53 Fever (pyrexia) of unknown origin (FUO); zoonoses

Case 54 Osteomyelitis; methicillin-resistant *Staphylococcus aureus* (MRSA)

Case 55 Leishmaniasis; arthropod-borne infectioins

Case 56 Blood-borne viruses and dialysis; cytomegalovirus (CMV) infection in a transplant recipient

Case 57 Needlestick injuries

Section 7 Pregnancy and the neonate

Case 58 Listeriosis; neonatal meningitis and bloodstream infection

Case 59 Rubella and parvovirus infection in pregnancy

Case 60 Hepatitis B virus (HBV); human immunodeficiency virus (HIV); and hepatitis C virus (HCV) in pregnancy

Case 61 Ophthalmia neonatorum

Case 62 Varicella-zoster virus infection in pregnancy; varicella embryopathy; neonatal varicella

Case 63 Herpes simplex virus infection in pregnancy; neonatal herpes

Case 64 Cytomegalovirus (CMV) in pregnancy; toxoplasmosis; toxoplasmosis in pregnancy

Section 8 Miscellaneous

Case 65 Mumps

Case 66 Human T-cell lymphotropic virus (HTLV)-1 and -2; adult T-cell leukaemia lymphoma (ATLL); tropical spastic paraparesis (TSP)

Case 67 Parvovirus-induced aplastic crisis, rash, and arthralgia

Case 68 Viral haemorrhagic fevers

Case 69 Yersiniosis; reactive arthropathy

Case 70 Nosocomial diarrhoea; hospital outbreak investigation

Answers to self-assessment

Answers to self-assessment

Section 1 Skin and mucous membranes

1. (e). All components of the MMR vaccine are live attenuated viruses.

2. (e). The encephalitis that may follow acute measles arises from an immunopathogenetic mechanism, not through spread of virus itself into the brain or meninges.

3. (a) (v); (b) (i); (c) (iv); (d) (iii); (e) (ii). Slapped cheek syndrome is also known as erythema infectiosum or fifth disease; German measles is the vernacular term for rubella; rubeola is the proper name for measles; chickenpox is also known as varicella; exanthem subitum is also known as roseola infantum or sixth disease.

4. (c). The common manifestations of adenovirus infection are in the upper respiratory tract (pharyngitis, tonsillitis, conjunctivitis), but virus can descend into the lower respiratory tract and cause pneumonia. Certain adenovirus serotypes (40 and 41) are a common cause of gastroenteritis in small children. Adenoviruses can rarely cause haemorrhagic cystitis, but urethritis is not described.

5. (b). A discharge that is frankly purulent suggests bacterial, not viral, infection.

6. (b). Reinfections are quite common, suggesting that the initial lesion does not induce a protective immune response.

7. (c). Primary viral pneumonia is the most common life-threatening complication. This is much more common in adults than in children.

8. (a)–(e), i.e. all five, are recognized features. The urinary retention may arise as a consequence of sympathetic nerve involvement.

9. (d). It is difficult to isolate dermatophytes from skin swabs and a nasal swab is inappropriate. Skin biopsies are not routine to diagnose tinea.

10. (b). Whitfield ointment may be used to treat tinea but all the others are antibacterial agents.

11. (b). The others may cause cellulitis or gangrene, especially *Cl. perfringens*, but *Proteus* species usually colonize only.

12. (e). Co-amoxyclav will cover staphylococci, streptococci, and anaerobes. Ampicillin will probably not be active against *Staph. aureus* as most strains are beta-lactamase-producing. Trimethoprim is mainly reserved for the treatment of urinary tract infection, ciprofloxacin, which has good anti-Gram-negative activity, is not optimal for Gram-positive infections such as those caused by staphylococci and streptococci, and metronidazole will only cover anaerobes.

13. (e). Bacteria (a) and (b) are beta-haemolytic and (c) or (d) may produce either form of haemolysis or, in the case of *Enterococcus faecalis*, may be non-haemolytic.

14. (d). This Gram-negative bacillus may be part of the normal flora of the mouth of dogs and a bite from a dog can cause wound infection at the site of the bite, cellulitis, or occasionally bacteraemia or bloodstream infection.

15. (c). TSST-1 or toxic shock syndrome toxin is a superantigen that can induce the major immune response that is part of toxic shock but many normal people may have been exposed to this toxin in the past and developed antibodies without clinical illness. Those who do not have antibodies are therefore more likely to get the syndrome. The syndrome was originally described in females whilst menstruating due to absorbent tampons, but female sex *per se* is not a risk factor. Bloodstream infection is unusual with toxic shock, underlying malignancy is not a risk factor, and methicillin-resistant strains of *Staph. aureus* are no more likely to produce TSST-1 than methicillin-sensitive strains.

16. (c). This especially applies in North America as some of the clinical features are similar. The other infections listed can be excluded on clinical grounds, e.g. characteristic vesicular rash with chickenpox.

17. (a). It is believed that the leprosy bacillus, which can be found in large numbers in the nose, is spread from nose to skin.

18. (e). This is caused by *Rickettsia conorii*, but all the others are viral in aetiology.

19. (a). Ceftriaxone is active against the aetiological agent of Lyme disease, *Borrelia burgdorferi*, penetrates well into the central nervous system, and, because it has a relatively long half-life, can be administered once a day unlike most of the other extended-spectrum cephalosporins such as cefotaxime. Although rifampicin penetrates into the central nervous system, it is not used in this context. Benzylpenicillin and tetracycline are used to treat Lyme disease but would not represent optimal therapy here.

20. (c). Especially if treating the tuberculous form. All the other regimens include agents with no activity against the leprosy bacillus, e.g. linezolid, or are more appropriate for the management of other forms of mycobacterial diseses, e.g. 6 months of rifampicin, isoniazid, and pyraxinamide for tuberculosis.

Section 2 Respiratory system

1. (d). Rhino- and coronaviruses usually cause a 'common cold'-like illness. RSV is associated with lower respiratory tract infection, especially in the first year of life. Enteroviruses can infect anywhere in the respiratory tract, but are not as common as the other viruses in this system.

2. (a). Ribavirin has a broad-spectrum antiviral effect *in vitro*, and *in vivo* has useful activity against RSV. Pleconaril inhibits enteroviruses, but is not licensed. Aciclovir is a viral DNA polymerase inhibitor, with activity only against HSV and VZV. Amantadine blocks the uncoating of influenza A viruses. Zanamivir is a neuraminidase inhibitor and therefore works only against influenza viruses.

3. (d). Virus-specific IgM is a marker of recent infection; IgG a marker of past infection. Atypical mononuclear cells may arise in a range of virus infections and are therefore not specific to EBV—likewise a raised bilirubin.

4. (b). The virus associated with Kaposi's sarcoma is human herpesvirus type 8 (HHV8), also known as Kaposi's sarcoma-associated herpesvirus.

5. (d). It is very difficult to demonstrate a viraemic phase in influenza (i.e. the presence of virus in the blood). The systemic manifestations of infection are believed to arise through the release of cytokines, e.g. interferon, which do circulate in the bloodstream.

6. (a), (b), (c), (d). All these patient groups are specifically targeted in the Department of Health guidance on influenza vaccination.

7. (a). Morbidity due to RSV infection is greatest in the first 12 or even the first 6 months of life.

8. (b). The technique depends on the presence of viral antigens in cells within which virus was

replicating *in vivo*. This is not affected by cell/virus death on the way to the laboratory.

9. (a). This condition is especially seen in patients with diabetes mellitus.

10. (e). Unlike non-capsulated strains, *H. influenzae* type b can cause invasive disease such as meningitis, cellulitis, bacteraemia or bloodstream infection, septic arthritis, and osteomyelitis. Otitis media, sinusitis, and bronchiolitis are caused by non-capsulated strains and *H. influenzae* is an unlikely cause of urinary tract infection.

11. (c). RSV as well as adenovirus, parainfluenzavirus, *B. parapertussis*, and *Mycoplasma pneumoniae* may cause a respiratory infection not unlike whooping cough.

12. (d). The other toxins/components of the vaccine are pertussis toxin and peractin.

13. (a). *Ps. aeruginosa* causes hospital-acquired pneumonia, especially in the ICU ventilated patient.

14. (b). But it is much higher in many other European countries where it is over 30%.

15. (e). This is an antigen detection technique where immunofluorescent antibodies bind to legionella antigen, present in the respiratory specimen, which is detectable under microscopy. It is quite specific but less sensitive than culture in diagnosing legionellosis.

16. (c). This can occur in various water systems, if these are poorly managed or maintained, and can contribute to the development or continuation of an outbreak.

17. (b). *Str. pneumoniae*, *Haemophilus influenzae*, and *Moraxella catarrhalis* are the most common causes of exacerbations of COPD. *Staph. saprophyticus* causes urinary tract infections, *Staph. aureus* is more likely to cause hospital-acquired respiratory infection, *B. parapertussis* may cause a whooping cough like clinical syndrome in children, and CMV causes respiratory infection in the immunocompromised patient.

18. (d). Benzylpenicillin is not active against *Haemophilus influenzae*; gentamicin must be administered parenterally and will not cover *Streptococcus pneumoniae*; cefotaxime has a broad spectrum of activity, but is expensive, must be administered parenterally, and may lead to antibiotic-associated diarrhoea; and ciprofloxacin is best reserved for Gram-negative infections, especially those caused by *Ps. aeruginosa*. Co-amoxyclav can be administered orally and parenterally and is active against the three common bacterial causes of acute exacerbation including beta-lactamase-producing *H. influenzae*.

19. (d). This bacterium may be found in the environment and is considered a low-grade or opportunist pathogen. However, it may colonize damaged lungs and cause exacerbations of airways infection in patients with cystic fibrosis. Whilst candida and enterococci may colonize the lungs, these two pathogens and the other two are not recognized respiratory pathogens.

20. (b). All the others are administerd parenterally—flucloxacillin for staphylococcal infection and the others for *Pseudomonas aeruginosa* infection. Nebulized tobramycin is less toxic than when administered parenterally.

Section 3 Gastrointestinal system

1. (b). Although the enteroviruses do enter and leave the human host through the gastrointestinal tract, clinical studies have failed to show a link between enteroviral infection and diarrhoeal illness.

2. (d). This is not a recognized feature of norovirus infection.

3. (a) (iii); (b) (ii); (c) (v); (d) (iv); (e) (i). The vaccine contains only HBsAg, so the only marker in vaccinated individuals is anti-HBs. IgM is a marker of recent infection; IgG a marker of past infection. The presence of

HBsAg indicates current infection, and HBeAg is a marker of highly active replication of virus.

4. (b). This is transmitted through blood contact, e.g. sharing of needles by injecting drug users, blood transfusion.

5. (e). The indicators of a good prognosis are: host factors—female, young (<40 years), no fibrosis evident on liver biopsy; viral factors—low viral load (<2 × 10^6 copies/ml) and non-genotype 1 infection.

6. (d). The vaccine for hepatitis A contains formaldehyde-inactivated whole virus.

7. (e). This is a cause of enteric fever, like *Salmonella typhi*, and is rarely acquired in the UK but usually from abroad. All the other species have been associated with food poisoning, including *S. dublin*, although originally described outside the UK!

8. (b). This might identify the likely source, e.g. food made from raw eggs. (c) and (d) might affect the proportion of patients that become ill but not identify the specific source and (a) and (e) are irrelevant.

9. (b). This is due to *Candida* spp., yeast-like fungi that are not susceptible to metronidazole.

10. (c). In some cases, no definite cause is ever identified but bacterial pathogens account for about 70% of all cases.

11. (c). Anaerobes outnumber facultative aerobes (i.e. (a), (b), (d), and (e)) by 1000–10 000 to 1. Yeast-like fungi are present usually only in small numbers in the normal large bowel.

12. (c). They have a narrow therapeutic index, do not penetrate well into CSF even when the meninges are inflamed, and regular blood assays are still required, although once-daily dosing results in less toxicity. The evidence suggesting that tobramycin is significantly less toxic than gentamicin is not convincing.

13. (e). (a) and (b) may suggest the diagnosis but are non-specific findings. The Widal test is unreliable, especially if the patient has been vaccinated in the past against enteric fever and there is no skin test.

14. (c). Ciprofloxacin is active against Gram-negative bacilli, has a good pharmacokinetic profile, and can penetrate inside cells unlike ampicillin. Gentamicin might be used in combination if the patient was very ill. Vancomycin is active against Gram-positive cocci only and flucloxacillin is used for the treatment of methicillin-sensitive staphylococcal disease. In some countries, chloramphenicol may be used, if isolates are susceptible, as it is cheaper than ciprofloxacin.

15. (c). (a) and (e) are possible causes but would not be as well recognized a cause as (c), which is important in many parts of the world. *Giardia lamblia* is usually confined to the bowel lumen and *Coxiella burnetti* causes Q fever.

16. (e). Suggestive but there are non-infective causes of an eosinophilia to be considered also.

17. (a). This is used in maximizing the possibility of isolating the *Vibrio cholerae* from stool samples. It does not grow on chocolate blood agar, which is usually used in the laboratory to isolate *Haemophilus* or *Neisseria*. Urease production is a feature of *Proteus* spp. and *Helicobacter pylori*, and many *Clostridia* produce lipase as do other bacteria.

18. (b). Good sanitary measures prevent spread, bacteraemia or bloodstream infection is unusual with cholera, antibiotics do not affect toxin production, and asymptomatic carriage of cholera is rare.

19. (c). The production of a cytotoxin is used to confirm a diagnosis, although the diarrhoea is induced by an enterotoxin. Overgrowth of the bowel with *C. difficile* of itself is not sufficient to cause diarrhoea and usually there is neither tissue nor bloodstream invasion, and the pancreas is not involved in the pathogenesis.

20. (c). Benzylpenicillin has a narrow spectrum and is least likely to disrupt the normal

protective anaerobic flora of the large bowel. Clindamycin followed by the cephalosporins are probably the most likely precipitating antibiotics but all broad-spectrum agents, including the newer quinolones, may cause *C. difficile*-associated diarrhoea.

Section 4 Genitourinary system

1. (e). Condylomata lata are a manifestation of secondary syphilis. Papillomaviruses cause condyloma acuminata.

2. (c). Aciclovir can only be activated by viruses that possess a thymidine kinase. Its spectrum of activity is therefore limited to certain herpesviruses only.

3. (b). Recurrent attacks are usually more benign than primary infections, i.e. the lesions are more localized and do not last as long.

4. (e). Trichomoniasis is associated with vaginal discharge and vaginal and vulval itching and erythema, but not ulceration.

5. (a). The characteristic lesion of primary syphilis is the chancre, a small, painless papule that rapidly ulcerates.

6. (d).

7. (a), (d), and (e). In addition to the features of glandular fever, patients with acute HIV seroconversion illness very often have an erythematous maculopapular rash. Anti-HIV may be negative at this stage, but HIV RNA will be present in blood. About three-quarters of HIV-infected patients give a history of a symptomatic seroconversion illness. There is usually a transient decrease in CD4 count at this stage of infection.

8. (d). There is no evidence that HIV can be transmitted via the faecal–oral route. It is to be hoped that Factor VIII is now safe due to proper screening of blood donors and heat inactivation, but this was a recognized route of infection in the early stages of the HIV epidemic.

9. (c). Trimethoprim is considered a 'urinary antiseptic', i.e. it is excreted in the urine in high concentrations and will cover most urinary pathogens. Erythromycin has little activity against Gram-negative bacteria, benzylpenicillin has none, metronidazole is only active against anaerobes, and gentamicin can only be administered parenterally.

10. (c). May suggest an underlying malignancy. *Staph. saprophyticus* is a common cause of urinary tract infection in females during the reproductive years, nocturia represents frequency at night, and, unless schistosomiasis was suspected (usually accompanied by haematuria), acquisition abroad has little clinical significance.

11. (c). Coagulase-negative staphylococcus species, such as *Staph. epidermidis*, are common commensals of the skin and hence likely to gain access to the peritoneum via the Tenckhoff catheter. In general, Gram-positive bacteria are the most common class, but infection due to *Staph. aureus* may require catheter removal and replacement. Infection caused by *Strep. pyogenes* may be associated with some systemic upset.

12. (d). *E. coli* is part of the normal flora of the bowel and is much less commonly found on the skin, the source of most cases of CAPD infection.

13. (c). There may also be skin lesions but the classical triad is urethritis, arthritis, and uveitis.

14. (b). Especially associated with *Schistosoma japonicum*. Other complications or features include skin rashes, Katayama fever, and liver fibrosis.

Section 5 Central nervous system

1. (c). Orolabial herpes may reactivate in seriously ill patients whatever the cause, and gives no indication as to the underlying disease process. The frontotemporal region is

the most common site for HSE. Whilst culture of CSF is very rarely positive, sensitive techniques such as PCR can detect the presence of HSV DNA in CSF. The lesions in HSE are almost always focal.

2. (a)–(e). The brain is the primary site of infection for West Nile and rabies viruses. Enteroviruses (including coxsackie B) may cause encephalitis especially in patients with immunodeficiency. There are a number of encephalitic complications of measles—this is the main reason for universal measles vaccination. Mumps usually causes meningitis, but virus can spread from the meninges into the brain substance.

3. (c). The vaccine used is rabies virus grown in tissue culture and then inactivated by beta-propiolactone.

4. (d). Spread to the brain is via the spinal cord, not the bloodstream.

5. (a)–(e). All of these modalities have transmitted CJD.

6. (a). Despite enormous efforts, no one has been able to demonstrate convincingly that the prion responsible for transmission of CJD contains any nucleic acid.

7. (b). PMLE is due to infection with JC virus, a polyomavirus. It is exclusively a disease of immunosuppressed patients, e.g. HIV-infected patients, where JC virus is able to reactivate and cause disease.

8. (c). Highly suggestive if not diagnostic of meningococcal meningitis. Some commensal neisseria might be seen in sputum or anaerobes from abdominal pus with similar appearances but this would usually be associated with the presence of other bacteria seen in the Gram film.

9. (e). Although *Leptospira* are bacteria, meningitis associated with leptospirosis is characterized by a lymphocytic picture. Other pathogens associated with a lymphocytic reaction in the CSF include those causing viral meningitis (e.g. enteroviruses), syphilis,

and tuberculosis. Bacterial meningitis (sometimes referred to as 'septic' compared with 'aseptic' or lymphocytic) typically produces increased neutrophils in the CSF.

10. (a). Usually as part of disseminated or metastatic staphylococcal disease. Septic emboli secondary to infective endocarditis are possible with the other bacteria but much less likely or even rare.

11. (c). Relatively high concentrations of beta-lactam antibiotics, especially the third-generation cephalosporins, are achieved in the brain and CSF, compared with many other classes of antibiotics including the aminoglycosides (e.g. gentamicin), macrolides (e.g. erythromycin), and quinolones (e.g. ciprofloxacin).

12. (b). *C. botulinum* produces a potent toxin that leads to neurological symptoms and signs including weakness, double vision, etc. Gastrointestinal symptoms are usually absent. *C. difficile* diarrhoea arises from exposure to antibiotics, *C. tetani* is acquired directly from the environment such as during trauma, and both *C. sporogenes* and *C. septicum* may cause opportunist infection arising from the patient's own flora or the environment.

13. (d). A dirty wound is more likely to be contaminated with *C. tetani* and, as it is probably 10 years or more since he was either vaccinated or received a booster of tetanus toxoid, immunoglobulin with toxoid is indicated.

Section 6 Systemic infections

1. (d) and (e). The decision to offer antiretroviral drugs as HIV post-exposure prophylaxis (PEP) is dependent on an assessment of the risk of HIV transmission. Most needlestick injuries do not arise from HIV-infected patients, and therefore PEP would not be necessary. It is not unreasonable to offer HBV vaccination in all needlestick recipients (if they haven't already been vaccinated), but the

use of HBIg is restricted to high-risk exposures in recipients who have not been vaccinated or are known to be vaccine non-responders. Of anti-HCV-positive individuals, 20% do not become chronic carriers, and therefore are not an infection risk. The EPP ban is on health-care workers who are shown to be HCV RNA-positive.

2. (b). Anyone who answered (a) needs urgent training in prevention of needlestick incidents! EPPs are those where the operator's blood may come into contact with the open tissues of the patient. It is not necessary to recheck anti-HBs levels at the time of needlestick injury, provided it is known that the individual was a responder to his/her initial course of vaccination. There are many more patients than health-care workers carrying blood-borne viruses.

3. (d). Whilst this is a manifestation of declining immune function, it is not categorized as an AIDS-defining illness. Oesophageal candidiasis is, however.

4. (c). HAART regimens may or may not contain a PI. Antiretroviral therapy should be monitored by serial viral load measurement. The decision to initiate HAART is dependent on a number of factors, not just HIV infection alone. The patient described in (e) does not warrant antiretroviral therapy at present and, in any case, monotherapy must be avoided if at all possible.

5. (b). The high-risk bone marrow transplant recipient is one who was CMV-seropositive pretransplant (and will therefore be harbouring latent CMV), who receives marrow from a CMV-seronegative donor (which will therefore not contain any CMV-specific T cells).

6. (e). All potential transplant recipients should be tested for evidence of current infection with HIV, HCV, and HBV, This involves initial testing for anti-HIV, anti-HCV, and HBsAg. If the patient is anti-HCV-positive, then HCV RNA testing should be performed to ascertain if the patient is chronically infected. The CMV serostatus of donor and recipient is important from the point of view of assessing the likelihood of posttransplant CMV disease. The presence or absence of immunity to VZV infection is useful to know, as the patient may be exposed to the virus posttransplantation when heavily immunosuppressed.

7. (a).

8. (b), (c), and (e). The malarial parasite is only transmitted to humans by the female mosquito. *P. vivax* and *P. ovale* have an exo-erythrocytic liver stage, but not *P. falciparum*. Antimalarial prophylaxis reduces the risk of acquiring malaria, but does not eliminate it completely. Typical tertian fevers are uncommon in falciparum malaria.

9. (b). With the most likely source being the urinary or gastrointestinal tracts. *Staph. saprophyticus* is a cause of urinary infection in females during the reproductive years and does not cause bacteraemia or bloodstream infection. (c)–(e) may all cause bacteraemia but less frequently than *E. coli*.

10. (c). This will cover Gram-negative bacilli and enterococci. Nitrofurantoin is a urinary antiseptic, useful in the management of urinary infection, but not when associated with bacteraemia or bloodstream infection. Clarithromycin and tetracycline are not optimal for the treatment of Gram-negative infection, flucloxacillin is an anti-staphylococcal agent, metronidazole is active only against anaerobes, and vancomycin has no activity against Gram-negative bacilli.

11. (a). Bloodstream infection or candidaemia is unusual in HIV patients whereas mucosal candidiasis is more common in patients with AIDS. Parenteral nutrition and not enteral nutrition is a risk factor, natural yogurt contains true yeasts and not yeast-like fungi, which is what *Candida* spp. are, and, unlike the situation with aspergillus, environmental

sources are not considered a major risk factor for systemic candida infection.

12. (c). Pneumonia in the immunocompromised patient, such as a patient with neutropenia, is amongst the most common presentations of aspergillosis. Encephalitis may occur as part of disseminated, often terminal, disease and endocarditis, caused by *A. fumigatus* or by another species such as *A. terreus*, may occur after prosthetic heart valve surgery.

13. (d). This suggests the presence of immune complex complications such as glomerulonephritis. (a)–(c) are non-specific findings *vis-á-vis* a diagnosis of endocarditis and (e) suggests recent myocardial infarction.

14. (b). Aminoglycosides disrupt protein synthesis and penicillins, like all beta-lactam agents, act on the cell wall. When used in combination, therefore, they act synergistically, which is important in treating endocarditis where bactericidal activity is essential for success. Unlike with most other indications, aminoglycosides are still administered twice or thrice daily to treat endocarditis. Gram-negative bacilli are not common causes of endocarditis. The clinical response, e.g. a fall in temperature, and repeat echocardiogram are how the antibiotic response to therapy is monitored. Finally, the aminoglycosides do not penetrate well into tissues including cardiac tissues.

15. (b). Skin tests should be positive if the patient has had tuberculosis recently or in the past. However, false-negative results can occur very early during the course of the disease, i.e. before an immune response has been mounted or if the infection overwhelms the immune system itself, as may occur in miliary tuberculosis. BCG should induce a positive result, not a negative result, and concurrent lobar pneumonia should not affect a skin test.

16. (c). Recent illness, unless likely to cause immune suppression, is not an indication *per*

se for chemoprophylaxis. The result of skin tests, especially if there is conversion from negative to positive in the absence of BCG, would be an indication for chemoprophylaxis but the absence of a history of BCG vaccination in the UK would not alone be an indication for prophylaxis. Neonates are especially vulnerable to disseminated disease.

17. (d). Although not common in the UK, unless acquired abroad such as in the USA, histoplasmosis should be considered in the differential diagnosis of pneumonia in the immunocompromised patient where appropriate. A positive skin test indicates exposure to the fungus.

18. (b). Usually diagnosed on serology (elevated phase 1 antibodies) or from examination of valve, e.g. PCR, taken at surgery.

19. (a). *H. influenzae* type b is a capsulated bacterium that, before the introduction of the Hib vaccine, was a major cause of invasive infection, e.g. bacteraemia or bloodstream infection, meningitis, etc., in children less than 5 years of age. Patients without a spleen are especially prone to severe infection by capsulated bacteria. All individuals, with or without an intact spleen, should receive tetanus and MMR. Hepatitis A is indicated for those individuals travelling abroad or those at particular risk of acquisition, e.g. certain occupational groups. Similarly, in the UK hepatitis B vaccine is only indicated for certain rish groups such as health-care workers.

20. (b). Fusidic acid or sodium fusidate penetrates well in to bone and joint tissue. However, if used alone, resistance may occur due to mutations. Erythromycin, although active against many strains of staphylococci, is not optimal for bone and joint infection. Gentamicin does not penetrate well into bone and joint tissue. Mupirocin can only be used topically and systemic antibiotics are required in this context, and, finally, metronidazole is active against anaerobes only.

Section 7 Pregnancy and the neonate

1. (d). Syphilis screening is by serological testing. Women found to be infected should be treated in order to reduce the risks of congenital syphilis. Rubella immunity screening is aimed at identifying susceptible women, who should then be offered post-partum vaccination. Screening for evidence of HBV or HIV infection is in order to allow proper management to reduce the risk of mother-to-baby infection. There is currently no rationale for antenatal HCV screening, as there is as yet no intervention that can be applied in order to reduce the risk of vertical transmission.

2. (a), (c), and (d). Pregnant women who lack IgG anti-rubella antibodies should be offered post-partum vaccination—the vaccine is live attenuated, and therefore should not be given to pregnant women. Breast-feeding does not influence the risk of mother-to-baby transmission of HBV, and therefore there is no reason to advise against breast-feeding in this instance.

3. (d). All babies of HIV carrier mothers will have anti-HIV in cord blood through passive transfer of maternal antibody. Tests for infection of the neonate should therefore involve virus detection (e.g. reverse transcriptase PCR) rather than serology.

4. (d). Adenoviruses are a very common cause of acute conjunctivitis in adults, but are not associated with neonatal infection.

5. (c). The organism is not susceptible to penicillin, gentamicin, or fusidic acid. Oral erythromycin should be given to treat the conjunctivitis, prevent the development of pneumonia, and eliminate nasopharyngeal carriage. Topical therapy provides no additional benefit.

6. (c). This is a live attenuated vaccine, and should therefore not be given to pregnant women. Vaccination should take place postnatally.

7. (a). Cataracts are a feature of the congenital rubella syndrome. Maternal parvovirus infection has not been associated with congenital abnormalities, so there is no such thing as a congenital parvovirus syndrome.

8. (c). Transplacental transfer of VZV may occur at any time in pregnancy. However, the congenital varicella syndrome is only described in babies of mothers with chickenpox in the first 20 weeks of pregnancy.

9. (a) and (b). Most women of child-bearing age have antibodies to VZV, even if they have no personal history of chickenpox. VZIg should be given to pregnant women who are anti-VZV-negative and have a contact with chickenpox or shingles. By the time the woman develops chickenpox it is too late to give the VZIg. Shingles is a reactivation of latent virus. Women with shingles will therefore already have antibodies to VZV, which will have crossed the placenta and will protect the neonate from infection.

10. (c). Most neonatal herpes arises from primary maternal infection in late pregnancy. Such women, by definition, will not have a history of recurrent genital herpes.

11. (a) (ii); (b) (iii); (c) (iv); (d) (v); (e) (i).

12. (b). The site of latency of CMV is not known with certainty, although it is *not* the B lymphocyte. The latter is the site of Epstein–Barr virus latency.

13. (b). Only about 5–10% of CMV-infected babies have evidence of disease at birth. Another 5–10% are normal at birth but have abnormalities detectable as the baby develops. The remaining 80–85% of CMV-infected babies are normal at birth and develop normally.

14. (e). *Ps. aeruginosa*, *A. baumanii*, and *Staph. arueus* are possible causes the longer the neonate remains in hospital, especially if requiring intensive care but *Strep. pneumoniae* would be an unusual cause. *Strep. agalactiae* is usually acquired during passage through the

birth canal and, with *E. coli*, is the most common cause of bacteraemia or neonatal meningitis.

15. (d). No source is usually identified even where investigations of food outlets occur, although soft cheeses are a well recognized source. Most affected patients are either pregnant, neonates, or have an underlying immune deficient state, e.g. lymphoma, but occasionally listeriosis occurs in the normal host.

Section 8 Miscellaneous

1. (b). The CD4 molecule on helper T cells is the primary receptor for HIV. The receptor for HTLV-1 has not been identified.

2. (b). The lifetime risk of developing ATLL or tropical spastic paraparesis is of the order of only 1–2%.

3. (c). Mumps encephalitis arises through direct spread of virus from the meninges into the brain substance. This is in contrast to the acute encephalitis associated with measles virus infection, which is believed to have an immunopathogenic basis.

4. (d). Mumps can cause orchitis in postpubertal males and oophoritis in postpubertal females, but the infection does not spread to cause pelvic inflammatory disease.

5. (e). Ross River virus is an alphavirus spread by *Aedes* mosquitoes in Australia and the Pacific Islands. Infection is associated with fever, a generalized maculopapular rash, and, most distinctively, a polyarthralgia of the small joints of the hands and feet. The arthritis can last from a few days to several months.

6. (b). Lassa fever virus is found from northern Nigeria to Guinea in west Africa. There are arenaviruses found in South America that can give rise to viral haemorrhagic fever (VHF), e.g. Junin virus (Argentine VHF), Machupo (Bolivian VHF), Guanarito (Venezualian

VHF), and Sabia (Brazilian VHF).

7. (a). Exanthem subitum (also known as roseola infantum, or sixth disease) is caused by human herpesvirus type 6.

8. (d). The skin rash and arthritis are manifestations of immune complex disease, which arises about a week after the viraemic phase of the disease. The arthritis is much more common in females than in males (also true of rubella arthritis). Chronic parvovirus infection is only described in immunodeficient hosts, e.g. those with HIV infection, leukaemia.

9. (b). Usually following an episode of gastroenteritis. All the others are possible causes of septic or infective arthritis with *Staph. aureus* being the most common cause, *Staph. epidermidis* being more likely in patients with prosthetic joints, *Strep. pneumoniae* occurring occasionally as part of a generalized septicaemic illness, and *Ps. aeruginosa* being possible after trauma.

10. (a). Often indistinguishable from appendicitis. Gastroenteritis and bacteraemia or bloodstream infection would be other well recognized clinical presentations of infection with *Yersinia* species.

11. (c), (d), (e). Electron microscopy can detect a variety of viruses, e.g. rotavirus, small round structured viruses, e.g. Norwalk virus, and adenovirus. PCR is not yet widely available in many centres, remains relatively expensive, and is usually used to confirm a likely cause with specific primers rather than used blindly. Culture for the main causes of viral gastroenteritis is difficult, and most of these infections do not result in a serological response as measured by serum antibodies. There are a few laboratory kits available for antigen detection.

12. (c). This is likely to prevent spread to other wards. However, hand-washing and the use of personal protective clothing such as aprons and gloves when directly caring for affected

patients remain the most important measures in limiting spread. Hospitalized food is not usually a likely source and all admissions should be restricted if possible and not just to any particular age group. If patients are well and can be cared for at home, discharge helps to reduce the pressure on nursing staff and the possibility that asymptomatic and otherwise well patients will become affected if they remain. Any reduction in nurses on a ward is likely to exacerbate the problem as staff shortages are known to be a risk factor for increased hospital-acquired infection.

Index